Understanding and Addressing Brain Injury and Repair Mechanisms After Intracerebral Hemorrhage

From Injury to Recovery: A Deep Dive into Brain Injury and Repair Post Intracerebral Hemorrhage

Gaiqing Wang
Jiachen Liu
Lirong Liu

Understanding and Addressing Brain Injury and Repair Mechanisms After Intracerebral Hemorrhage

From Injury to Recovery: A Deep Dive into Brain Injury and Repair Post Intracerebral Hemorrhage

ELIVA PRESS

ISBN: 978-99993-1-832-7

Cover Design: Eliva Press
Cover Image: www.ingimage.com
Email: info@elivapress.com
Website: www.elivapress.com

This Eliva Press imprint is published by the registered company Eliva Press Global Ltd. part of Eliva Press S.R.L. Publishing Group

The registered company address is: Pope Hennessy Street Level 2, Hennessy Tower Port Louis, Mauritius
Eliva Press S.R.L. Publishing Group legal address is: Bd. Cuza-Voda 1/4 of. 21, Chisinau, Moldova, Europe

Understanding and Addressing Brain Injury and Repair Mechanisms After Intracerebral Hemorrhage

Table of Contents

Understanding and Addressing Brain Injury and Repair Mechanisms

After Intracerebral Hemorrhage

ABSTRACT:

Intracerebral hemorrhage (ICH) is a devastating form of stroke associated with high morbidity and mortality rates. Understanding the mechanisms of brain injury and repair following ICH is crucial for developing effective therapeutic strategies. This review summarizes recent advances in our research on endogenous hematoma clearance mechanisms, focusing on processes such as red blood cell phagocytosis, heme clearance, and iron metabolism modulation. Additionally, the role of phagocytes, scavenger receptors, neurovascular units and lymphatic system in mediating these processes is discussed. Insights into these mechanisms offer promising avenues for the development of novel treatments aimed at reducing brain injury and promoting recovery after ICH.

KEY WORDS: Intracerebral   hemorrhage (ICH); Hematoma clearance; Endogenous   clearance   system;   Scavenger   receptors;   Phagocytosis; Neurovascular units

CHAPTER 1:

The Influence and Decision-making on Outcome of Spontaneous Intracerebral Hemorrhage

ABSTRACT:

Aim: To explore the influence on short-term prognosis of intracerebral hemorrhage (ICH) and make decision for ameliorating the clinical outcome.

Methods: 252 ICH cases were diagnosed by CT , then all patients were filled in the case data questionnaire and Analyzed data with SAS6.12 statistics software.

Results: The lower GCS and blood potassium and higher serum glucose value and mean blood pressure at admission, past history of ICH, smoking and coronary heart disease, non-lobar ICH are in line with the lower value of 30-day Glasgow—Pittsberg score.

Conclusion: The above variables were the independent predictors of 30-day outcome in ICH patients and intervening them maybe improve prognosis of ICH.

KEY WORDS: Intracerebral hemorrhage (ICH); Short-term outcome; Influence factors; Decision-making

1. **Introduction:**

Intracerebral hemorrhage (ICH) is one of the important events threatening human health and quality of life, with extremely high mortality and disability rates. ICH accounts for approximately 20% of stroke incidence, and although long-term prognosis is similar, its mortality is higher than that of cerebral infarction. At present, there are no specific effective treatments for cerebral hemorrhage. This study analyzes the relevant factors that may affect the prognosis of cerebral hemorrhage, aiming to provide possible decision analysis for evaluating the prognosis of cerebral hemorrhage and intervening in its modifiable influencing factors as much as possible to improve clinical outcomes for patients.

2. Subjects and Methods

A total of 252 patients aged 32 to 89 years, diagnosed with acute ICH (onset to hospital admission time <3 days) from June 2001 to September 2003 at the Neurology Department of Taiyuan Central Hospital in Shanxi Province, were included in the study. Patients with intracranial hemorrhage due to brain tumors, post-anticoagulant therapy, traumatic brain injury, and multi-site bleeding were excluded. All cases were clinically and by cranial CT confirmed as cerebral hemorrhage.

Data collection was done using a self-designed case information survey form, including family history, past medical history (hypertension, previous cerebral hemorrhage, diabetes, coronary heart disease, smoking, alcohol consumption, regular medication), long-term use of aspirin, general condition upon admission (age, consciousness, body temperature, pulse, respiration, blood pressure), Glasgow Coma Scale (GCS) score upon admission, location and volume of hemorrhage, laboratory tests (routine blood tests, liver and kidney function, blood glucose, blood lipids, electrolytes), treatment methods (conservative treatment and surgery), presence of complications, and whether tracheotomy was performed.

Glasgow-Pittsburgh Scale scores were assessed at one month (for those who died within one month, the score was calculated as if they had survived for one month). Mean arterial pressure was calculated, and the volume of hemorrhage was calculated using the formula by Maudsley for cerebral parenchymal hemorrhage, and the Graeb score multiplied by 4 was roughly calculated for intraventricular hemorrhage.

The above data were truthfully filled out by neurology physicians and entered into the SAS database. Statistical analysis was performed using SAS 6.12 software. The Glasgow-Pittsburgh Scale (GPS) score at one month after the onset was used as the short-term prognostic evaluation index (ranging from 7 to 35 points, with lower scores indicating poorer prognosis). T-tests, Q-tests, and multiple stepwise regression analyses were conducted separately.

3. **Results:**

3.1 Examination of Factors Influencing Short-Term Prognosis of Cerebral Hemorrhage Using GPS Score

Statistical analysis was conducted on the factors investigated after admission, and the one-month GPS scores were analyzed. The results showed that a history of previous cerebral hemorrhage, coronary heart

Impact Factor	Patients	GPS Score	p Value
Gender			>0.05
Male	153	21.3 ± 2.4	
Female	99	23.4±3.21	
Age			>0.05
≤65 (years)	134	22.3 ± 1.86	
> 65 (years)	118	24.6 ± 2.65	
Site of hemorrhage			<0.01
basal ganglia	203	21.2±1.36	
lobar	17	28.6±0.98	
cerebellum	13	26.9±1.67	
brainstem	7	16.7±2.56	
ventricle	12	18.4±2.95	
Volume of hemorrhage			<0.05
≤30 ml	78	23.8±2.19	
30–50 ml	105	21.4±3.57	
>50 ml	69	16.5±2.08	
Hypertension history			>0.05
No	58	22.6 ± 3.52	
Yes	194	20.1 ± 2.43	
Coronary heart disease history			<0.05
No	122	25.5 ± 1.63	
Yes	130	18.7 ±2.66	
Diabetes history			>0.05
No	184	21.8 ± 3.46	
Yes	68	19.4 ± 2.31	
Intracerebral hemorrhage history			<0.01
No	193	28.1 ± 3.87	
Yes	59	17.9 ± 2.62	
Cerebral infarct history			>0.05
No	190	21.1 ± 3.05	
Yes	62	19.3 ± 2.31	
Smoking history			<0.05
No	156	23.6 ± 2.41	
Yes	96	18.5 ± 3.88	
Drinking history			<0.05
No	216	22.6 ± 3.97	
Yes	36	17.2 ± 3.54	
GCS scores at admission			<0.01
≤6	168	25.8 ± 1.64	
>6	84	17.1 ± 2.33	
Blood glucose at admission			<0.05
<7.8mmol/L	135	22.0 ± 3.49	
≥7.8mmol/L	117	17.6± 2.52	
Serum triglyceride at admission			>0.05
≥1.7 mmol/L	95	23.7 ± 2.54	
<1.7 mmol/L	157	21.9 ±3.46	
Serum sodium at admission			>0.05
≥135 mmol/L	149	23.2 ± 2.69	
<135 mmol/L	103	20.9 ±3.62	
Serum potassium at admission			<0.05
≥3.5 mmol/L	87	24.3 ± 2.64	
<3.5 mmol/L	165	19.1 ± 1.37	
Mean artery pressure at admission			<0.05
≥14.6kpa	191	19.6 ± 2.55	
<14.6kpa	61	24.7 ± 3.22	
Mean heart rate at admission)			>0.05
<100 次/分 (bpm)	96	21.5 ± 3.16	
≥100 次/分 (bpm)	156	23.1 ± 3.22	
Body temperature at admission			>0.05
<37.5°C	130	25.7 ± 3.01	
≥37.5°C	122	26.4 ± 2.56	
Mean respiratory rate at admission			>0.05
<22 次/分 (bpm)	154	25.6 ± 2.68	
≥22 次/分 (bpm)	98	24.5 ± 3.42	
Therapeutic methods			>0.05
microsurgery	39	24.5 ± 2.61	
medication	213	22.9 ± 2.54	
Taking aspirin			<0.05
≥1 year	120	20.6± 3.12	
<1 year	132	25.9 ± 2.98	
Complication			<0.05
No	117	23.9 ± 2.99	
Yes	135	18.6 ±3.21	
Trachea incision			<0.01
No	209	21.3 ± 2.01	
Yes	43	15.9 ±2.03	

disease, smoking, and alcohol consumption, as well as the location and volume of hemorrhage, low GCS score upon admission, low blood potassium, high blood glucose, high mean arterial pressure, non-lobar hemorrhage, long-term use of aspirin, tracheotomy, and presence of complications were associated with lower GPS scores at one month, indicating poorer short-term prognosis (see Table 1).

3.2 Variable Selection and Optimal Regression Equation by Variance Analysis

The significant variables mentioned above were introduced into multiple stepwise regression analysis in relation to short-term prognosis. The dependent variable was GPS score (see Tables 2 and 3). The variance analysis showed $P < 0.0001$, indicating that the model was statistically significant. The main effect model that finally entered the regression equation comprised eight variables (see Table 3). The multiple linear regression equation obtained was:

$CPS = -3.125+5.482A+3.32lB -1.992C+5.153D-0.568E+3.480F-0.186G +0.085H$ (P <0.001)

The results indicate that lower GCS scores upon admission, lower blood potassium levels, higher blood glucose levels, higher mean arterial pressure, non-lobar hemorrhage, a history of previous cerebral hemorrhage, smoking, and coronary heart disease are associated with lower Glasgow-Pittsburgh scores at 30 days, suggesting poorer short-term prognosis.

Tab 2 Analysis of variance

Source	DF	Sum of squares	Mean square	F value	P value
Model	8	969.394	107.71	3658.24	0.0001
Error	243	0.0008	0.00003		
Total	251	969.395			

Tab 3 Parameter estimates

Variable	Parameter Estimate	Standard Error	Sum of Squares	F Value	P Value
Intercept	-3.215	0.022	0.631	214.407	0.0001
GCS scores at admission(A)	5.482	0.002	173.128	58800.45	0.0001
Intracerebral hemorrhage history(B)	3.321	0.005	13.721	4660.051	0.0001
smoking history(C)	1.912	0.003	3.54	1202.47	0.0001
Coronary heart disease history(D)	5.133	0.004	44.789	15211.95	0.0001
Blood sugar at admission(E)	-0.568	0.006	11.264	3825.54	0.0001
Mean heart rate at admission(F)	3.48	0.002	102.041	34656.84	0.0001
Volume of hemorrhage(G)	-0.186	0.001	0.571	193.83	0.0001
Blood potassium at admission(H)	0.085	0.006	0.008	2.693	0.0001

4. Discussion

The results of this study demonstrate that lower GCS scores upon admission, lower blood potassium levels, higher blood glucose levels, higher mean arterial pressure, non-lobar hemorrhage, a history of previous cerebral hemorrhage, smoking, and coronary heart disease are associated with poorer short-term prognosis in patients with cerebral hemorrhage. These factors may serve as independent predictors of short-term prognosis in cerebral hemorrhage patients.

Recent studies have identified independent risk factors associated with 30-day mortality following cerebral hemorrhage, including age, GCS score upon admission, hemorrhage volume, intraventricular extension, blood glucose levels upon admission, and previous antiplatelet drug use. The relationship between GCS score and prognosis in cerebral hemorrhage has been widely reported in literature. Our findings indicate that higher blood glucose levels upon admission are associated with poorer short-term prognosis, independent of diabetes history, suggesting that high blood glucose may serve as an indicator of the severity and outcome of cerebral hemorrhage.

Coronary heart disease history may be associated with poorer short-term prognosis in cerebral hemorrhage patients due to the increased risk of acute cardiac events following stress. The mortality rate for recurrent cerebral hemorrhage is significantly higher than that for first-time hemorrhage, with survivors facing a 10% to 16% risk of recurrent stroke in the first year, decreasing by 5% each subsequent year. Survivors also face a twofold increase in relative risk of death compared to the general population, which persists for many years. Many individuals succumb to other vascular issues such as ischemic heart disease or peripheral arterial disease, making a history of previous cerebral hemorrhage a major adverse factor for short-term prognosis.

Smoking is known to increase the incidence of cerebral hemorrhage, but there are currently no reports on its association with short-term prognosis after cerebral hemorrhage. Higher mean arterial pressure upon admission is associated with poorer short-term prognosis, possibly due to the increased risk of rebleeding and hematoma expansion caused by extremely high blood pressure.

This study found that short-term prognosis is significantly better for lobar and cerebellar hemorrhages compared to other locations, possibly due to differences in hemorrhage severity caused by the location of bleeding. Additionally, low blood potassium upon admission was found to worsen clinical outcomes following cerebral hemorrhage. Animal studies have shown that a high-potassium diet can enhance vascular wall damage in cerebral arteries under sustained high pressure, thereby reducing mortality. This suggests that potassium supplementation may counteract cerebral hemorrhage, although there are currently no reports on the association between low potassium and short-term prognosis after cerebral hemorrhage. The specific mechanism of potassium's action remains unclear and requires further confirmation through basic and clinical research.

This study did not find age, gender, history of hypertension, history of diabetes, body temperature, pulse, respiratory rate, or treatment method to have an impact on short-term prognosis. However, hemorrhage volume, complications, and long-term use of antiplatelet drugs were found to have some influence on short-term prognosis, though they were ultimately eliminated as significant variables in regression analysis. Nonetheless, their potential impact on the dependent variable cannot be completely ruled out, warranting further confirmation through increased sample size or further stratified analysis.

REFERENCES:

1. Irimia-Sieira P, Moya-Molina M, Martínez-Vila E. Aspectos clínicos y factores pronósticos en la hemorragia intracerebral [Clinical aspects and prognostic factors

of intracerebral hemorrhage]. Rev Neurol. 2000;31(2):192-8

2. Hu Changlin, Lv Yongtao, Li Zhichao, et al. Minimally Invasive Evacuation Technique Standardization Treatment Guidelines for Intracranial Hematomas [M]. China Union Medical University Press, 2003;75, 210

3. Roquer J, Rodríguez Campello A, Gomis M, et al. Previous antiplatelet therapy is an independent predictor of 30-day mortality after spontaneous supratentorial intracerebral hemorrhage. J Neurol. 2005;252(4):412-6

4. Rincon F, Mayer SA. Novel therapies for intracerebral hemorrhage. Curr Opin Crit Care. 2004;10(2):94-100

5. Fogelholm R, Murros K, Rissanen A, et al. Admission blood glucose and short term survival in primary intracerebral haemorrhage: a population based study. J Neurol Neurosurg Psychiatry. 2005;76(3):349-53

6. Bilińska M, Swierkocka-Miastkowska M, Dobrzyńska L. Krwawienia dokomorowe pierwotne i wtórne--analiza kliniczna [Primary and secondary intraventricular hemorrhage--clinical analysis]. Neurol Neurochir Pol. 1999;32 Suppl 6:141-7

7. Davenport R, Dennis M. Neurological emergencies: acute stroke. J Neurol Neurosurg Psychiatry. 2000;68(3):277-88

8. Kurth T, Kase CS, Berger K, Schaeffner ES, et al. Smoking and the risk of hemorrhagic stroke in men. Stroke. 2003;34(5):1151-5

9. Rasool AH, Rahman AR, Choudhury SR, et al. Blood pressure in acute intracerebral haemorrhage. J Hum Hypertens. 2004;18(3):187-92

10. Inagawa T, Ohbayashi N, Takechi A, et al. Primary intracerebral hemorrhage in Izumo City, Japan: incidence rates and outcome in relation to the site of hemorrhage. Neurosurgery. 2003;53(6):1283-97

11. Tobian L, Lange JM, Johnson MA, et al. High-K diets reduce brain haemorrhage and infarcts, death rate and mesenteric arteriolar hypertrophy in stroke-prone spontaneously hypertensive rats. J Hypertens Suppl. 1986;4(5): S205-7

DECLARATION: This chapter was authored by Gaiqing Wang, Qidong Yang, Qingping Tang et al and published as "The Relationship Between Admission-Related Factors and Prognosis in Spontaneous Intracerebral Hemorrhage and Decision Analysis" in "Chinese Clinical Neuroscience", 2005;13(4):396-398

CHAPTER 2:

Progress on the secondary brain damage by the decomposition products of red blood cells after Intracerebral Hemorrhage (ICH)

ABSTRACT:

After intracerebral hemorrhage (ICH), the brain damage caused by the decomposition products of red blood cells is closely related to several molecules and pathways, including:

HO-1 (Heme Oxygenase-1): HO-1 is an important antioxidant enzyme that can break down free hemoglobin into bilirubin, carbon monoxide, and free iron. After ICH, the expression of HO-1 significantly increases, possibly to counteract the oxidative stress response caused by hemoglobin release. However, excessive activation of HO-1 may also lead to cellular toxicity, exacerbating brain damage.

AQP4 (Aquaporin 4): AQP4 is primarily distributed on the foot processes of astrocytes surrounding the brain ventricles and serves as the main channel for water molecules in the blood-brain barrier and brain interstitium. After ICH, the expression and activity of AQP4 may be affected, leading to the occurrence and exacerbation of brain edema.

Ferritin and Transferrin: After cerebral hemorrhage, large amounts of hemoglobin are released and decomposed, resulting in the release of large amounts of iron ions into surrounding tissues. Iron ions are crucial for the generation of oxygen free radicals, thereby exacerbating oxidative stress and cell damage. Additionally, iron can bind to transferrin, further promoting its transport and accumulation within neuronal cells, leading to intracellular iron overload and subsequent cellular toxicity reactions.

Therefore, understanding and intervening in the activity of molecules and pathways such as HO-1, AQP4, ferritin, and transferrin may help alleviate the secondary brain damage caused by red blood cell products after ICH.

KEY WORDS: Intracerebral   hemorrhage (ICH); Secondary brain injury; Brain edema; Erythrolysis; Hematoma clearance; AQP4

Introduction:

Intracerebral hemorrhage (ICH) is one of the significant events threatening human health and quality of life, with high mortality and disability rates. Early prediction and intervention of brain damage shortly after cerebral hemorrhage are challenging, while delayed brain damage often determines clinical outcomes. Delayed brain damage includes the formation of cerebral edema, neuronal loss, degeneration, or death. The peak period of brain tissue swelling and edema after cerebral hemorrhage occurs around three days later, and clinical studies indicate that neurological function deterioration in many patients reaches its peak several days after the hemorrhage, gradually improving thereafter. Therefore, studying the mechanisms and interventions for delayed brain damage after cerebral hemorrhage is of great significance. It is particularly important to alleviate or control the formation of secondary brain damage to improve patient prognosis. The disruption of the blood-brain barrier, the formation of brain edema, and oxidative damage to neuronal cells caused by the hydrolysis of red blood cells after cerebral hemorrhage are delayed processes, typically occurring around three days after the hemorrhage, consistent with the peak deterioration observed clinically. Thus, preventing and reducing brain damage during this period is crucial for improving clinical outcomes and is the most feasible time for intervention. This article summarizes recent advances in understanding the mechanisms of brain damage caused by the hydrolysis of red blood cells after hemorrhage, aiming to provide possible insights for new treatment strategies.

Wherever red blood cells are destroyed, the hemoglobin released from their rupture is broken down into globin and heme. Globin participates in the general metabolic processes of the body. Heme is further decomposed into iron and biliverdin, which can be converted into bilirubin under the action of enzymes.

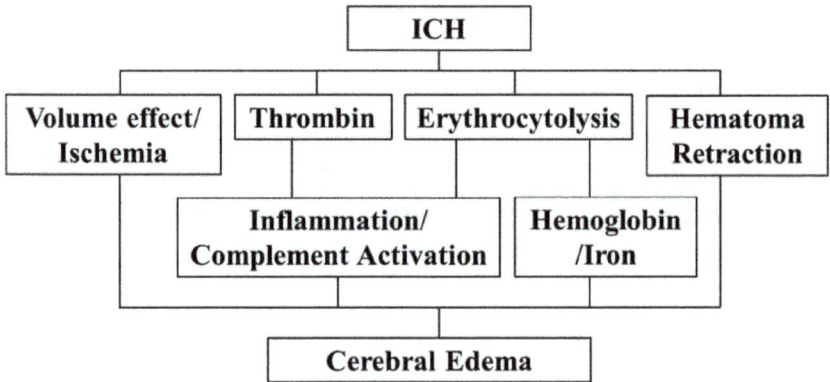

Figure 1: Schematic diagram of the stage model of edema formation after ICH

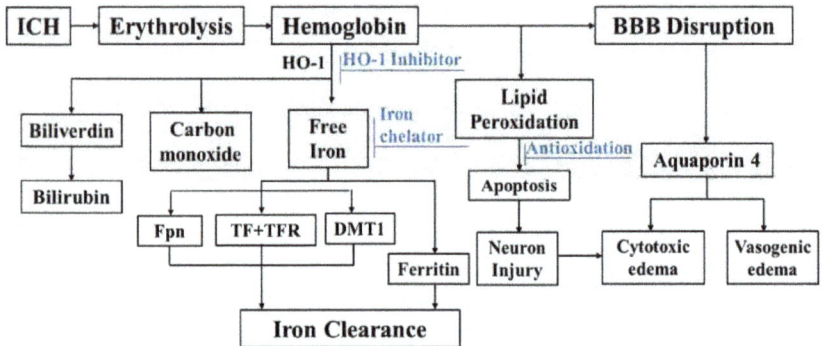

Figure2: Secondary brain damage and anti-damage model by hemolysis post- ICH

Annotation:

ICH: Intracerebral Hemorrhage; **BBB:** Blood-brain barrier; **HO-1:** Heme oxidase-1; **Fpn:** Ferroportin; **TF:** Transferritin; **TFR:** Transferritin Receptor; **DMT-1:** Divalent Metal Transporter 1

1. Hemolysis of red blood cells and generation of its products: After cerebral hemorrhage, a large number of red blood cells enter the brain parenchyma. Hemolysis and subsequent release of hemoglobin result in the production of hematin, which can be degraded into iron, carbon monoxide, and bilirubin by heme oxygenase (HO). Iron is eventually converted into ferritin and iron-containing hemosiderin. Research has shown that the toxic effects of red blood cell hydrolysis products, such as hemichrome, on neuronal cells are iron-dependent, oxidative, and primarily necrotic in nature. Red blood cell hemolysis occurs approximately 3 days after bleeding, consistent with the peak period of clinical hematoma. The toxic effects of red blood cell hemolysis and its decomposition products can induce severe neurological deficits and significant cerebral edema. Intracerebral injection of concentrated red blood cells can cause more pronounced disruption of the blood-brain barrier compared to dissolved red blood cells, occurring 72 hours after injection rather than 24 hours. Moreover, hemolysis can induce strong expression of HSP-70 in the brain, which is a marker of cellular stress. Injection of dissolved red blood cells into the brain leads to a significant increase in peri-hematomal water content, which is associated with decreased potassium ion levels and increased sodium ion levels in the brain. The increase in blood-brain barrier permeability induced by injection of dissolved blood is far greater than that induced by thrombin, suggesting that red blood cell-induced edema is primarily vasogenic edema, accompanied by damage to neuronal cells. Neurological deficits may be related to the formation of edema and brain damage caused by oxidative stress. Injection of red blood cells and their products into the brain can significantly induce the formation of cerebral edema, but nearby cerebral blood flow remains close to normal, suggesting that edema is unrelated to ischemia.

1.1 Hemoglobin and its breakdown product generation and toxic effects: The mechanism of brain damage caused by red blood cell hemolysis is not entirely clear, but hemoglobin and its breakdown products (oxyhemoglobin, deoxyhemoglobin, methemoglobin) play a major role in it. Intracerebral injection of hemoglobin can lead to chronic focal spike waves and proliferation of neuroglial cells at the injection site. Hemoglobin can inhibit sodium-potassium ATPase activity, activate lipid peroxidation, exacerbate excitotoxic damage in cortical cell cultures, and induce depolarization of neurons in the hippocampal CA1 region. Exposure of cultured mouse spinal cord cells to hemoglobin can result in concentration-dependent cytotoxic effects. Hemoglobin can activate lipid peroxidation and kill cultured neurons. Oxyhemoglobin can induce apoptosis in cultured endothelial cells, a process already observed in cerebral hemorrhage. Research on the molecular mechanisms of hemoglobin-induced cell damage or even death mainly focuses on its toxic effects resulting from oxidative stress responses in cells. Hemoglobin consists of heme and globin, and free heme is usually sequestered by plasma proteins and does not reach toxic levels. However, during cerebral hemorrhage, a large amount of hemoglobin is released from lysed red blood cells, leading to the production of excessive hematin which saturates plasma proteins, thereby exposing surrounding neurons to hematin. Hematin is a significant source of oxidants and free radicals, disrupting the balance between oxidation and antioxidation and exerting specific oxidative toxicity on cells. Additionally, hematin is an iron-containing porphyrin, with two-thirds to four-fifths of the total iron in the body existing in hematin, which releases a significant amount of reactive iron, and free iron has significant tissue toxicity. Furthermore, studies have shown that hemoglobin-induced cerebral edema formation is partly caused by its degradation products and can be alleviated by intraperitoneal injection of deferoxamine.

1.2 Heme Oxygenase Forms, Characteristics, and Functions: Heme oxygenase (HO) is the rate-limiting enzyme in heme catabolism, a protein enzyme found in the microsomes of mammalian tissue cells. It degrades heme in the cytoplasm to produce biliverdin, free iron ions, and carbon monoxide. Free iron ions exhibit tissue toxicity. There are three isoforms of HO, with HO-1 being the most extensively studied. Under normal conditions, HO-1 is primarily present in peripheral tissues and is difficult to detect in the brain. It can be induced and activated by factors such as heme, metal elements, oxidative stress, ultraviolet irradiation, chemical substances, high heat, certain drugs, depletion of glutathione, trauma, subarachnoid hemorrhage, and ischemia, thus it is also referred to as inducible HO. HO-1 contains sites that can be mediated by many physiological stressors, including heme, heat shock, oxidative stress, hypoxia, and immediate early factors. HO-1 is mainly distributed in the mononuclear phagocyte system (spleen, liver, and bone marrow) and is activated by oxidative stress reactions, participating in heme metabolism, with the highest activity found in the spleen. Tissue content decreases in the order of lung > liver > brain > heart, with the spleen showing the highest HO-1 activity. Studies using cDNA probes have found that the human HO-1 gene is approximately 14 kb in size, containing 4 introns and 5 exons, encoding 288 amino acid residues with a molecular weight of 32 kDa, while rat HO-1 contains 289 amino acids, with a high homology of up to 80%, indicating the gene's high stability. Its 5'-untranslated region contains regulatory binding sites such as activator protein 1 (AP-1), metal responsive element (MRE), c-myc/max heterodimer binding site (Myc/Max), antioxidant response element (ARE), and glucocorticoid box binding (Sp1) site, heat shock factor (HSF), and nuclear factor-κB (NF-κB) hemoglobin response element. Thus, multiple stimuli can induce its production, such as heat shock, blood loss, inflammation, various metals (Fe, Ni, Co, Al, Cd, etc.), glutathione reductase deficiency, radiation injury, hypoxia, oxygen poisoning, cellular transport disorders, and various cytokines can all increase its expression. It has a similar structure to heat shock protein 70 (HSP70) and stress protein P32, so it is classified into the HSP family and referred to as HSP32. The increased activity of HO-1 is due to increased expression of the HO-1 gene. Current research suggests that HO-1 not only functions in the physiological state of the body but also plays a major role in other abnormal or stressful states of the body. HO-1 is mainly expressed in small glial cells in the cerebral hemorrhage model. HO is the rate-limiting enzyme in heme metabolism, with HO-1 protein levels in the dissolved red blood cell model group being 14 times higher than in the control group. The biological significance of its upregulation is currently unclear. Upregulation of HO-1 can lead to excessive accumulation of heme degradation and free iron in the brain, stimulate free radical generation, and promote oxidative damage. This mechanism is evidenced by the detection of superoxide dismutase (SOD) levels in the brain. SOD is a scavenger of reactive oxygen species (ROS) and protects brain tissue from damage after ischemia and hypoxia. Studies have shown that copper-zinc superoxide dismutase (Cu-Zn-SOD) and manganese superoxide dismutase (Mn-SOD) are significantly reduced in the ipsilateral striatum of the cerebral hemorrhage model, indicating impaired free radical clearance system, which may increase oxidative stress damage in the brain, thereby exacerbating post-hemorrhagic brain damage. ROS-induced brain damage can occur through various pathways, one of which is direct DNA damage, which is caused by at least two pathways: endonuclease-mediated DNA cleavage and oxidative stress damage. ROS directly attack DNA, causing oxidative damage and single-strand breaks. Compared to endonuclease-mediated DNA cleavage, oxidative single-strand cleavage occurs relatively early. Significant exacerbation of DNA damage caused by ROS occurs in the presence of free iron. Additionally, the increased content of protein carbonyls (a marker of oxidative stress) in the brain is correlated with DNA damage, reflecting the damage of oxidative stress in the brain.

HO-1 is mainly expressed in microglial cells in the cerebral hemorrhage model. Research by Matz et al. has shown that injection of whole blood or dissolved blood into the striatum and cortex can induce expression of HO-1 in microglial cells in the ipsilateral striatum, cortex, hippocampus, and thalamus. It suggests that glial cells play a major role in the metabolism of hemoglobin released into the brain parenchyma after cerebral hemorrhage. Hematin is a potent inducer of HO-1. During cerebral hemorrhage, extravasated hematin can directly bind to the hematin factor on HO-1, inducing its expression. HO-1 expression appears to be a good marker of oxidative stress associated with brain cell damage and is also an important protein for iron efflux from cells. TNF-α and IL-1β can induce expression of HO-1 in endothelial cells through protein kinase-C, calcium ions, and phospholipase A2. Depletion of glutathione can induce expression of HO-1 in the brain, possibly mediated by NF-Kappa B sites on the HO-1 gene. NF-Kappa B specifically regulates the expression of IL-1β and TNF-α, promoting perihematomal edema and cell death. Antioxidants can reduce the production of HO-1. The expression of HO-1 peaks at 3 days after hemorrhage and lasts for a long time, indicating that hemoglobin released from red blood cells may be the main inducer of HO-1, while plasma proteins, especially thrombin, may also induce early expression of HO-1.

HO-2, also known as constitutive heme oxygenase, is mainly expressed in the vast majority of neurons in the brain and is not inducible. Neuronal HO-2 is induced by glucocorticoids and may affect brain growth and development by inducing HO-2 expression in motor neurons and the cognitive system during development. HO-2 has a protective effect against ischemic damage and partly exhibits antioxidant characteristics. However, research by Matz et al. suggests that the immune response of HO-2 in the cerebral hemorrhage model is similar to that of the control, indicating that the expression of HO-2 is not affected by oxidative stress and is not a known stress protein.

HO-3 is a heme-binding protein gene that lacks HO activity, and its role in the brain is unclear. It may act as an intracellular transporter and chaperone protein, accompanying hematin to HO-1, HO-2, or entering mitochondria.

Increased expression of HO-1 in the perihematomal area can

accelerate the degradation of iron and accumulation of free iron in the brain, thereby promoting the formation of brain edema. Inhibition of HO can reduce the formation of cerebral edema in pigs and mice. However, there is also research showing that overexpression of HO-1 can protect neurons from oxidative damage. Increased expression of HO-1 promotes the chelation of catalytic iron into ferritin and increases the generation of biliverdin by degrading hematin. Increased local concentrations of bilirubin and biliverdin protect cells from oxidative damage, thereby exerting a protective effect on neurons. CO, as a degradation product of hematin, produces effects similar to nitric oxide (NO). As a regulator of endothelial cell function after hemorrhage/oxidative damage, CO is also a vasodilator. It can counteract the vasoconstrictive effects of hemoglobin and methemoglobin along with other vasodilators. This contradictory result may be due to the different functions and concentrations of hematin degradation products, indicating that exacerbation or alleviation of oxidative stress in the brain depends mainly on the concentration and environment of degradation products. A moderate increase in HO-1 (less than 5-fold) can prevent neuronal damage, while a significant upregulation (more than 15-fold) is associated with pronounced oxidative toxicity. Application of HO inhibitors can reduce the extent of edema and damage. Current data suggest that HO-1 may have a dual role in exacerbating and alleviating brain damage mechanisms.

1.3 The Role of Iron and Iron-Handling Proteins: Iron is a fundamental component of many cellular functions and has some specific functions in the nervous system, such as the synthesis of dopamine, serotonin, and norepinephrine, possibly also including the synthesis of γ-aminobutyric acid (GABA) and the formation of myelin sheaths. Iron is distributed throughout the entire brain, including the white matter, but the highest levels of iron are found in the basal ganglia of the brain, with biochemical and histochemical studies indicating that the entire white matter of the brain is the main site of iron accumulation. Intracellular iron reactions are a source of free radicals and promote lipid peroxidation, leading to damage to lipid-rich structures such as brain tissue. Iron plays a crucial role in generating powerful oxidants. Increasing iron levels can increase oxidative stress, while removing iron can reduce this stress. As iron concentration increases in cultured cells, the levels of reactive oxygen species (ROS) increase, accompanied by protein degradation. Iron toxicity mediated by ROS can cause apoptosis and cell death, possibly involving both cytochrome-C (Cyt-C) and caspase-3-independent apoptotic pathways. Iron can also induce DNA modification by forming 8-OH-2'-deoxyguanosine, causing chromatin oxidation damage, thus affecting cell survival and normal function. Iron-induced oxidative damage may be associated with neurodegeneration and the cascade of events leading to cell death.

In the central nervous system (CNS), iron transport is generally believed to occur through two main pathways: transferrin-mediated and non-transferrin-mediated pathways. Iron-handling proteins include transferrin (Tf), transferrin receptor (TfR), and ferritin, all of which participate in maintaining the iron homeostasis in the brain. Tf is an 80 kDa protein mainly expressed in monosynaptic cells, serving as the primary distributor of iron in the brain by binding iron to TfR to facilitate iron uptake by brain cells. TfR, also known as CD71, consists of two 95 kDa glycoprotein subunits. Tf and TfR are involved in the transport of iron across biological membranes. Under pathological conditions, the levels of Tf and TfR can vary. Much evidence suggests that the Tf-TfR pathway may be the major route for iron transport across the capillary endothelial basement membrane. Under normal physiological conditions, oligodendrocytes release iron-free transferrin and uptake extracellular iron through the blood-brain barrier into cells. Therefore, extracellular iron in the brain parenchyma after hemorrhage is most likely taken up by oligodendrocytes via transferrin. Iron fragments bound to non-transferrin proteins significantly increase in circulation. Substantia nigra cells rich in divalent cation iron transporter (DMT-1) in the ventricles can also clear free iron in the cerebrospinal fluid. After hemorrhage, transferrin becomes fully saturated, and other components in the cerebrospinal fluid, including citrates and vitamin C, may also participate in iron transport. Cultured astrocytes, characterized by reactive astrocytes, also express DMT-1, and iron transport pathways have been identified in cultured astrocytes. Therefore, the expression of DMT-1 in reactive astrocytes may facilitate the uptake of metals after injury. Astrocytes around the hematoma area are activated after hemorrhage and are highly likely to participate in iron clearance. However, the fate of extracellular iron and the cellular, protein, and molecular mechanisms involved in iron clearance after hemorrhage are still unclear.

Ferritin, with a molecular weight of 45 kDa, is highly stable and has a hollow spherical structure composed of 24 subunits, exhibiting ferroxidase activity. In the form of O-OH microclusters, it can contain up to 4500 iron atoms. Ferritin is mainly located in the cytoplasm and mitochondria. Cytoplasmic ferritin is widely present in mammals, while mitochondrial ferritin is only found in testes, neurons, and pancreatic islets, with similar functions. In bacteria, the DNA-binding protein family (Dps) has ferritin-like activity in starving cells, serving as an iron storage and detoxification agent and reducing the generation of ROS products, a view that has been recognized. Therefore, ferritin has a high binding capacity for iron, serving as the main storage site for iron released from hemoglobin metabolism, a naturally occurring iron chelator related to iron utilization and storage. It is normally present in neurons and glial cells in the brain. Most ferritins around hematomas are expressed in small glial cells and astrocytes. Hemoglobin is a physiological inducer of ferritin synthesis, stimulating the expression of ferritin mRNA after hemorrhage. Iron ions produced by HO activation and TNF-α can also stimulate ferritin biosynthesis. Ferritin can store and detoxify iron, thus also known as inducible iron detoxification protein. Application of ferric citrate ammonium in astrocyte culture medium can increase cellular ferritin content, indicating that iron accumulation can regulate ferritin synthesis in astrocytes, which is necessary to prevent iron-mediated astrocyte toxicity. The ferritin content in cerebrospinal fluid is about 10% of that in plasma, and it can also clear free iron in the cerebrospinal fluid. Since the cerebrospinal fluid is replaced approximately every 8 hours, cerebrospinal fluid ferritin has the mechanism to clear iron after cerebral hemorrhage. Ferritin synthesized and released locally by choroid plexus cells may provide ferritin in cerebrospinal fluid.

Ferritin is normally synthesized in small glial cells, which depends on local iron levels and the presence of iron-regulatory proteins. Immunoreactivity of ferritin around hemorrhagic brain tissue 24-48 hours post-hemorrhage is significantly higher than histological staining of iron in small glial cells. Additionally, whole blood elicits a greater ferritin response compared to pure red blood cells, suggesting a role of plasma proteins derived from clotting in stimulating ferritin expression. Uncontrolled biosynthesis of ferritin occurs in the area of hemorrhagic damage post-bleeding. Excessive accumulation of ferritin may involve two mechanisms: 1) Loss of iron response protein (IRP); 2) Cytokine stimulation of ferritin biosynthesis. Since IRP is localized in astrocytes in the brain, iron must be transported to small glial cells to control ferritin biosynthesis. Therefore, disruption of connections between astrocytes and small glial cells caused by hematoma and surrounding edema may lead to uncontrolled ferritin biosynthesis independent of iron levels. As ferritin is a precursor of heme, these events may promote heme aggregation. Excessive iron must be promptly cleared from the brain after intracerebral hemorrhage to prevent further oxidative stress, with ferritin being the executor of this function. Thus, elucidating the intracellular responses of ferritin and its distribution after brain damage is crucial. The relationship between ferritin, iron, and small glial cells increases in importance with the discovery of ferritin receptors in oligodendrocytes.

Increased activity of HO-1 is closely associated with pathological iron accumulation in astrocytes. When the brain is overloaded with iron after cerebral hemorrhage, levels of Tf and TfR significantly increase, with Tf facilitating iron clearance from the brain through the blood-brain barrier. Ferritin serves as a natural iron chelator, associated with iron utilization and storage. It is normally present in neurons and glial cells in the brain, with most ferritin expressed in small glial cells and astrocytes around hematomas. Iron ions and TNF-α can promote ferritin synthesis. Iron content in the brain rapidly peaks after red blood cell lysis. Since iron can react with hydrogen peroxide and oxygen, excessive iron can initiate lipid peroxidation, leading to membrane damage and ultimately cell death, thus promoting acute cerebral edema (within 1 week) and delayed cerebral atrophy (within 1 month). Increased HO-1 activity is closely associated with pathological iron accumulation in astrocytes. Non-heme iron around the hematoma area increases more than threefold after cerebral hemorrhage. The peak accumulation of non-heme iron occurs 1-2 weeks after cerebral hemorrhage, delayed compared to the peak of HO-1, possibly reflecting delayed erythrocyte hydrolysis post-hemorrhage. Iron overload can lead to lipid peroxidation and free radical formation, causing brain damage. Overexpression of HO-1 increases the release of free iron, further exacerbating the brain's oxidative stress response, leading to a vicious cycle of secondary neuronal damage. Antioxidants such as superoxide dismutase (SOD) can mitigate neuronal toxicity caused by hemoglobin and iron. Iron chelators such as deferoxamine or heme oxygenase-1 inhibitors such as tin protoporphyrin can alleviate cerebral edema formation caused by inhibition of Na+-K+-ATPase activity and iron release by hemoglobin, as well as reduce lipid peroxidation and free radical formation-induced brain damage. This suggests a critical role of iron in cerebral edema formation post-cerebral hemorrhage. In summary, iron overload and upregulation of iron-handling proteins post-cerebral hemorrhage indicate that iron could be a potential target for future therapies for cerebral hemorrhage.

2. Secondary Ischemia and Edema: There is ongoing debate regarding whether post-hemorrhagic ischemia contributes to edema formation and to what extent it impacts. Although significant edema can be induced by intracranial injection of red blood cell lysate, cerebral blood flow in the perihematomal region remains close to normal. Unlike ischemic damage, edema formation after cerebral hemorrhage is associated with marked blood-brain barrier disruption caused by the toxic effects of erythrocyte hydrolysis. Experiments have shown mild reductions in cerebral blood flow around the hematoma, lasting for at most around 1 hour and returning to normal control levels within 3-4 hours. This suggests that the level and duration of this decrease in blood flow are insufficient to cause hypoperfusion after hemorrhage, and ischemia is unrelated to perihematomal brain edema formation. Qureshi et al. also reported the absence of ischemic penumbra around cerebral hematomas in dogs. However, reports on post-hemorrhagic cerebral blood flow reduction in humans vary. Carhuapoma et al. reported no widespread ischemia around hematomas using diffusion-weighted MRI and perfusion magnetic resonance spectroscopic imaging. In contrast, Zazulia et al. found decreased oxygen metabolism and cerebral blood flow around hematomas in patients with cerebral hemorrhage, leading to reduced oxygen extraction fractions. This suggests that significant reductions in cerebral blood flow may result from decreased metabolic rates around the hematoma. The differences in blood flow data between human and animal models may be due to variations in the absolute amount and location of hemorrhage.

3. Blood-Brain Barrier and Edema: Unlike ischemia, the formation of edema around hematomas may involve damage to the vascular endothelium. Iron serves as a potent catalyst for lipid peroxidation, and the release of iron after erythrocyte hydrolysis may promote dysfunction of the blood-brain barrier. Additionally, oxyhemoglobin can induce apoptosis in cultured endothelial cells, possibly through free radical damage to the endothelial vessel wall. Significant disruption of the blood-brain barrier occurs after intracranial injection of concentrated erythrocytes, corresponding to the time of erythrocyte hydrolysis occurring in vivo, typically around 72 hours post-hemorrhage. Erythrocyte hydrolysis-induced disruption of the blood-brain barrier can even lead to the entry of large molecules such as fibrinogen into brain parenchyma, and thrombin precursor may also enter the brain. If factor X activator (possibly entering the brain from the bloodstream) is present, thrombin precursor may generate thrombin, which also contributes to the formation of brain edema. The ability of erythrocyte hydrolysis and thrombin to cause blood-brain barrier disruption differs, with erythrocyte hydrolysis being much more potent than thrombin in inducing blood-brain barrier disruption, and its peak increase in blood-brain barrier permeability occurs around 2 days post-hemorrhage, significantly later than the formation of edema caused by thrombin.

4. Aquaporins and Brain Edema: Brain edema, including cellular swelling and vasogenic edema, mainly occurs around hematomas and can extend to distant areas. It is a key factor contributing to clinical deterioration and prognosis. The formation of edema in brain tissue around hematomas involves a series of reactions, including clot retraction, thrombin formation, erythrocyte destruction and lysis, hemoglobin toxicity, complement activation, volume effects, and blood-brain barrier disruption. Experimental evidence shows no association between perihematomal brain edema and ischemia, and there is no correlation between the extent of edema and hematoma size. One class of proteins particularly important in the mechanism of brain edema formation is the aquaporin family, which facilitates water movement across various cell membranes. Various factors contributing to brain edema formation may ultimately act through inducing aquaporin expression. Secondary neuronal damage and edema formation following erythrocyte hydrolysis may be related to aquaporin expression.

The aquaporin family comprises 11 subtypes (AQP0-AQP10) with a molecular weight of approximately 30 kDa, each subtype having different extracellular glycosylation patterns. They are ubiquitously distributed in various tissues and organs. So far, six subtypes have been described in the mouse brain, namely AQP1, 3, 4, 5, 8, and 9.

Aquaporin-4 (AQP4) plays a major role in the transport of water in brain tissue and the formation of brain edema. Under physiological conditions, AQP4 mainly maintains the homeostasis of the brain's internal environment and regulates the permeability between the central nervous system and the bloodstream. Control of aquaporin expression and distribution can induce and organize water movement, facilitating edema formation following ischemia and injury. AQP4 is primarily located in astrocytes and ependymal cells. AQP4 protein is enriched in the perivascular end-feet of astrocytes. Polarization of perivascular astrocyte end-feet around blood vessels is a prominent feature of AQP4 immunolabeling. AQP4 expression during brain development may be related to the formation of the blood-brain barrier. The distribution of AQP4 corresponds to the phenotype of the blood-brain barrier. Disruption of the blood-brain barrier can lead to decreased AQP4 expression, although the exact mechanism is unclear. The distribution of AQP4 is remarkably similar to that of connexin-43 and connexin-43 mRNA. Connexin-43 is a major component of gap junctions between astrocytes, suggesting that brain regions rich in this protein may have strong potassium spatial buffering capabilities. In these regions, AQP4 may assist astrocytes in removing excess potassium to allow for rapid water transport, which may promote the formation of cellular edema under pathological conditions.

Although the cause of cellular toxic edema remains unclear, it is primarily associated with swelling of perivascular astrocyte end-feet. During ischemia, astrocytes take up osmotic substances such as sodium, potassium, chloride, and neurotransmitters from the extracellular space into the intracellular space through water channels, participating in the formation of cellular edema by affecting water balance and blood-brain barrier integrity. AQP4 may play a key role in this process. An increase in AQP4 content around blood vessels in the perivascular space reflects the need for rapid movement of water, maintaining water balance and normal intercellular connections by rapidly removing excess water. Mechanical injury or injection of quinolinic acid into the mouse brain can induce increased expression of AQP4 mRNA in the lesion area, suggesting that induced expression of AQP4 is related to blood-brain barrier disruption. The expression of AQP4 is time-dependent, with reduced AQP4 immunostaining observed 24 hours after brain injury, especially in the region of blood-brain barrier disruption, while AQP4 expression increases in the border zone 3 days after injury. These contradictory results suggest that the decrease in AQP4 expression after brain injury may be related to a protective effect against the formation of vasogenic edema. AQP4 knockout mice show reduced brain edema (without cytotoxic edema caused by blood-brain barrier disruption) and promote neurological recovery after acute water intoxication and middle cerebral artery occlusion-induced ischemic stroke. The role of AQP4 in the formation of brain edema remains controversial, whether it plays a protective or harmful role, and its relationship with secondary brain damage following erythrocyte hydrolysis has not been reported in the literature. There are currently no AQP4 blockers or inducers used in experimental studies on the mechanisms of intervention in brain hemorrhage-induced edema.

In summary, the cascade of events triggered by erythrocyte hydrolysis is crucial for the delayed formation of brain edema following hemorrhagic stroke. Brain ischemia does not play a major role in edema formation after hemorrhage. Specifically, the toxic effects of erythrocyte and/or hemoglobin breakdown products lead to blood-brain barrier disruption and subsequent edema formation, with lipid peroxidation potentially causing neuronal damage and cytotoxic edema formation. Moreover, blood-brain barrier disruption and edema formation induced by erythrocyte breakdown products are delayed, thus holding significant implications for later-stage neurological recovery.

The poor prognosis associated with intracerebral hemorrhage appears closely related to the toxic effects of blood components within the brain, raising the question of whether hematoma evacuation is the optimal treatment. However, some clinical trials have not provided sufficient evidence to support the efficacy of hematoma evacuation. This may be due to the potential blood-brain barrier disruption caused by surgery itself, while the release of hemoglobin, iron, and other factors following hematoma evacuation may counteract its effects. Thrombin intervention appears impractical, not only due to its very short therapeutic window but also because thrombin itself has protective effects, preventing hematoma expansion in the early stages. Intervention targeting inflammatory reactions is limited by its lack of specificity and significant side effects, restricting its effective application. The mechanisms of brain damage induced by erythrocyte lysis products following intracerebral hemorrhage suggest that interventions targeting iron and lipid peroxidation may be potential targets for future drug therapies.

REFERENCES:

1   Mayer SA, Rincon F. Treatment of intracerebral haemorrhage. *Lancet Neurol* 2005; 4(10):662-72

2   Mayer SA, Sacco RL, Shi T, Mohr JP. Neurologic deterioration in noncomatose patients with supratentorial intracerebral hemorrhage. *Neurology* 1994; 44: 1379 - 84.

3   Goldstein L, Teng ZP, Zeserson E,et al. Hemin induces an iron-dependent, oxidative injury to human neuron-like cells. *J Neurosci Re* 2003;73(1):113-21

4   Xi G, Hua Y, Bhasin R,et al. Mechanisms of Edema Formation After Intracerebral Hemorrhage: Effects of Extravasated Red Blood Cells on Blood Flow and Blood-Brain Barrier Integrity. *Stroke* 2001;32(12):2932-2938

5   Matz PG, Weinstein PR, Sharp FR. Heme oxygenase-1 and heat shock protein 70 induction in glia and neurons throughout rat brain after experimental intracerebral hemorrhage. *Neurosurgery* 1997; 40（1）: 152–160.

6   Hua Y, Schallert T,Keep RF,et al. Behavioral Tests After Intracerebral Hemorrhage in the Rat. *Stroke* 2002; 33(10): 2478-2484

7   Wagner, Kenneth R.; Sharp, Frank R.; Ardizzone, Timothy D.. Heme and Iron Metabolism Role in Cerebral Hemorrhage. *J Cereb Blood Flow Metab 2003;23 (6):* 629-652

8   Xi G, Hua Y, Bhasin RR, et al. Mechanisms of Edema Formation After Intracerebral Hemorrhage: Effects of Extravasated Red Blood Cells on Blood Flow and Blood-Brain Barrier Integrity. *Stroke* 2001; 32(12) : 2932-2938

9   Gong C, Boulis N, Qian J, et al. Intracerebral hemorrhage-induced neuronal death. *Neurosurgery* 2001; 48: 875–883.

10 Huang FP, Xi G, Keep RF,et al. Brain edema after experimental intracerebral hemorrhage: role of hemoglobin degradation products. *J Neurosurg* 2002; 96(2):287-93

11 JF Ewing, SN Haber, MD Maines.Normal and heat-induced patterns of expression of heme oxygenase-1(HSP32) in rat brain: hyperthermia causes rapid induction of mRNA and protein. *J Neurochem* 1992; 58:1140-1149

12 JF Ewing, MD Maines.Glutathione depletion induces heme oxygenase-1(HSP32) mRNA and protein in rat brain. *J Neurochem* 1993; 60:1512-1519

13 Fukuda K, Richmon JD, Sato M, et al. Induction of heme oxygenase-1 (HO-1) in glia after traumatic brain injury. *Brain Res* 1996;736(1-2):68-75.

14 Turner CP, Bergeron M, Matz P, et al. Heme oxygenase-1 is induced in glia throughout brain by subarachnoid hemoglobin. *J Cereb Blood Flow Metab* 1998;18(3):257-73.

15 Attuwaybi BO, Kozar RA, Moore-Olufemi SD, et al. Heme oxygenase-1 induction by hemin protects against gut ischemia/reperfusion injury. *J Surg Res* 2004;118(1):53-7.

16 Bidmon HJ, Emde B, Oermann E, et al. Heme oxygenase-1 (HSP-32) and heme oxygenase-2 induction in neurons and glial cells of cerebral regions and its relation to iron accumulation after focal cortical photothrombosis. *Exp Neurol* 2001;168(1):1-22.

17 Bergeron M, Ferriero DM, Sharp FR. Developmental expression of heme oxygenase-1 (HSP32) in rat brain: an immunocytochemical study. *Brain Res Dev*

Brain Res 1998;105(2):181-94.

18 Jimin Wu , Ya Hua , Richard F. Keep ,et al. O xidative brain injury from extravasated erythrocytes after intracerebral hemorrhage. *Brain Res* 2002; 953:45–52

19 Peluffo H, Acarin L, Faiz M, et al. Cu/Zn superoxide dismutase expression in the postnatal rat brain following an excitotoxic injury. *J Neuroinflammation* 2005; 2(1):12.

20 Shimizu K, Rajapakse N, Horiguchi T, et al. Neuroprotection against hypoxia-ischemia in neonatal rat brain by novel superoxide dismutase mimetics. *Neurosci Lett* 2003; 346:41–44.

21 Wagner KR, Sharp FR, Ardizzone TD, et al. Heme and Iron Metabolism: Role in Cerebral Hemorrhage. *J Cereb Blood Flow Metab* 2003; 23(6):629-652

22 Wu J, Hua Y, Keep RF, et al. Iron and Iron-Handling Proteins in the Brain After Intracerebral Hemorrhage. *Stroke* 2003; 34 (12): 2964-2969

23 Matz PG, Weinstein PR,Sharp FR. Heme Oxygenase-1 and Heat Shock Protein 70 Induction in Glia and Neurons throughout Rat Brain after Experimental Intracerebral Hemorrhage. Neurosurgery 1997; 40(1): 152-162

24 Barron KD. The microglial cell. A historical review. *J Neurol Sci* 1995; 134 (Suppl): 57-68.

25 David H. Haile. Regulation of SLC11A3 by inflammation. *BioMetals* 2003;16: 225–241

26 Cederbaum AI. Iron and CYP2E1-dependent oxidative stress and toxicity.*Alcohol* 2003;30(2):115-20

27 Liu R, Liu W, Doctrow SR, et al. Iron toxicity in organotypic cultures of hippocampal slices: role of reactive oxygen species. *J Neurochem* 2003;85(2):492-502

28 Zhong Ming Qian , Xun Shen. Brain iron transport and neurodegeneration. *Trends Mol Med* 2001; 7 (3): 103-8

29 Bradbury M W B. Transport of iron in the blood–brain–cerebrospinal fluid system.. *J Neurochem* 1997; 69: 443–451

30 Moos T, Morgan EH. Evidence for low molecular weight, non-transferrin-bound iron in rat brain and cerebrospinal fluid. *J Neurosci Res* 1998; 54:486–494

31 Burdo JR, Menzies SL, Simpson IA, et al. Distribution of divalent metal transporter 1 and metal transport protein 1 in the normal and Belgrade rat. *J Neurosci Res* 2001; 66:1198–1207

32 Levi S, Arosio P. Mitochondrial ferritin. *Int J Biochem Cell Biol* 2004; 36(10):1887-9.

33 Chiancone E, Ceci P, Ilari A, et al. Iron and proteins for iron storage and detoxification. *Biometals* 2004;17(3):197-202

34 Suzuki H, Muramatsu M, Kojima T, et al. Intracranial heme metabolism and cerebral vasospasm after aneurysmal subarachnoid hemorrhage. *Stroke* 2003; 34(12):2796-800.

35 Hoepken HH, Korten T, Robinson SR, et al. Iron accumulation, iron-mediated toxicity and altered levels of ferritin and transferrin receptor in cultured astrocytes during incubation with ferric ammonium citrate. *J Neurochem* 2004; 88(5):1194-202

36 Earley CJ, Connor JR, Beard JL, et al. Abnormalities in CSF concentrations of ferritin and transferrin in restless legs syndrome. *Neurology* 2000;54:1698–1700

37 Koeppen AH, Dickson AC, McEvoy JA . The cellular reactions to experimental intracerebral hemorrhage. *J Neurol Sci* 1995;134:102–112

38 Koeppen AH, Dickson AC, Smith J. Heme oxygenase in experimental intracerebral hemorrhage: the benefit of tin-mesoporphyrin. *J Neuropathol Exp Neurol* 2004; 63(6):587-97.

39 Nakamura T, Keep RF, Hua Y, et al. Deferoxamine-induced attenuation of brain edema and neurological deficits in a rat model of intracerebral hemorrhage. *J Neurosurg* 2004; 100(4):672-8.

40 Hua Y, Keep RF, Hoff JT. Thrombin Preconditioning Attenuates Brain Edema Induced by Erythrocytes and Iron. *J cereb Blood Flow Metab* 2003; 23(12): 1448-1454

41 Qureshi AI, Wilson DA, Traystman RJ. No evidence for an ischemic penumbra in

massive experimental intracerebral hemorrhage. *Neurology* 1999; 52: 266–272.

42 Carhuapoma JR, Wang PY, Beauchamp NJ, et al. Diffusion-weighted MRI and proton magnetic resonance spectroscopic imaging in the study of secondary neuronal injury after intracerebral hemorrhage. *Stroke* 2000; 31: 726–732.

43 Zazulia AR, Diringer MN, Videen TO, et al. Hypoperfusion without ischemia surrounding acute intracerebral hemorrhage. *J Cereb Blood Flow Metab* 2001; 21: 804–810.

44 Hoff JT, Xi G. Brain edema from intracerebral hemorrhage. *Acta Neurochir Suppl* 2003;86:11-15.

45 Badaut J, Lasbennes F, Magistretti PJ, et al. Aquaporins in Brain: Distribution, Physiology, and Pathophysiology. *J Cereb Blood Flow Metab* 2002; 22 (4): 367-378

46 Rash JE, Yasumura T. Direct immunogold labeling of connexins and aquaporin-4 in freeze-fracture replicas of liver, brain, and spinal cord: factors limiting quantitative analysis. *Cell Tissue Res* 1999; 296(2):307-21.

47 Lo AC, Chen AY, Hung VK, et al. Endothelin-1 overexpression leads to further water accumulation and brain edema after middle cerebral artery occlusion via aquaporin 4 expression in astrocytic end-feet. *J Cereb Blood Flow Metab* 2005; 25(8):998-1011.

48 Taniguchi M, Yamashita T, Kumura E , et al. Induction of aquaporin -4 water channel mRNA after focal cerebral ischemia in rat. *Brain Res Mol Brain Res* 2000;78 (1 - 2) :131 – 137

49 Nico B, Frigeri A, Nicchia GP, et al. Role of aquaporin - 4 waterchannel in the development and integrity of the blood - brain barrier. J Cell Sci 2001;114 (pt7) :1297 -1307

50 Ke C, Poon WS, Ng HK, et al. Heterogeneous responses of aquaporin-4 in oedema formation in a replicated severe traumatic brain injury model in rats. *Neurosci Lett* 2001; 301:21–24

51 Regan RF, Rogers B. Delayed treatment of hemoglobin neurotoxicity. *Neurotrauma* 2003;20(1):111-20.

52 Manley GT, Fujimura M, Ma T, et al. Aquaporin-4 deletion in mice reduces brain edema after acute water intoxication and ischemic stroke. *Nat Med* 2000;6:159–163

53 Xi G, Keep RF, Hoff JT. Mechanisms of brain injury after intracerebral haemorrhage. *Lancet Neurol* 2006; 5(1):53-63.

54 Qureshi AI, Tuhrim S, Broderick JP, Batjer HH, Hondo H,Hanley DF. Spontaneous intracerebral hemorrhage. *N Engl J Med* 2001; 344: 1450–60.

55 Hankey GJ, Hon C. Surgery for primary intracerebral hemorrhage:is it safe and effective? A systematic review of case series and randomized trials. *Stroke* 1997; 28: 2126–32.

56 Mendelow AD, Gregson BA, Fernandes HM, et al. Early surgery versus initial conservative treatment in patients with spontaneous supratentorial intracerebral haematomas in the International Surgical Trial in Intracerebral Haemorrhage (STICH): a randomised trial. *Lancet* 2005; 365: 387–97

57 Morgenstern LB, Demchuk AM, Kim DH, et al. Rebleeding leads to poor outcome in ultra-early craniotomy for intracerebral hemorrhage. *Neurology* 2001;56: 1294–1299.

58 Morgenstern LB, Frankowski RF, Shedden P, Pasterur WJCG. Surgical treatment for intracerebral hemorrhage (STICH): a single-center, randomized clinical trial. *Neurology* 1998; 51: 1359–1363.

59 Zuccarello M, Brott T, Derex L, Kothari R, Sauerbeck L, Tew J, Van Loveren H, Yeh HS, Tomsick T, Pancioli A, Khoury J, Broderick J. Early surgical treatment for supratentorial intracerebral hemorrhage: a randomized feasibility study. *Stroke* 1999; 30: 1833–1839.

60 Thiex R, Kuker W, Jungbluth P, et al. Minor inflammation after surgical evacuation compared with fibrinolytic therapy of experimental intracerebral hemorrhages. *Neurol Res* 2005; 27(5):493-8

61 Kitaoka T, Hua Y, Xi G, Hoff JT, Keep RF. Delayed argatrobantreatment reduces edema in a rat model of intracerebral hemorrhage. *Stroke* 2002; 33: 3012-18

62 Gong C, Hoff JT, Keep RF. Acute inflammatory reaction following experimental intracerebral hemorrhage. *Brain Res* 2000; 871: 57–65.

DECLARATION: This chapter was authored by Gaiqing Wang and published as "The Mechanisms and Deferoxamine Intervention of Delayed Brain Injury After Experimental Intracerebral Hemorrhage in Rats" in Doctoral Dissertation of Central South University, 2006

CHAPTER 3:

Hematoma Expansion: Clinical and Molecular Predictors and Corresponding Pharmacological Treatment

ABSTRACT:

Hematoma expansion is a detrimental event of intracerebral hemorrhage (ICH) which results in progressive neurologic deteriorations and poor outcomes. Although the exact mechanism of hematoma expansion is unclear, accumulating evidences suggest that multiple clinical markers such as coagulation/hemostasis dysfunction, higher blood pressure and BRAIN scores, higher serum glucose and/or glycosylated hemoglobin A1c, serum creatinine, Factor XIII and international normalized ratio (INR), lower serum cholesterol or LDL cholesterol, and fibrinogen, may be correlated with incidents of hematoma expansion. Furthermore, activation of several molecular pathways (i.e. plasma kallikrein, von Willebrand factor, N-methyl-D-aspartate and its receptor, cytokines/ adipokines, cellular fibronectin and apolipoprotein $E_\varepsilon 2$ allele) may lead to hematoma expansion. We searched MEDLINE with the keywords "hematoma expansion", "hematoma enlargement", "hematoma growth", "rebleeding", "secondary bleeding", "recurrent bleeding" and "rehemorrhage". We excluded hemorrhage from SAH, aneurysm and trauma. Four papers about hematoma expansion and corresponding intervention published in English were reviewed. Articles were selected for their conceptual importance and primacy. Where issues are controversial, evidence on both sides of the issue is given. In this review, we summarized the current understanding of the mechanisms underlying hematoma expansion. The potential approaches of treatment and prevention will also be discussed.

KEY WORDS: Hematoma expansion; Predictors; Molecular mechanism; Pharmacological treatment; Molecular intervention; Prevention; Intracerebral hemorrhage

INTRODUCTION

Hematoma expansion is the primary cause of neurologic deterioration after intracerebral hemorrhage (ICH) [1-3] and remains one of the few remediable risk factors for poor outcome [4, 5]. Hematoma expansion occurs in about one third of patients with cerebral hemorrhage [1, 3, 6]. In a study by Brott and colleagues, hematoma growth was defined by an increase in hematoma volume by 33% of the baseline volume [7], i.e. a 10% increase in diameter [8-10]. An almost linear association between hematoma expansion and the probability of poor outcome has been reported: a 1 mL additional hematoma expansion yields a 5% increased risk of death and dependency [11, 12]. Hematoma expansion is a significant, independent predictor of adverse outcomes after ICH, over and above established baseline prognostic indicators [11, 13]. Therefore, effective therapy directed at stopping rebleeding in acute ICH patients could potentially decrease mortality and improve the neurological outcome [6]. Therefore, additional information on the precise underlying mechanisms of hematoma expansion and its potential

therapeutic interventions are required. This review focuses on the current understanding of the mechanisms underlying hematoma expansion and proposes potential strategies for clinical prevention and intervention.

PREDICTORS OF HEMATOMA EXPANSION

Many predictors of hematoma expansion (Fig. 1) have been proposed, but some of them e.g., fibrinogen [14, 15], blood pressure [6, 13, 14, 16-18], blood glucose [3, 13, 19, 20], and IVH [10, 16, 21, 22] remain controversial. In patients with medical histories of bleeding and/or coagulation abnormalities [23], who suffered from liver disease 3 and/or were alcoholics [14], who were under treatment of anticoagulants [23-29] or antiplatelets [19, 29, 30] (i.e, for valvular heart disease, venous thromboembolism and/or atrial fibrillation [31-33], and brain infarction [3]) or where there was prior ICH, the odds of hematoma expansion were higher. A coagulation/ hemostasis dysfunction appears to contribute to hematoma growth.

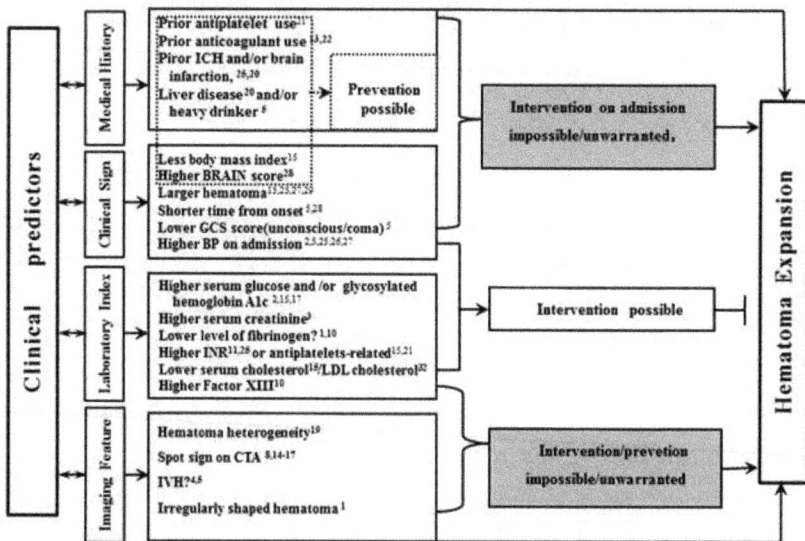

Fig.1. Clinical markers (including medical history, clinical signs on admission, laboratory and imaging findings) for predicting hematoma expansion, then selected some possible interventions after intracerebral hemorrhage.

Other clinical predictors include higher blood pressure (BP) on admission (systolic BP¯160-200mmHg) [3, 14, 33-37], higher BRAIN scores [16] based on Baseline ICH volume, Recurrent ICH, Anticoagulation with warfarin at onset, Intraventricular extension, and the Number of hours to baseline CT from symptom onset [38, 39]. The larger volume of ICH [19, 33, 36, 37], the shorter time period from symptom onset to CT [14, 16], as well as Recurrent ICH, Anticoagulation with warfarin at onset, Intraventricular extension [1, 9, 16, 25, 39, 40], predicted a higher risk of hematoma expansion [16]. The BRAIN scores can be easily assessed and implemented by clinicians and, in particular, can be used for shared clinical decision-making where CTA is not readily available or routinely performed for acute ICH [16]. In addition, it was reported that consciousness disturbance on admission14 and less mass index [19] were more likely to cause hematoma growth. Where laboratory indices included higher serum glucose [3, 19, 20, 41] and/or glycosylated hemoglobin A1c [3], higher serum creatinine [19], Factor XIII [15] and international normalized ratio (INR) [6, 27, 33], lower serum cholesterol [19] or LDL cholesterol [42], and fibrinogen [14], the chances of expanding hematomas were greater.

Patients with imaging characteristics displaying irregularly shaped hematoma [14], hematoma heterogeneity [36], spot sign on computed tomography angiography (CTA) [11,43-47], and intraventricular hemorrhage (IVH) and/or extension [10, 16] were at an increased risk of hematoma expansion. The so-called "spot-sign", which reflects contrast extravasation into the hematoma, has increasingly gained attention, and many studies have included this parameter to promote recognition of a potential target population in hematoma expansion prevention [7, 43-45].

CURRENT CLINICAL PREVENTION OF HEMATOMA EXPANSION

Risk of hematoma expansion may be alleviated by premorbid management of liver disease, alcohol consumption, and prior infarct [3]. Controlling daily alcohol consumption or abstaining from alcohol may serve to lower the risk of hematoma growth. It is known that controlling blood pressure (BP) is beneficial for preventing recurrent stroke (hemorrhagic and ischemic) [6, 48-52]. However, because there are many other etiologies that cause ICH and ischemic stroke, only controlling BP is not enough to prevent stroke recurrence. Current guidelines recommend antiplatelet therapy for non-cardioembolic ischemic stroke or TIA, with aspirin, clopidogrel, or their combination for prevention of stroke recurrence [52-56]. Clopidogrel may be used as an alternative to aspirin– dypiridamole for secondary stroke prevention [52, 53, 55, 56]. For decades warfarin has been used to lower the risk of stroke in patients with atrial fibrillation. Previous studies indicated that dose-adjusted warfarin significantly reduced the incidence of stroke, but its use is associated with risk of bleeding57and/or rebleeding [6, 57-59]. Paradoxically, warfarin may be a way to prevent brain ischemic stroke and cause lower hematoma expansion, because hematoma expansion is common in the setting of anticoagulant-related [23-29] and antiplatelets-related [19, 29,30] ICH. It is necessary that patients on warfarin or antiplatelets therapy be periodically monitored with dose adjustments.

Another preventable index is body mass index (BMI), with patients having higher BMIs at a lesser risk of hematoma expansion [19]. The author explained that this may be due to a volume-based dose relationship of rFVIIa, which was administered based on estimated body weight [19, 60]. It may also be related to the reduced lipid level [19, 42] from the lower BMI. This phenomenon may demonstrate that an improved nutritional status and energy reservoirs serve as protections against mortality, and that following a healthy lifestyle may reduce adverse outcomes associated with obesity in patients with higher BMIs [61].

POTENTIAL CLINICAL INTERVENTION FOR HEMATOMA EXPANSION

Some of the clinical signs and nearly all of the laboratory findings indicate that hematoma expansion can be intervened (Fig. 1 and Fig. 2).

Higher blood pressures [3, 6, 14, 33, 35-37, 62] have been recognized to increase hematoma expansion [3, 6, 14,33, 35-37, 62], although precise data on the risks and benefits of acute BP lowering remain limited [13, 16-18, 63]. The INTERACT I and ATACH I pilot studies revealed a safety profile and lower risk of hematoma expansion when aggressive systolic BP lowering to levels between 110–140 mmHg was achieved [62-64]. More specifically, the Intensive Blood Pressure Reduction in INTERACT II has evaluated the safety and efficacy of intensive BP reduction [65] (with a target systolic level of <140 mm Hg within 1 hour) in comparison to guideline-recommended BP treatment (with a target systolic level of <180 mm Hg) [66] and has shown a favorable trend toward improved functional outcomes with intensive BP reduction [6, 66]. Moreover, intensive BP reduction appears to be associated with a greater attenuation of absolute hematoma growth at 24 hours [65, 67].

Serum glucose reduction is another possible clinical intervention. Although high levels of fasting plasma glucose may represent stress hyperglycemia caused by large hematomas or dense neurological deficits [3, 11], HbA1c would provide an estimate of control of diabetes mellitus or blood glucose level for the preceding three months period [3]. In addition to aggravating atherosclerosis and arteriolosclerosis [3, 68], hyperglycemia may precipitate hemorrhage expansion by the analogy with hemorrhagic infarction [3]. Some studies have reported evidence of hematoma growth from bleeding into an ischemic penumbra zone surrounding the hematoma, while other reports have not confirmed the existence of ischemia at the hypoperfused area in the periphery of the hematoma [69-71]. Decline in serum glucose concentration associated with a decrease in the proportion of subjects with hematoma expansion and poor clinical outcome [41]. The results provide a standard for a randomized, controlled clinical trial to evaluate the efficacy of aggressive serum glucose reduction in lessening mortality and disability

among patients with ICH [41]. Creatinine is a recognized marker of long-standing hypertension with accumulated vascular injury and increased fragility of small vessels. Elevated creatinine levels may reflect severe renal dysfunction, which is associated with impaired platelet function [72] and uncontrolled hypertension or diabetes mellitus [3]. Additional factors may be accelerative of creatinine increases, such as patient hydration status and diabetes history. The monitoring of appropriate drug therapy, especially drugs which are cleared by the kidneys to prevent rise of serum creatinine, is more important than therapy for lowering creatinine. The adoption of maintenance dialysis was the first step that improved the bleeding tendency in uremia, although not fully satisfactorily [72], and heparin administration could induce hematoma expansion [26, 29]. The regular administration of erythropoietin has minimized the frequency and severity of bleeding symptoms in patients with end-stage renal insufficiency beyond the benefits obtained by dialysis [72]. In handling the management and prevention of spontaneous bleeding, some drugs have been found to shorten the prolonged bleeding time (i.e., desmopressin with a short-lasting effect and conjugated estrogens with a more prolonged effect) [72]. Because these medications cannot be administered prophylactically for prolonged periods of time, long-lasting prevention of the bleeding tendency in uremia remains unsettled [72].

There is a systemic activation of hemostasis after acute ICH. However, most of the changes in hemostatic protein levels were common to patients with or without hematoma expansion, and only the activity of factor XIII increased in those with hematoma expansion [15]. The investigators interpreted that patients with higher factor XIII activity were able to have faster and/or better-stabilized clots with enhanced resistance to endogenous lysis. Because of this increased utilization of factor XIII, its activity in peripheral blood decreased with time, whereas it was stable or increased in hematoma expansion patients [15]. It is possible that the increased activity of factor XIII possibly reflects the potentiated hemostasis to prevent the hematoma expansion and works as a self-compensatory or self-protective mechanism. As such, it is not advisable to intervene aggressively in the activity of factor XIII.

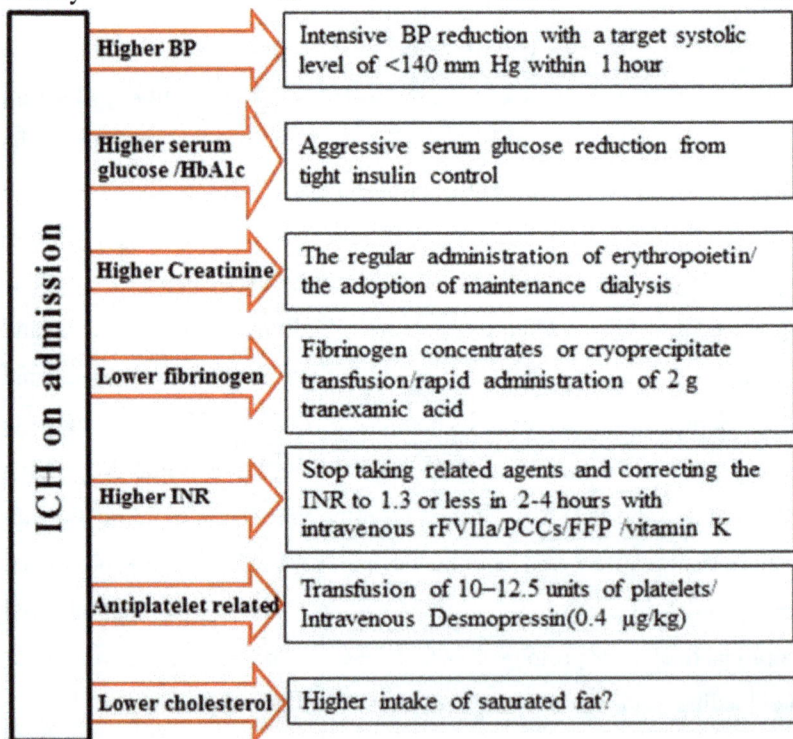

ICH on admission		
	Higher BP	Intensive BP reduction with a target systolic level of <140 mm Hg within 1 hour
	Higher serum glucose /HbA1c	Aggressive serum glucose reduction from tight insulin control
	Higher Creatinine	The regular administration of erythropoietin/ the adoption of maintenance dialysis
	Lower fibrinogen	Fibrinogen concentrates or cryoprecipitate transfusion/rapid administration of 2 g tranexamic acid
	Higher INR	Stop taking related agents and correcting the INR to 1.3 or less in 2-4 hours with intravenous rFVIIa/PCCs/FFP /vitamin K
	Antiplatelet related	Transfusion of 10–12.5 units of platelets/ Intravenous Desmopressin(0.4 µg/kg)
	Lower cholesterol	Higher intake of saturated fat?

Fig.2. A point-by-point available clinical intervention strategies for risk factors of hematoma expansion among ICH patients admitted to the hospital.

Fibrinogen is cross-linked with each other in the presence of factor XIII to become fibrin polymers, which are the final products of the coagulation cascade (the secondary hemostasis). Fibrinogen also takes part in primary hemostasis, i.e., platelet aggregation. Fibrinogen levels may represent the function of both blood coagulation and platelet aggregation [14]. Fibrinogen is a critical protein for hemostasis and clot formation. Fibrinogen concentrates or cryoprecipitate (containing fibrinogen, factor VIII, von Willebrand factor, and FXIII) are more effective at fibrinogen repletion than transfusing plasma [73, 74]. Furthermore, rapid administration of antifibrinolytic, intravenous administration of 2g tranexamic acid over a period of 10 minutes, was recommended for prevention of hematoma growth in patients with ICH [75, 76].

International normalized ratio (INR) is the marker of coagulation. Impaired coagulation can potentially facilitate hematoma expansion [26], so its rapid reversal should be one of the main targets for this condition. The hemostatic impairment may be due to the intake of anticoagulants, antiplatelet agents, or inherited or acquired abnormalities in the coagulation system [26]. The first consideration for emergency management of anticoagulant and antiplatelet-related hematoma expansion is to stop taking these agents. Correcting the INR to 1.3 or less within 2-4 hours has been shown to decrease hematoma expansion [33, 58, 71]. Rapid reversal of coagulopathy is desirable to prevent ICH expansion. The most promising agents for rapid INR reversal to prevent hematoma expansion include recombinant activated factor VIIa (rFVIIa), fresh frozen plasma (FFP), intravenous vitamin K, and activated and inactivated prothrombin complex concentrates (PCCs) [24, 26, 29, 58, 59, 68, 77, 78]. Recombinant factor VIIa is effective for immediate INR reversal and prevention of hematoma expansion, but is also associated with increased thrombotic complications such as myocardial infarction, pulmonary embolism, and deep venous thrombosis (DVT). Recombinant factor VIIa has not been shown to improve survival or functional outcome and is generally not recommended for reversal in anticoagulant-related ICH [26,29, 71]. FFP (the historical standard of care) is relatively deficient in factor IX, requires large volume infusion and a slow thawing time, and can lead to transfusion-related complications such as infections, pulmonary edema and delayed reversal of INR [29, 58, 59]. Vitamin K is essential but does not have a rapid effect, often taking 24 hours for INR reversal [59]. PCCs are increasing in popularity as low-volume, rapid-reversal agents and have been reported to be superior to FFP and vitamin K in several studies [63, 79-81]. Individualized dosing of PCC may be the most effective method of reversal. In one study, individualized dosing of PCC based on the patient's body weight and initial INR was superior at reaching the target INR 15 minutes after dosing compared with the standard dosage of PCC [80]. Similar data has led to support for PCC as the standard of care at many institutions [28, 29, 63]. However, increasing concentrations of PPC can carry a risk of thromboembolic complications and disseminated intravascular coagulation [63]. As such, the optimal dosing and infusion rates of PCC to rapidly but safely reverse INR are not clearly defined.

Another possible strategy for reducing hematoma growth is to reverse the effect of antiplatelet medications by administering a platelet transfusion [30, 82]. Transfusion of 10-12.5 units of platelets has been shown to restore normal platelet function in patients on aspirin and clopidogrel [83]. Desmopressin (0.4 μg/kg IV) has been known to improve platelet reactivity in patients treated with aspirin by releasing a greater number of von Willibrand multimers [84].

Lower cholesterol levels have been related to the development of medial smooth muscle cell necrosis [42, 85], thus decreasing the resistance to rupturing of the vascular wall. Moreover, cholesterol levels modify platelet aggregability by their action on the platelet activating factor, so that lower cholesterol levels may decrease platelet aggregation [86], thus predisposing the individual to ICH growth [42]. However, no relationship was found between lipid-lowering agents and hematoma expansion [42, 87]. Higher intake of saturated fat, which leads to higher LDL cholesterol concentrations, was shown to be associated with reduced risk of intraparenchymal hemorrhage for both Japanese and American patients [88, 89]. A high fat diet may be beneficial to patients suffering from hematoma expansion. The role of serum cholesterol is to maintain the integrity of vascular vessels.

NEW MOLECULAR PREDICTORS AND HEMATOMA EXPANSION

Function and Inhibition of Plasma Kallikrein

The role of plasma kallikrein (PK) in cerebral hematoma expansion with hyperglycemia has been reported [20]. Plasma kallikrein is activated during hemorrhage by the contact system and plays a key role in innate inflammation, vascular function, the intrinsic coagulation cascade, and the fibrinolytic system [20, 90, 91]. Hyperglycemia promotes ICH through PK-mediated inhibition of the platelet-vessel wall interaction. PK exerts potent anti- hemostatic function in diabetic rodent models, and this effect is greatly enhanced in hyperglycemic blood [20, 90, 91]. Adhesion of PK to collagens blocks binding sites for platelet glycoprotein VI receptors (GPVI) and inhibits platelet aggregation on collagen fibers at the injury site, leading to sustained bleeding and hematoma expansion [20, 90, 91]. These findings suggest targeting PK for prevention of brain hematoma in hyperglycemic patients [20, 90, 91]. Further studies are required to verify this confusing hypothesis in animals and patients with ICH [90].Systemic administration of a small molecule PK inhibitor, ASP-440 [92, 93], reduced hematoma expansion in DM rats [20], which is similar to the effects of PK-deficiency in humans [94]. Treatment of DM rats with ASP-440 increased aPTT and tail bleeding time, while reducing hematoma expansion induced by autologous blood. ASP-440 is believed to reduce hematoma expansion by suppressing the formation of PK from prekallikrein, possibly mediated by inhibition of the contact activation system [20]. The mechanism for PK inhibition of collagen-induced platelet aggregation requires further experiments to confirm.

Von Willebrand Factor and Intervention

Von Willebrand factor (vWF) is a plasma protein that is involved in thrombosis and hemostasis [95, 96]. VWF mediates the adhesion of platelets to sites of vascular injury and forms [96] an adhesive bridge between platelets and vascular subendothelial structures, as well as between adjacent platelets at sides of endothelial injury [96]. Increased platelet aggregation and pathological thrombus formation strongly rely on endothelial vWF accumulation and plasma vWF adhesion [70]. Recent research results showed the role of vWF genetic variant in increasing risk for hematoma expansion after ICH [4]. This research suggested that vWF rs216321 SNP genotype independently predicted relative hematoma enlargement, even when controlling known risk factors for hematoma growth [4], and confirmed the role of hemostatic polymorphism on hematoma expansion [4]. VWF dysfunction was thought to be an important culprit in bleeding disorders. A target therapy for vWF in hematoma expansion has been reported. Desmopressin is a vasopressin agonist used as first-line therapy for mild-to-moderate vWF deficiency or hemophilia [97, 98]. Desmopressin is widely used in the management of bleeding disorders and improves primary hemostasis through up-regulation of plasma vWF and factor VIII, while having possible direct effects on platelet reactivity [98]. Desmopressin leads to the release of vWF and reduces clinical bleeding [84]. Desmopressin improved platelet activity, increased vWF antigen levels, and hematoma expansion was muted in the subset of patients treated within 12 hours of ICH symptom onset [84]. Given its safety, low cost, and reduction in clinical bleeding, desmopressin is an attractive pharmacological treatment for acute ICH [84]. Cryoprecipitate (a plasma product rich in vWF) should be considered for patients with vWF genetic variation and/or patients unresponsive to desmopressin in hematoma expansion.

N-methyl-D-aspartate (NMDA) and its Receptor Antagonist

Overactivation of the extra synaptic N-methyl-D-aspartate (NMDA)- type receptor is a major route for excessive $Ca2+$ influx in triggering excitotoxic neuronal cell damage or death [99, 100]. Glutamate stimulation of the metabotropic glutamate receptors leads to a vertiginous increase in neuronal tPA synthesis [101]. Some reports suggest that tPA cleaves the NR1 subunit of the NMDAR and strengthens NMDA toxicity via the magnification of NMDA calcium currents [102, 103]. Thus, this cascade of reactions, which involves glutamate, NMDAR, and tPA, constitutes a vicious cycle which ends in catastrophic neurotoxicity [104] (Fig. 3). Memantine, which is known to be a moderate-affinity, uncompetitive NMDA receptor antagonist, was found to reduce hemorrhagic extension and to exert a complicated inhibitory effect on glutamate overstimulation, tissue plasminogen activator (tPA) upregulation, and matrix metalloproteinase (MMP)-9 increment in hemorrhagic rat brains [105]. Memantine (20 mg/kg/day) was intraperitoneally administered 30 min after the induction of ICH, and at daily intervals afterwards, for either 3 or

14 days [105]. The mechanisms underlying NMDA's association with hematoma expansion are not fully understood but warrant further consideration.

Inflammatory Markers and Possible Intervention

Inflammatory responses participate in the pathophysiological processes of brain injury following ICH [106]. They can result in disruption of the blood–brain barrier, elicit brain edema, and contribute to cell death after hemorrhage via cytotoxic mediators [106-109]. Activation of innate immunity and inflammatory responses also contributes to progression of brain edema and hematoma expansion after ICH (Fig.4) [22, 110-112].

Interleukin-6 (IL-6) represents a keystone cytokine in infection, cancer and inflammation, in which it speeds up disease progression or supports the maintenance of immunological reactions [111, 113]. IL-6 can induce amplification of gap junctions of endothelial cells and enlarge vascular permeability by altering actin filaments and by transforming the shape of endothelial cells [112, 114]. Binding of IL-6 to its receptor induces the phosphorylation of receptor associated Janus kinases (JAK), allowing the recruitment of signal transducer and activator of transcription STAT1 and STAT3 [110, 115]. STAT3 can bind to NF-κB then facilitate NF-κB activation and nuclear entry [116, 117]. NF-κB, known to stimulate inflammatory cytokine production, inflammatory cell function, and endothelial injury, ultimatelycaused increased injury [118] after ICH. One study showed that IL-6 levels >24 pg/mL increased 16-fold the risk of early hematoma expansion after controlling for other markers of inflammation [22]. Tocilizumab, which targets the receptor for IL-6 (IL-6R) in the treatment of inflammatory arthritis and a subset of other immunological conditions, has been identified [113] as an effective intervention. Tocilizumab may exert possible protective effects on hematoma expansion and block this vicious cycle, but there are no reports as yet on its efficacy in treating ICH.

C-reactive protein (CRP), an acute-phase reactant induced by IL-6, was associated with hematoma expansion as well as IL-6 in ICH patients [110, 115]. One study demonstrated that plasma CRP>10 mg/L within the first few hours of spontaneous ICH was independently predictive of both early hematoma expansion and early neurological worsening, both of which are associated with increased mortality [111]. It is likely that both inflammatory factors impair coagulation function and vessel wall pathophysiology and contribute to a persistent vessel leak [111, 119].

Visfatin is a novel adipokine with different functions. Visfatin can accelerate up -regulation of inflammatory cytokines and chemokines and has an link with a proinflammatory state that may contribute to poor clinical outcomes after acute ICH [108, 120]. Visfatin is also released by IL-6 in cells involving innate immunity [116], and plasma visfatin level was highly correlated with plasma CRP [108, 110,120]. Visfatin has been demonstrated to positively correlate with ICH severity and inflammatory biomarkers such as CRP and also hematoma expansion at 24 hours, supporting an inflammatory role of visfatin in progression of hematoma expansion after ICH [110].

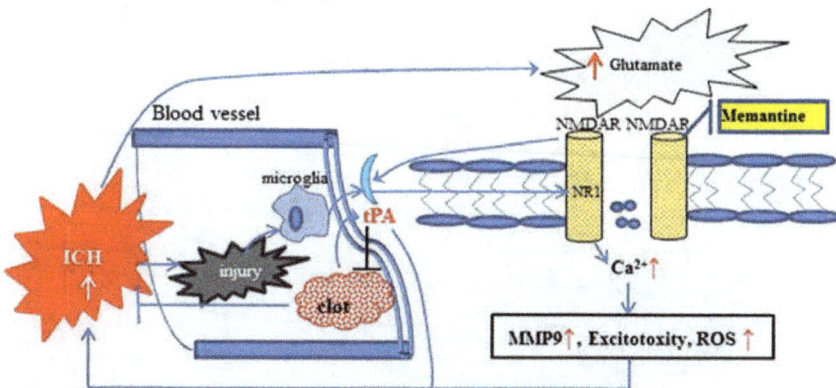

Glutamate

Blood vessel

NMDAR NMDAR   Memantine

microglia

tPA

NR1

ICH

injury

clot

Ca²⁺↑

MMP9↑, Excitotoxity, ROS ↑

Fig.3. The detrimental role of N-methyl-D-aspartate receptor (NMDAR) in hematoma expansion after ICH and the corresponding intervention.

Leptin, another important adipokine,is not only an energy regulator but also a novel mediator of inflammation [118]. Leptin promotes phagocytosis by monocytes/ macrophages and their secretion of proinflammatory cytokines [118] such as IL-6 and tumor necrosis factor-α (TNF-α) [121]. This detrimental effect of leptin on ICH is mediated by the STAT3 signaling pathway in inflammatory cells [121]. As previously mentioned, a connection between STAT3 and hematoma expansion has been demonstrated [116]. Similarly to visfatin, Plasma leptin levels were positively correlated and independently associated with hematoma expansion, ICH severity, and CRP [109, 112, 120].

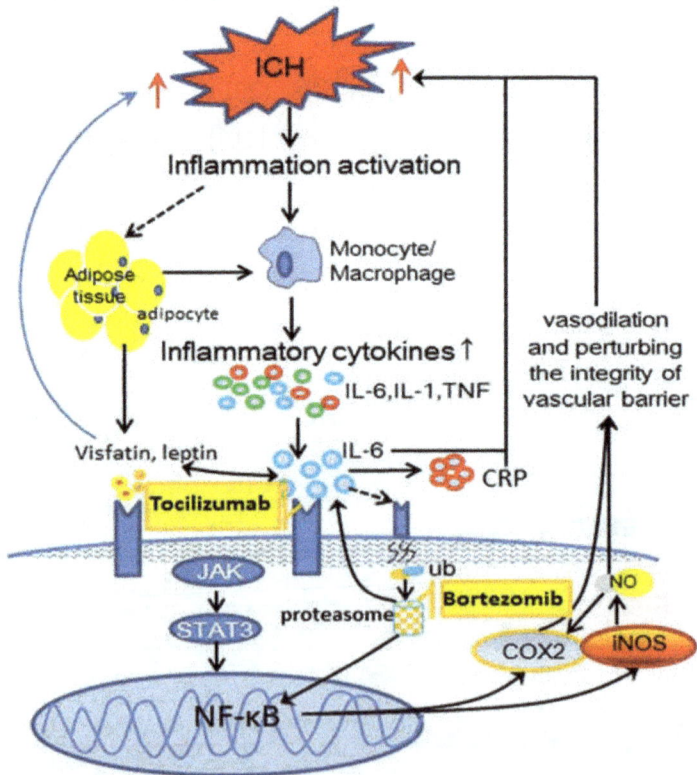

Fig.4. Schematic representation and mechanism of various inflammatory cytokines and adipokines on hematoma expansion in ICH and available clinical blockers.

The ubiquitin-proteasome system (UPS) regulates inflammatory response via the up-regulation of several proinflammatory molecules (NF-κB and IL-6) [120, 122]. The relation of IL-6, NF-κB and hematoma expansion has been discussed previously [114, 118]. Bortezomib, a proteasome inhibitor, has anti-inflammatory effects in reducing both hematoma expansion and brain edema during the early period of ICH [120, 123]. The mechanism of proteasome inhibition was thought to be associated with the reduction of COX2 and iNOS after ICH, resulting in the attenuation of vasodilation and perturbing the integrity of the vascular barrier induced by COX2 [120, 123, 124], also protecting against oxidative injury, abnormal mitochondrial respiration and DNA damage induced by Inos [125]. A single intravenous 0.2mg/kg dose of bortezomib inhibited the early hematoma growth occurring within 24 hours and diminished hematoma volume after 72 hours [123]. Because bortezomib is now used in human treatment, with few side effects, its therapeutic application for ICH seems available, although its precise mechanism and validity in inhibiting hematoma growth after ICH requires further confirmation. The signaling cassette that controls the activity of IL-6/ CRP/visfatin/leptin is complicated (Fig. 4), and more research on the underlying mechanism is required to determine potential intervention strategies.

MOLECULAR VASCULAR INJURY AND HEMATOMA EXPANSION

Cellular Fibronectin

Cellular fibronectin (c-Fn), as a basal membrane component, is a glycoprotein especially important for the adhesion of platelets to fibrin, a function necessary for the blockage of bleeding [126]. One research study demonstrated that plasma c-Fn levels >6 µg/mL were associated with a 92 -fold increase in the risk of early hematoma expansion, and c-Fn levels showed a high correlation with the percentage of the ICH growth. This study suggested c-Fn was the most powerful predictor of ICH enlargement [22]. C-Fn is largely confined to the vascular endothelium, and high plasma levels of C-Fn might be indicative of endothelial damage and loss of microvascular integrity [22]. As c-Fn plays a key role in blood clot formation by mediating the adhesion of platelets to fibrin [22, 126], the disappearance of c-Fn in the vascular endothelium might compromise this clotting mechanism and facilitate ICH expansion [22]. Plasma c-Fn is a marker of vascular injury, and there is no better way to intervene in this process except by preventing its occurrence and maintaining vascular integrity. Improving or modulating the function of platelet plug formation is a potential means to preserve the structural integrity of intact blood vessels [127] in the future.

Apolipoprotein EƐ Alleles

Apolipoprotein E (APOE) Ɛ2 and Ɛ4 alleles are independent risk factors for spontaneous ICH in the lobar brain regions [126, 128], most likely a reflection of their role in cerebral amyloid angiopathy (CAA) [127, 129]. The Ɛ4 allele increases the severity of vascular amyloid deposition, whereas the Ɛ2 allele appears to cause increased vasculo-pathic changes that lead to vessel rupture [127, 129, 130]. A multicenter genetic association study showed that larger ICH volume is associated with the

APOE ε2, but not ε4, allele. APOE ε2 carriers are at disproportionately increased risk of mortality and poor outcome after ICH127. One study demonstrated that the APOE ε2 allele is associated with hematoma expansion in patients with lobar ICH [127, 129, 131]. There are no available interventions for the APOE ε2 allele, but APOE ε2 allele knock-out may be introduced into animal experiment protocols in the next few years.

CONCLUSION

Taking together, most studies of hematoma expansion were in the clinical environment where intervention was difficult. However, there remain some indexes that should be considered for prevention and treatment. In this review, available information from clinical signs to molecular mechanisms are provided and potential intervention strategies discussed. Prospective study for hematoma expansion How to predict the patients who are at highest risk of hematoma expansion is more challengeable than restricting hematoma expansion itself following acute ICH.

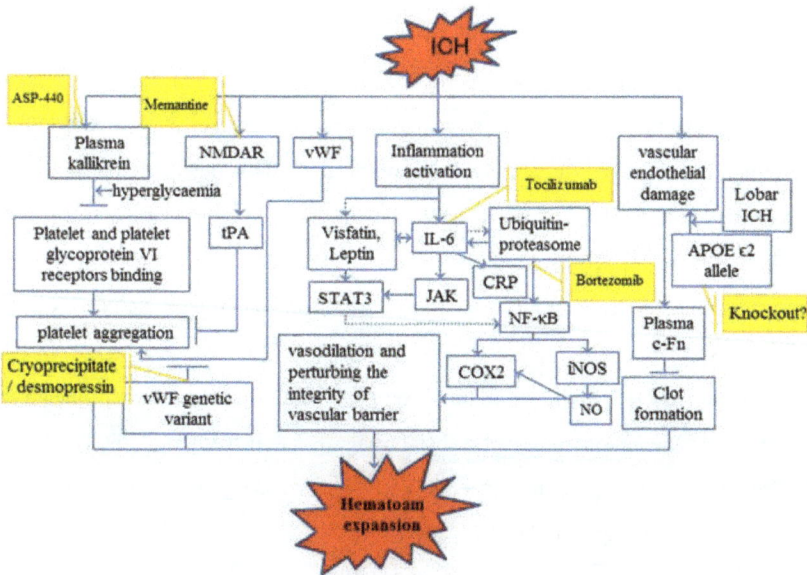

Fig.5. Summary of current understanding from molecular pathways and risk predictors to the potential intervention strategies of hematoma expansion after ICH.

So seeking and detecting risk markers in plasma that can be intervened appropriately is meaningful for patients with potential hematoma expansion, which may contribute to improve clinical outcomes in patients suffering from ICH.

REFERENCES:

[1] Xi G, Keep RF, Hoff JT. Mechanisms of brain injury after intracerebral haemorrhage. Lancet Neurol 2006; 5: 53-63.

[2] Sahni R, Weinberger J. Management of intracerebral hemorrhage. Vasc Health Risk Manag 2007; 3: 701-9.

[3] Kazui S, Minematsu K, Yamamoto H, Sawada T, Yamaguchi T. Predisposing factors to enlargement of spontaneous intracerebral hematoma. Stroke 1997; 28: 2370-5.

[4] Appelboom G, Piazza M, Han JE, et al. Von - 60 -ccluding- 60 - factor genetic variant associated with hematoma expansion after intracerebral hemorrhage. J Stroke Cerebrovasc Dis 2013; 22: 713-7.

[5] Tsai Y-H, Hsu L-M, Weng H-H, Lee M-H, Yang J-T, Lin C-P. Voxel-based analysis of apparent diffusion coefficient in perihaematomal oedema: Associated factors and outcome predictive value for intracerebral haemorrhage. BMJ Open 2011; 1:e000230.

[6] Pandey AS, Xi G. Intracerebral hemorrhage: A multimodality approach to improving outcome. Transl Stroke Res 2014; 5: 313-5.

[7] Morotti A, Jessel MJ, Brouwers HB, et al. CT angiography spot sign, hematoma expansion, and outcome in primary pontine intracerebral hemorrhage. Neurocrit Care 2016; 25(1):79-85

[8] Li Q, Huang YJ, Zhang G, et al. Intraventricular hemorrhage and early hematoma expansion in patients with intracerebral hemorrhage. Sci Rep 2015; 5: 11357.

[9] Brott T, Broderick J, Kothari R, et al. Early hemorrhage growth in patients with intracerebral hemorrhage. Stroke 1997; 28: 1-5.

[10] Cheung RT. Predictors of hematoma growth? Stroke 1998; 29: 2442-3.

[11] Ovesen C, Havsteen I, Rosenbaum S, Christensen H. Prediction and observation of post-admission hematoma expansion in patients with intracerebral hemorrhage. Front Neurol 2014; 5: 186.

[12] Delcourt C, Huang Y, Arima H, et al. Hematoma growth and outcomes in intracerebral hemorrhage: The interact1 study. Neurology 2012; 79: 314-9.

[13] Davis SM, Broderick J, Hennerici M, et al. Hematoma growth is a determinant of mortality and poor outcome after intracerebral hemorrhage. Neurology 2006; 66: 1175-81.

[14] Fujii Y, Takeuchi S, Sasaki O, Minakawa T, Tanaka R. Multivariate analysis of predictors of hematoma enlargement in spontaneous intracerebral hemorrhage. Stroke 1998; 29: 1160-6.

[15] Marti-Fabregas J, Borrell M, Silva Y, et al. Hemostatic proteins and their association with hematoma growth in patients with acute intracerebral hemorrhage. Stroke 2010; 41: 2976-8.

[16] Wang X, Arima H, Al-Shahi Salman R, et al. Clinical prediction algorithm (brain) to determine risk of hematoma growth in acute intracerebral hemorrhage. Stroke 2015; 46: 376-81.

[17] Gioia LC, Kate M, Dowlatshahi D, Hill MD, Butcher K. Blood pressure management in acute intracerebral hemorrhage: Current evidence and ongoing controversies. Curr Opin Crit Care 2015; 21:99-106.

[18] Jauch EC, Lindsell CJ, Adeoye O, et al. Lack of evidence for an association between hemodynamic variables and hematoma growth in spontaneous intracerebral hemorrhage. Stroke 2006; 37: 2061-5.

[19] Broderick JP, Diringer MN, Hill MD, et al. Determinants of intracerebral hemorrhage growth: An exploratory analysis. Stroke 2007; 38: 1072-5.

[20] Liu J, Gao BB, Clermont AC, et al. Hyperglycemia-induced cerebral hematoma expansion is mediated by plasma kallikrein. Nat Med 2011; 17: 206-10.

[21] Albright KC, Burak JM, Chang TR, et al. The impact of left ventricular hypertrophy and diastolic dysfunction on outcome in intracerebral hemorrhage patients.

ISRN stroke 2013; 2013.

[22] Silva Y, Leira R, Tejada J, Lainez JM, Castillo J, Davalos A. Molecular signatures of vascular injury are associated with early growth of intracerebral hemorrhage. Stroke 2005; 36: 86-91.

[23] Schlunk F, Schulz E, Lauer A, et al. Warfarin pretreatment reduces cell death and mmp-9 activity in experimental intracerebral hemorrhage. Transl Stroke Res 2015; 6: 133-9.

[24] Yaghi S, Eisenberger A, Willey JZ. Symptomatic intracerebral hemorrhage in acute ischemic stroke after thrombolysis with intravenous recombinant tissue plasminogen activator: A review of natural history and treatment. JAMA Neurol 2014; 71: 1181-5.

[25] Huttner HB, Schellinger PD, Hartmann M, et al. Hematoma growth and outcome in treated neurocritical care patients with intracerebral hemorrhage related to oral anticoagulant therapy: Comparison of acute treatment strategies using vitamin k, fresh frozen plasma, and prothrombin complex concentrates. Stroke 2006; 37: 1465-70.

[26] Emiru T, Bershad EM, Zantek ND, et al. Intracerebral hemorrhage: A review of coagulation function. Clin Appl Thromb Hemost 2013; 19: 652-62.

[27] Le Roux P, Pollack CV, Jr., Milan M, Schaefer A. Race against the clock: Overcoming challenges in the management of anticoagulant associated intracerebral hemorrhage. J Neurosurg 2014; 121 Suppl:1-20.

[28] Hanger HC, Geddes JA, Wilkinson TJ, Lee M, Baker AE. Warfarin-related intracerebral haemorrhage: Better outcomes when reversal includes prothrombin complex concentrates. Intern Med J 2013; 43: 308-16.

[29] James RF, Palys V, Lomboy JR, Lamm JR, Jr., Simon SD. The role of anticoagulants, antiplatelet agents, and their reversal strategies in the management of intracerebral hemorrhage. Neurosurg Focus 2013; 34: E6.

[30] Naidech AM, Jovanovic B, Liebling S, et al. Reduced platelet activity is associated with early clot growth and worse 3-month outcome after intracerebral hemorrhage. Stroke 2009; 40: 2398-401.

[31] Stampfli SF, Asmis LM, Tanner FC. [mechanism of action of old and new anticoagulants]. Herz. 2008; 33: 4-12.

[32] Ruff CT, Giugliano RP, Braunwald E, et al. Association between edoxaban dose, concentration, anti-factor xa activity, and outcomes: An analysis of data from the - 63 -ccluding- 63 -, double-blind engage af-timi 48 trial. Lancet 2015; 385: 2288-95.

[33] Kuramatsu JB, Gerner ST, Schellinger PD, et al. Anticoagulant reversal, blood pressure levels, and anticoagulant resumption in patients with anticoagulation-related intracerebral hemorrhage. Jama 2015; 313: 824-36.

[34] Rodriguez-Luna D, Pineiro S, Rubiera M, et al. Impact of blood pressure changes and course on hematoma growth in acute intracerebral hemorrhage. Eur J Neurol 2013; 20: 1277-83.

[35] Lim JK, Hwang HS, Cho BM, et al. Multivariate analysis of risk factors of hematoma expansion in spontaneous intracerebral hemorrhage. Surg Neurol 2008; 69: 40-45; discussion 45.

[36] Takeda R, Ogura T, Ooigawa H, et al. A practical prediction model for early hematoma expansion in spontaneous deep ganglionic intracerebral hemorrhage. Clin Neurol Neurosurg 2013; 115: 1028-31.

[37] Ohwaki K, Yano E, Nagashima H, Hirata M, Nakagomi T, Tamura A. Blood pressure management in acute intracerebral hemorrhage: Relationship between elevated blood pressure and hematoma enlargement. Stroke 2004; 35: 1364-7.

[38] Chan S, Hemphill JC, 3rd. Critical care management of intracerebral hemorrhage. Crit Care Clin 2014; 30: 699-717.

[39] Morawo AO, Gilmore EJ. Critical care management of intracerebral hemorrhage. Semin Neurol 2016; 36: 225-32.

[40] Yaghi S, Dibu J, Achi E, Patel A, Samant R, Hinduja A. Hematoma expansion in spontaneous intracerebral hemorrhage: Predictors and outcome. Int J Neurosci 2014; 124: 890-3.

[41] Qureshi AI, Palesch YY, Martin R, et al. Association of serum glucose concentrations during acute hospitalization with hematoma expansion, perihematomal edema, and three month outcome among patients with intracerebral hemorrhage. Neurocrit Care 2011; 15: 428-35.

[42] Rodriguez-Luna D, Rubiera M, Ribo M, et al. Serum low-density lipoprotein

cholesterol level predicts hematoma growth and clinical outcome after acute intracerebral hemorrhage. Stroke 2011; 42:2447-52.

[43] Radmanesh F, Falcone GJ, Anderson CD, et al. Risk factors for computed tomography angiography spot sign in deep and lobar intracerebral hemorrhage are shared. Stroke 2014; 45: 1833-5.

[44] Goldstein JN, Fazen LE, Snider R, et al. Contrast extravasation on ct angiography predicts hematoma expansion in intracerebral hemorrhage. Neurology 2007; 68: 889-94.

[45] Wada R, Aviv RI, Fox AJ, et al. Ct angiography "spot sign" predicts hematoma expansion in acute intracerebral hemorrhage. Stroke 2007; 38: 1257-62.

[46] Demchuk AM, Dowlatshahi D, Rodriguez-Luna D, et al. Prediction of haematoma growth and outcome in patients with intracerebral haemorrhage using the ct-angiography spot sign (predict): A prospective observational study. Lancet Neurol 2012; 11: 307-14.

[47] Delgado Almandoz JE, Yoo AJ, Stone MJ, et al. The spot sign score in primary intracerebral hemorrhage identifies patients at highest risk of in-hospital mortality and poor outcome among survivors. Stroke 2010; 41: 54-60.

[48] Steiner T, Al-Shahi Salman R, Beer R, et al. European stroke - 64 - ccluding - 64 -- 64 - n (eso) guidelines for the management of spontaneous intracerebral hemorrhage. Int J Stroke 2014; 9: 840-55.

[49] Rashid P, Leonardi-Bee J, Bath P. Blood pressure reduction and secondary prevention of stroke and other vascular events: A systematic review. Stroke 2003; 34: 2741-8.

[50] De Lima LG, Saconato H, Atallah AN, da Silva EM. Beta-blockers for preventing stroke recurrence. Cochrane Database Syst Rev 2014: Cd007890.

[51] Fuentes B, Ortega-Casarrubios MA, Martinez P, Diez-Tejedor E. Action on vascular risk factors: Importance of blood pressure and lipid lowering in stroke secondary prevention. Cerebrovasc Dis 2007; 24 Suppl 1: 96-106.

[52] Sherzai AZ, Elkind MS. Advances in stroke prevention. Ann N Y Acad Sci 2015; 1338: 1-15.

[53] Kernan WN, Ovbiagele B, Black HR, et al. Guidelines for the prevention of stroke in patients with stroke and transient ischemic attack: A guideline for healthcare professionals from the American heart association/American stroke association. Stroke 2014; 45: 2160-236.

[54] Albers GW, Amarenco P. Combination therapy with clopidogrel and aspirin: Can the cure results be extrapolated to cerebrovascular patients? Stroke 2001; 32: 2948-9.

[55] Aw D, Sharma JC. Antiplatelets in secondary stroke prevention: Should clopidogrel be the first choice? Postgrad Med J 2012; 88: 34-7.

[56] Shulga O, Bornstein N. Antiplatelets in secondary stroke prevention. Front Neurol 2011; 2: 36

[57] Hsu JC, Hsieh CY, Yang YH, Lu CY. Net clinical benefit of oral anticoagulants: A multiple criteria decision analysis. PloS One 2015; 10: e0124806.

[58] Turpie AG. New oral anticoagulants in atrial fibrillation. Eur Heart J 2008; 29: 155-165.

[59] Cairns JA, Connolly S, McMurtry S, Stephenson M, Talajic M. Canadian cardiovascular society atrial fibrillation guidelines 2010: Prevention of stroke and systemic thromboembolism in atrial fibrillation and flutter. Can J Cardiol 2011; 27: 74-90.

[60] Ribo M, Grotta JC. Latest advances in intracerebral hemorrhage. Curr Neurol Neurosci Rep 2006; 6: 17-22.

[61] Bagheri M, Speakman JR, Shabbidar S, Kazemi F, Djafarian K. A dose-response meta-analysis of the impact of body mass index on stroke and all-cause mortality in stroke patients: A paradox within a paradox. Obes Rev 2015; 16: 416-23.

[62] Anderson CS, Huang Y, Wang JG, et al. Intensive blood pressure reduction in acute cerebral haemorrhage trial (interact): A - 65 -ccluding- 65 - pilot trial. Lancet Neurol 2008; 7: 391-9.

[63] Kuramatsu JB, Huttner HB, Schwab S. Advances in the management of intracerebral hemorrhage. J Neural Transm (Vienna) 2013; 120 Suppl 1: S35-41.

[64] Kawanishi M, Kawai N, Nakamura T, Luo C, Tamiya T, Nagao S.Effect of delayed mild brain hypothermia on edema formation after intracerebral hemorrhage in rats. J

Stroke Cerebrovasc Dis 2008;17: 187-95.

[65] Tsivgoulis G, Katsanos AH. Intensive blood pressure reduction in acute intracerebral hemorrhage: A meta-analysis. Neurology 2015;84: 2464.

[66] Anderson CS, Heeley E, Huang Y, et al. Rapid blood-pressure lowering in patients with acute intracerebral hemorrhage. N Engl J Med. 2013; 368: 2355-65.

[67] Tsivgoulis G, Katsanos AH, Butcher KS, et al. Intensive blood pressure reduction in acute intracerebral hemorrhage: A meta-analysis. Neurology 2014; 83: 1523-9.

[68] Waje-Andreassen U, Naess H, Thomassen L, et al. Biomarkers related to carotid intima-media thickness and plaques in long-term survivors of ischemic stroke. Transl Stroke Res 2015; 6: 276-83.

[69] Rincon F, Mayer SA. Clinical review: Critical care management of spontaneous intracerebral hemorrhage. Crit Care 2008; 12: 237.

[70] Li TT, Fan ML, Hou SX, et al. A novel snake venom-derived gpib antagonist, anfibatide, protects mice from acute experimental ischaemic stroke and reperfusion injury. Br J Pharmacol 2015; 172:3904-16.

[71] Rincon F, Mayer SA. Intracerebral hemorrhage: Clinical overview and pathophysiologic concepts. Transl Stroke Res 2012; 3: 10-24.

[72] Mannucci PM, Tripodi A. Hemostatic defects in liver and renal dysfunction. Hematology / the Education Program of the American Society of Hematology. Hematology 2012; 2012: 168-73.

[73] Levy JH, Goodnough LT. How I use fibrinogen replacement therapy in acquired bleeding. Blood 2015; 125: 1387-93.

[74] Collis RE, Collins PW. Haemostatic management of obstetric haemorrhage. Anaesthesia 2015; 70 Suppl 1: 78-86, e27-78.

[75] Sorimachi T, Fujii Y, Morita K, Tanaka R. Rapid administration of antifibrinolytics and strict blood pressure control for intracerebral hemorrhage. Neurosurg 2005; 57: 837-44.

[76] Meretoja A, Churilov L, Campbell BC, et al. The spot sign and tranexamic acid on preventing ich growth—australasia trial (stopaust): Protocol of a phase ii randomized, placebo-controlled, double-blind, multicenter trial. Int J Stroke 2014; 9: 519-24.

[77] Zhou W, Schwarting S, Illanes S, et al. Hemostatic therapy in experimental intracerebral hemorrhage associated with the direct thrombin inhibitor dabigatran. Stroke 2011; 42: 3594-9.

[78] Zhou W, Zorn M, Nawroth P, et al. Hemostatic therapy in experimental intracerebral hemorrhage associated with rivaroxaban. Stroke 2013; 44: 771-8.

[79] Pabinger I, Brenner B, Kalina U, Knaub S, Nagy A, Ostermann H. Prothrombin complex concentrate (beriplex p/n) for emergency anticoagulation reversal: A prospective multinational clinical trial. J Thromb Haemost 2008; 6: 622-31.

[80] van Aart L, Eijkhout HW, Kamphuis JS, et al. Individualized dosing regimen for prothrombin complex concentrate more effective than standard treatment in the reversal of oral anticoagulant therapy: An open, prospective randomized controlled trial. Thromb Res 2006; 118: 313-20.

[81] Yasaka M, Oomura M, Ikeno K, Naritomi H, Minematsu K. Effect of prothrombin complex concentrate on inr and blood coagulation system in emergency patients treated with warfarin overdose. Ann Hematol 2003; 82: 121-3.

[82] Beshay JE, Morgan H, Madden C, Yu W, Sarode R. Emergency reversal of anticoagulation and antiplatelet therapies in neurosurgical patients. J Neurosurg 2010; 112: 307-18.

[83] Vilahur G, Choi BG, Zafar MU, et al. Normalization of platelet reactivity in clopidogrel-treated subjects. J Thromb Haemost 2007; 5: 82-90.

[84] Naidech AM, Maas MB, Levasseur-Franklin KE, et al. Desmopressin improves platelet activity in acute intracerebral hemorrhage. Stroke 2014; 45: 2451-3.

[85] Ooneda G, Yoshida Y, Suzuki K, et al. Smooth muscle cells in the development of plasmatic arterionecrosis, arteriosclerosis, and arterial contraction. Blood vessels 1978; 15: 148-56.

[86] Chui DH, Marotta F, Rao ML, Liu DS, Zhang SC, Ideo C. Cholesterol-rich ldl perfused at physiological ldl-cholesterol concentration induces platelet aggregation and paf-acetylhydrolase activation. Biomedicine & pharmacotherapy 1991; 45: 37-42.

[87] Priglinger M, Arima H, Anderson C, Krause M. No relationship of lipid-lowering agents to hematoma growth: Pooled analysis of the intensive blood pressure reduction

in acute cerebral hemorrhage trials studies. Stroke 2015; 46: 857-9.

[88] Noda H, Iso H, Irie F, et al. Low-density lipoprotein cholesterol concentrations and death due to intraparenchymal hemorrhage: The - 68 -ccludi prefectural health study. Circulation 2009; 119: 2136-45.

[89] Iso H, Sato S, Kitamura A, Naito Y, Shimamoto T, Komachi Y. Fat and protein intakes and risk of intraparenchymal hemorrhage among middle-aged - 68 -ccludin. Am J Epidemiol 2003; 157: 32-9.

[90] Liu J, Gao BB, Feener EP. Proteomic identification of novel plasma kallikrein substrates in the astrocyte secretome. Transl Stroke Res 2010; 1: 276-86.

[91] Bjorkqvist J, Jamsa A, Renne T. Plasma kallikrein: The bradykinin producing enzyme. Thromb Haemost 2013; 110: 399-407.

[92] Clermont A, Chilcote TJ, Kita T, et al. Plasma kallikrein mediates retinal vascular dysfunction and induces retinal thickening in diabetic rats. Diabetes 2011; 60: 1590-8.

[93] Phipps JA, Clermont AC, Sinha S, Chilcote TJ, Bursell SE, Feener EP. Plasma kallikrein mediates angiotensin ii type 1 receptor-stimulated retinal vascular permeability. Hypertension 2009; 53: 175-81.

[94] Asmis LM, Sulzer I, Furlan M, Lammle B. Prekallikrein deficiency: The characteristic normalization of the severely prolonged aptt following increased preincubation time is due to autoactivation of factor xii. Thromb Res 2002; 105: 463-70.

[95] Sadler JE. Biochemistry and genetics of von - 68 -ccluding- 68 - factor. Annu Rev Biochem 1998; 67: 395-424.

[96] Arslan Y, Yoldas TK, Zorlu Y. Interaction between vwf levels and aspirin resistance in ischemic stroke patients. Transl Stroke Res 2013; 4: 484-7.

[97] Mannucci PM, Ruggeri ZM, Pareti FI, Capitanio A. 1-deamino-8-d-arginine vasopressin: A new pharmacological approach to the management of haemophilia and von willebrands' diseases. Lancet 1977; 1: 869-72.

[98] Teng R, Mitchell PD, Butler K. The effect of desmopressin on bleeding time and platelet aggregation in healthy volunteers administered ticagrelor. J Clin Pharm Ther 2014; 39: 186-91.

[99] Song M, Yu SP. Ionic regulation of cell volume changes and cell death after ischemic stroke. Transl Stroke Res 2014; 5: 17-27.

[100] Lipton SA. Pathologically-activated therapeutics for neuroprotection: Mechanism of nmda receptor block by memantine and s-nitrosylation. Curr Drug Targets 2007; 8: 621-32.

[101] Shin CY, Kundel M, Wells DG. Rapid, activity-induced increase in tissue plasminogen activator is mediated by metabotropic glutamate receptor-dependent mrna translation. J Neurosci 2004; 24: 9425-33.

[102] Gravanis I, Tsirka SE. Tissue plasminogen activator and glial function. Glia. 2005; 49: 177-83.

[103] Nicole O, Docagne F, Ali C, et al. The proteolytic activity of tissue-plasminogen activator enhances nmda receptor-mediated signaling. Nat Med 2001; 7: 59-64.

[104] Liu D, Cheng T, Guo H, et al. Tissue plasminogen activator neurovascular toxicity is controlled by activated protein c. Nat Med 2004; 10: 1379-83.

[105] Lee ST, Chu K, Jung KH, et al. Memantine reduces hematoma expansion in experimental intracerebral hemorrhage, resulting in functional improvement. J Cereb Blood Flow Metab 2006; 26: 536-44.

[106] Chen S, Yang Q, Chen G, Zhang JH. An update on inflammation in the acute phase of intracerebral hemorrhage. Transl Stroke Res 2015; 6: 4-8.

[107] Di Napoli M, Parry-Jones AR, Smith CJ, et al. C-reactive protein predicts hematoma growth in intracerebral hemorrhage. Stroke 2014; 45: 59-65.

[108] Gu SJ, Xuan HF, Lu M, et al. Admission plasma visfatin level strongly correlates with hematoma growth and early neurologic deterioration in patients with acute spontaneous basal ganglia hemorrhage. Clinica chimica acta 2013; 425: 85-9.

[109] Du Q, Yang DB, Shen YF, et al. Plasma leptin level predicts hematoma growth and early neurological deterioration after acute intracerebral hemorrhage. Peptides 2013; 45: 35-9.

[110] Mingam R, Moranis A, Bluthe RM, et al. Uncoupling of interleukin-6 from its signalling pathway by dietary n-3-polyunsaturated fatty acid deprivation alters sickness behaviour in mice. Eur J Neurosci 2008; 28: 1877-86.

[111] Hunter CA, Jones SA. Il-6 as a keystone cytokine in health and disease. Nat Immunol 2015; 16: 448-57.

[112] Osuka K, Watanabe Y, Usuda N, et al. Activation of jak-stat3 signaling pathway in chronic subdural hematoma outer membranes. Neurosci Lett 2013; 534: 166-70.

[113] Grivennikov SI, Karin M. Dangerous liaisons: Stat3 and nf-kappab collaboration and crosstalk in cancer. Cytokine & growth factor reviews 2010; 21: 11-9.

[114] Gonzalez-Moreno EI, Camara-Lemarroy CR, Gonzalez-Gonzalez JG, Gongora-Rivera F. Glycemic variability and acute ischemic stroke: The missing link? Transl Stroke Res 2014; 5: 638-46.

[115] Di Napoli M, Godoy DA, Campi V, et al. C-reactive protein in intracerebral hemorrhage: Time course, tissue localization, and prognosis. Neurology 2012; 79: 690-9.

[116] Huang Q, Dai WM, Jie YQ, Yu GF, Fan XF, Wu A. High concentrations of visfatin in the peripheral blood of patients with acute basal ganglia hemorrhage are associated with poor outcome. Peptides 2013; 39: 55-8.

[117] Yao X, Zhu F, Zhao Z, Liu C, Luo L, Yin Z. Arctigenin enhances chemosensitivity of cancer cells to cisplatin through inhibition of the stat3 signaling pathway. J Cell Biochem 2011; 112: 2837-49.

[118] Kim CK, Ryu WS, Choi IY, et al. Detrimental effects of leptin on intracerebral hemorrhage via the stat3 signal pathway. J Cereb Blood Flow Metab 2013; 33: 944-53.

[119] Nandi D, Tahiliani P, Kumar A, Chandu D. The ubiquitin proteasome system. J Biosci 2006; 31: 137-55.

[120] Sinn DI, Lee ST, Chu K, et al. Proteasomal inhibition in intracerebral hemorrhage: Neuroprotective and anti-inflammatory effects of bortezomib. Neurosci Res 2007; 58: 12-8.

[121] Gong C, Ennis SR, Hoff JT, Keep RF. Inducible cyclooxygenase-2 expression after experimental intracerebral hemorrhage. Brain Res 2001; 901: 38-46.

[122] Keynes RG, Garthwaite J. Nitric oxide and its role in ischaemic brain injury. Curr Mol Med 2004; 4: 179-91.

[123] Makogonenko E, Tsurupa G, Ingham K, Medved L. Interaction of fibrin(ogen)

with fibronectin: Further characterization and localization of the fibronectin-binding site. Biochemistry 2002; 41: 7907-13.

[124] Ho-Tin-Noe B, Demers M, Wagner DD. How platelets safeguard vascular integrity. J Thromb Haemost 2011; 9 Suppl 1: 56-65.

[125] Lei B, Mace B, Bellows ST, et al. Interaction between sex and apolipoprotein e genetic background in a murine model of intracerebral hemorrhage. Transl Stroke Res 2012; 3: 94-101.

[126] Biffi A, Sonni A, Anderson CD, et al. Variants at apoe influence risk of deep and lobar intracerebral hemorrhage. Ann Neurol 2010; 68: 934-43.

[127] Brouwers HB, Biffi A, Ayres AM, et al. Apolipoprotein e genotype predicts hematoma expansion in lobar intracerebral hemorrhage. Stroke 2012; 43: 1490-5.

[128] Biffi A, Anderson CD, Jagiella JM, et al. Apoe genotype and extent of bleeding and outcome in lobar intracerebral haemorrhage: A genetic association study. Lancet Neurol 2011; 10: 702-9.

[129] Rannikmae K, Kalaria RN, Greenberg SM, et al. Apoe associations with severe caa-associated vasculopathic changes: Collaborative meta-analysis. J Neurol Neurosurg Psychiatry 2014; 85: 300-5.

[130] Montanola A, de Retana SF, Lopez-Rueda A, et al. Apoa1, apoj and apoe plasma levels and genotype frequencies in cerebral amyloid angiopathy. Neuromolecular Med 2016; 18: 99-108.

[131] Chen S, Zeng L, Hu Z. Progressing haemorrhagic stroke: Categories, causes, mechanisms and managements. J Neurol 2014; 261: 2061-78.

CONFLICT OF INTEREST

The author(s) confirm that this article content has no conflict of interest.

ACKNOWLEDGEMENTS

Declared none.

DECLARATION: This chapter was authored by Gaiqing Wang and John

H. Zhang published as " Hematoma Expansion: Clinical and Molecular Predictors and Corresponding Pharmacological Treatment " in " Current drug targets ", 2017; 18 (12):1367-1376

CHAPTER 4:

Mechanisms of oxidative stress and therapeutic targets following intracerebral hemorrhage

ABSTRACT:

Oxidative stress (OS) is induced by the accumulation of reactive oxygen species (ROS) following intracerebral hemorrhage (ICH) and plays an important role in secondary brain injury caused by the inflammatory response, apoptosis, autophagy, and blood-brain barrier (BBB) disruption. This review summarizes the current state of knowledge regarding the pathogenic mechanisms of brain injury after ICH, markers for detecting OS, and therapeutic strategies that target OS to mitigate brain injury.

KEY WORDS: Intracerebral hemorrhage; Oxidative stress; Brain damage

5. Introduce

ICH is a type of stroke characterized by spontaneous and nontraumatic bleeding in the brain that is associated with high morbidity and mortality rates [1]. ICH can be classified as primary and secondary. While treatment options for the former are limited, various strategies have been proposed for managing the latter [1]. Hematomal and perihematomal regions are biochemically active environments that sustain oxidative damage following ICH [2]. OS is defined as an imbalance between the formation of strong oxidants and physiologic antioxidant capacity [3]. ROS such as oxygen free radicals (e.g., superoxide (O_2-) and hydroxyl radicals ($OH-$)) and nonradical compounds (e.g., hydrogen peroxide (H_2O_2) and hypochlorous acid), as well as reactive nitrogen species (RNS; e.g., nitric oxide (NO)) and a variety of nitrogenous compounds produced as metabolic byproducts, are the major drivers of oxidative damage [4] to proteins, lipids, and nucleic acids, which can induce inflammation, autophagy, apoptosis, and destruction of the BBB. OS is associated with dysregulation of cellular oxidation and reduction (redox) mechanisms; redox sensitive thiols that are easily oxidized by nonradical oxidants such as H_2O_2 after ICH are essential for transcription factor regulation (e.g., nuclear factor erythroid 2-related factor (Nrf) 2 and nuclear factor- (NF-) Kb) [5].

The Kelch-like ECH-associated protein (Keap) 1/Nrf2/antioxidant response element (ARE) signaling pathway is the main regulatory system protecting cells against oxidative damage. Nrf2 is a master regulator of the cellular response to oxidative stress, which is associated with the expression of antioxidant and detoxification enzymes and factors such as NAD(P)H: quinone oxidoreductase (NQO) 1, catalase (CAT), superoxide dismutase (SOD), heme oxygenase (HO-) 1, glutathione peroxidase (GPX), and glutathione-S-transferase (GST) [6]. Nrf2 was shown to mitigate early brain injury after ICH by translocating to the nucleus following activation and binding to AREs to activate the transcription of genes encoding antioxidant enzymes [7].

2. ROS Production after ICH

2.1. Production of ROS by Activated Phagocytes and Nonphagocytic Cells following ICH.

Activated neutrophils, microglia, and macrophages are the main sources of ROS following ICH. Nicotinamide adenine dinucleotide phosphate (NADPH) oxidase (NOX) is expressed on the surface of neutrophils and macrophages and stimulates the production of ROS in response to extracellular signals such as hormones and cytokines [8]. Nonphagocytic cells such as neurons, microglia, astrocytes, and cerebrovascular endothelial cells also express NOX [8–10]. To date, 7 NOX isozymes have been identified in nonphagocytic cells that use NADH or NADPH as an electron donor for ROS production [11]. While NOX activity is generally low in these cells, they continuously produce O2− even in the absence of external stimulation [11]. Hypoxia after ICH induces conformational changes in gp91phox, the heme-binding subunit of NOX, which activates the protein and leads to the formation of NOX complexes and increased ROS production [12] The activation of NOX was also reported to be the main mechanism underlying ROS generation in a rabbit model of intraventricular hemorrhage (IVH) [13], and OS resulting from NOX activation was shown to contribute to collagenase induced ICH and brain injury [14]. NOX2 protein level was upregulated in the striatum of mice 12 h after ICH, which peaked at 24 h [15], and another study found that gp91phox was primarily expressed in activated microglia and colocalized with peroxynitrite (ONOO−) 24 h after ICH in the injured hemisphere [16]. However, following ICH, activated leukocytes release myeloperoxidase (MPO), which catalyzes lipid peroxidation and causes OS at the site of injury [17]. Additionally, increased expression of inducible NO synthase (Inos) in M1 microglia in conjunction with the release of proinflammatory mediators and cytotoxic substances caused significant tissue damage after ICH [18].

2.2. Increased ROS Production in Mitochondria following ICH.

Another important ROS is O_2^- produced by mitochondria, which is generated as a byproduct of biological oxidation during mitochondrial respiration under physiologic conditions [19]. In most cells, the electron transport chain consumes 90% of cellular oxygen; 2% of this is transformed into oxygen free radicals in the mitochondrial inner membrane and matrix [20, 21]. Electrons that leak from the respiratory chain react with oxygen to form O_2^-. Mitochondrial O_2^- is detoxified to H_2O_2 by SOD, then to O_2 and H_2O by antioxidant enzymes such as CAT and GPX. However, O_2^- that elude antioxidant mechanisms can damage proteins, lipids, and DNA [21]. There are 7 known sources of O_2^- in mammalian mitochondria: the ubiquinone-binding sites in complex I (site IQ) and complex III (site IIIQo), glycerol 3-phosphate dehydrogenase, complex I flavin (site IF),electron-transferring flavoprotein: Q oxidoreductase in fatty acid beta oxidation, pyruvate, and 2-oxoglutarate dehydrogenase,with site IQ and site IIIQo having the highest production capacities [21].

Mitochondria are storage sites for calcium ions ($Ca2+$). Under ischemia/reperfusion (I/R), excessive glutamate levels can cause an influx of $Ca2+$ into neurons via N-methyl-daspartic acid receptor (NMDAR), a ligand-gated ion channel [22]. Activation of the NMDAR leads to further $Ca2+$ influx,with increased levels in the cytosol and mitochondrial $Ca2+$ loading. Thrombin produced after ICH leads to Src kinase activation by activating protease-activated receptor 1(PAR1), which phosphorylates and activates NMDAR. PARs are a subfamily of G protein-coupled receptors (GPCRs) with four members, namely, PAR1, PAR2, PAR3, and PAR4. PAR1 is highly expressed in many different cell types. PAR1 plays an important role in astrocyte proliferation, stimulus-induced long-term potentiation (LTP), and nerve growth factor (NGF) secretion. PAR1 enhances Src mediated tyrosine phosphorylation of NMDA receptor in ICH [23]. Activation of α-amino-3-hydroxy-5-methyl-4-isoxazolepropionic acid (AMPA) receptor by glutamate after ICH in motor neurons also increased $Ca2+$ and $Na+$ influx and mitochondrial $Ca2+$ loading [22]. Following ICH, $Ca2+$ stored in the endoplasmic reticulum

(ER) is thought to be sequestered by mitochondria. Mitochondrial Ca2+ loading reduces mitochondrial membrane potential (MMP) and opens the mitochondrial permeability transition pore (MPTP), resulting in mitochondrial damage and disruption of the mitochondrial respiratory chain; together, these processes result in the release of excess ROS [22].

2.3. Increased ROS Production by the ER following ICH.

The ER is the site of protein synthesis, posttranslational modification, folding, and trafficking. ICH can cause ER stress (ERS), which is characterized by protein misfolding, accumulation of abnormal proteins, and Ca2+ imbalance, all of which trigger the unfolded protein response (UPR) [24]. Glutamate excitotoxicity and the inflammatory response can result in ERS. When ICH causes ERS, ROS are generated by NOX4 in the internal membrane. ROS then acts as a signaling intermediate that subsequently mitigates ERS via the UPR. If ERS is not alleviated, the delayed expression of proteins such as C/EBP homologous protein (CHOP) causes a secondary increase in ROS levels [25]. Additionally, disulfide bonds in proteins translated in the ER are highly sensitive to changes in redox balance; thus, both reducing and oxidizing conditions can disrupt protein folding and cause ERS. On the other hand, oxidative protein folding is a major source of intracellular ROS production [26]; during this process, thiol groups on the cysteines of peptides are oxidized and form disulfide bonds [26]. After accepting electrons from protein disulfide isomerase (PDI), ER oxidoreductin (ERO) 1 transfers electrons to molecular oxygen to generate H2O2, the major type of ROS formed in the ER lumen [26]. In the ERS following ICH, disruption of disulfide bond formation leads to ROS accumulation and OS [26]. Inositol 1,4,5-trisphosphate receptor and voltage-dependent anion channel-which are located in the ER and mitochondria, respectively-form a complex with the chaperone protein glucose-regulated protein (GRP) 75, thus physically connecting the 2 organelles [22]. Upon ERS, Ca2+ transfer at the contact points between the ER and mitochondria leads to mitochondrial dysfunction, thereby increasing mitochondrial ROS production, resulting in cellular stress or neuronal death. Although there have been few studies investigating the relationship between ERS and ICH, given the interaction between ERS and microglial activation [27], neuroinflammation, and autophagy after ICH, clarification of this point can inspire new avenues for ICH treatment.

2.4. Hemoglobin (Hb) Toxicity after ICH.

Hb toxicity is induced by free radicals generated via Fenton-type reactions and by oxidative damage to proteins, nucleic acids, and lipids [28]. During its conversion to methemoglobin, oxyhemoglobin releases O2 −, which in turn forms OH− and contributes to ROS production [29]. Hb, a major component of erythrocytes, is a heterotetramer composed of α and β globin subunits that each bind a heme molecule. Hb induces the expression of Inos by M1 microglia and neutrophils after ICH. NOS is expressed by endothelial cells, macrophages, neurophagocytes, and nerve cells; there are 2 isoenzymes besides Inos—namely, neural and endothelial NOS [30]. Overexpression of Inos or endothelial NOS and the consequent overproduction of NO lead to changes in tight junction proteins and can potentially disrupt the BBB [31]. Following ICH, heme is released by Hb and decomposed into bilirubin, free iron, and carbon monoxide.

2.5. Increased ROS Production by Heme following ICH.

Heme (ferrous protoporphyrin IX) is a reactive, low molecular weight form of iron that participates in Fenton-type oxygen radical reactions in neurons, microglia, and neutrophils [32]. Hemin, the oxidized form of heme, accumulates in intracranial hematomas and is a potent oxidant [33]. Hemin is bound by hemopexin in serum, and the complex is translocated into the cell via lipoprotein receptor-related protein (LRP) 1. Intracellular hemin is degraded into bilirubin, Fe^{2+}, and carbon monoxide. Fe^{2+} derived from hemin can generate OH—the most reactive oxygen radical-via the Fenton reaction, leading to an increase in ROS levels [22].

2.6. Increased ROS Production from Ferrous Iron and Ferritin following ICH.

Ferrous iron is one of the main contributors to OS following ICH. Free iron catalyzes the conversion of O_2^- and H_2O_2 into OH^- via the Fenton reaction while oxidizing iron from a divalent to a trivalent form [34]. Ferrous iron is

transported into the cell through divalent metal transporter (DMT) 1 and into mitochondria by ATP-binding cassette-(ABC-) 7 [22], resulting in OS. Ferritin functions as a source of iron in lipid peroxidation; the release of iron from ferritin is mediated by O2− [34] (Figure 1). Knowledge of the mechanisms and dynamics of ROS generation following ICH can guide the development of drugs for the treatment of ICH that act by mitigating OS.

3. OS-Induced Brain Damage following ICH

3.1. Organelle Damage by OS.

Oxidative damage in DNA includes base modifications and hydrogen bond breakage [35]; in proteins, it can include amino acid modifications, peptide chain fractures, and protein cross-linking [36]. Free radicals cause cellular membrane damage by promoting lipid peroxidation (especially of polyunsaturated fatty acids); the binding of free radicals to membrane receptors also leads to the destruction of membrane integrity [37].

3.2. OS-Induced Autophagy in ICH.

Autophagy is a cellular process for the clearance of damaged organelles and proteins that are misfolded or no longer required. Autophagy is triggered by ICH-induced OS [38]. Studies have indicated that superoxide is the major form of ROS regulating autophagy [39].

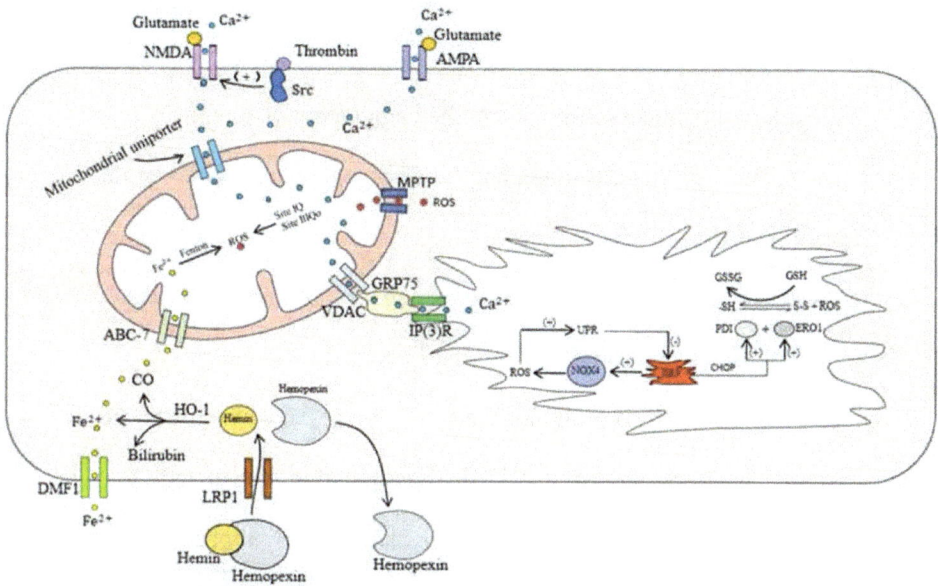

Figure 1: The production of reactive oxygen species after cerebral hemorrhage: hemin and divalent iron ions enter the cell through the corresponding receptors on the cell membrane, and further, Fenton reaction occurs in the mitochondria, thereby generating excess ROS; glutamate and thrombin activate ion channel receptors on the cell membrane to promote Ca2+ influx; in addition, the VDAC and IP(3)R located in the mitochondria and the endoplasmic reticulum are connected through GRP75, so that the Ca2+ in the endoplasmic reticulum flows into the mitochondria, and the Ca2+ in the mitochondria is further overloaded, and the MPTPA channel on the mitochondria is opened and released. The H2O2 produced at the two sites of site IQ and site IIIQo in the mitochondria generates ROS when it encounters Fe(III). Endoplasmic reticulum UPR can reduce ERS. When ERS cannot be relieved, certain UPR components (such as C/EBP homologous protein CHOP) may cause oxidative stress; in addition, in the stressed ER, the imbalance of disulfide bond formation and breaking may lead to the accumulation of reactive oxygen species (ROS) and cause oxidative stress. ROS: reactive oxygen species; Fe2+: ferrous iron; AMPA: α-amino-3-hydroxy-5-methyl-4-isoxazole-propionic acid receptor; NMDA: N-methyl-D-aspartic acid receptor; HO-1: heme oxygenase-1; DMT: divalent metal transporter 1; MPTP: mitochondrial permeability transition pore; VDAC: voltage-dependent anion channel; ER: endoplasmic reticulum; IP3R: inositol 1,4,5-trisphosphate receptor; ERO1: ER oxidase 1; CHOP: C/EBP homologous protein; UPR: unfolded protein response; PDI: protein disulfide isomerases; LRP1: lipoprotein receptor-related protein; NOX4: adenine dinucleotide phosphate oxidase 4.

A hallmark of the process is the reversible conjugation of autophagy-related protein (Atg) 8 to the autophagosome membrane.Under conditions of serum starvation, ROS (especially H2O2) induces the inactivation of Atg4 during autophagosome formation, which promotes the lipidation of Atg8. As the autophagosome matures and fuses to a lysosome,the reduction in H2O2 levels promotes the activation of Atg4 along with the delipidation and recycling of Atg8 [39]. The regulation of autophagy is closely related to p62/Keap1/Nrf2 redox signaling. The autophagy-related factor p62 binds to ubiquitinated protein aggregates, and its affinity for Keap1 is increased upon phosphorylation at Ser351 [40]. This induces the degradation of Keap1 via autophagy and releases Nrf2, which accumulates and translocates to the nucleus where it binds to AREs to activate the transcription of genes encoding antioxidant enzymes and p62 as well as other autophagy-related factors [40]. ROS produced as a result of ICH act on the mammalian target of rapamycin complex (Mtorc) 1/UNC51-like kinase (ULK) 1 and AMP-activated protein kinase (AMPK)/ULK1 signaling pathways that regulate autophagy. AMPK activation and Mtorc1 inhibition in response to ROS lead to ULK1 activation and induction of autophagy [40]. Activated ULK1 phosphorylates its interaction partners Atg13 and FAK family-interacting protein of 200 kDa (FIP200), resulting in the activation of the class III phosphoinositide 3-kinase (PI3K) complex via activating molecule in

BECN1-regulated autophagy (AMBRA) 1, thus initiating the nucleation of autophagosomes from the ER or mitochondria [40]. Some research data suggest that oxidative stress induces autophagy activation, which may make ICH-induced brain injury disappear [41]. This may also reduce early brain damage in SAH [42]. However, others believe that under- or overactivation of autophagy may lead to cell damage and death.

The potential role of selective autophagy in the clinical treatment of hemorrhagic stroke has been recognized. The mechanism of autophagy activation mediated by mitochondrial and ERS induced by OS after ICH remains to be studied.

3.3. Apoptosis Induced by OS following ICH.

Severe OS and a high intracellular concentration of Ca2+ following ICH induces MPTP opening and a reduction in MMP, with subsequent release of cytochrome C and other proapoptotic proteins from the mitochondrial membrane into the cytosol, which activates the intrinsic neuronal apoptosis pathway in mitochondria [43]. After cerebral hemorrhage (ICH), oxidative stress leads to DNA and protein damage, which leads to neuronal apoptosis.

3.4. Matrix Metalloproteinase (MMP) Activation by OS after ICH.

Following ICH, O2− and NO levels are increased as a result of endothelial NOS and Inos activities, respectively. In the context of cerebral I/R, NO reacts with O2− produced by gp91phox to form ONOO−. The activation of MMP-9 and MMP-2 by ONOO− results in the degradation of the tight junction proteins claudin-5 and - 84 -ccluding as well as the extracellular matrix, leading to disruption of the BBB [44].

ONOO− induces other forms of cellular damage including protein oxidation, DNA damage, lipid peroxidation, tyrosine nitration, and mitochondrial dysfunction. Notably, tyrosine nitration leads to the modification of functional proteins and vascular endothelial cell injury [45]. Following ICH, Hb induced OS resulting from MMP activation disrupted the BBB and induced cell apoptosis, which was reversed by overexpression of SOD1 [29].

3.5. OS Mediates the Inflammatory Response following ICH.

ROS-induced activation of the NACHT, LRR, and PYD domain-containing protein (NLRP) 3 inflammasome following ICH results in the release of interleukin- (IL-) 1β, which promotes neutrophil infiltration, inflammation, and brain edema [46]. ROS and RNS produced by neutrophils regulate the inflammatory response after ICH by modulating phagocytosis, cellular function, gene expression, and apoptosis [47]. In the context of ICH, MPO from activated white blood cells catalyzes the oxidation of chloride ions by H2O2, producing the strong oxidant hypochlorous acid (HOCl), which can cause further tissue damage and promote inflammation [48]. Thiol redox circuits are a normal part of cell signaling and physiologic regulation; their destruction in vascular disease causes OS, leading to the activation of a proinflammatory signaling cascade [5]. The net effect of NOX activation may be proinflammatory, as evidenced by its activation in phagocytes after ICH and the resultant generation of reactive oxygen intermediates that enhance inflammation and tissue damage [8] and further increase OS. The infiltration of inflammatory cells induces an influx of Ca2+, increasing free radical production, and lipid peroxidation. After ICH, M1 phenotypic microglia can be activated by thrombin to release proinflammatory cytokines and chemokines such as interleukin-1β (IL-1β), tumor necrosis factor-α (TNF-α), and ROS, thereby attracting surrounding inflammatory mediators. In addition, microglia strongly express HO-1, which converts heme into iron, carbon monoxide (CO), and biliverdin [45] (Figure 2).

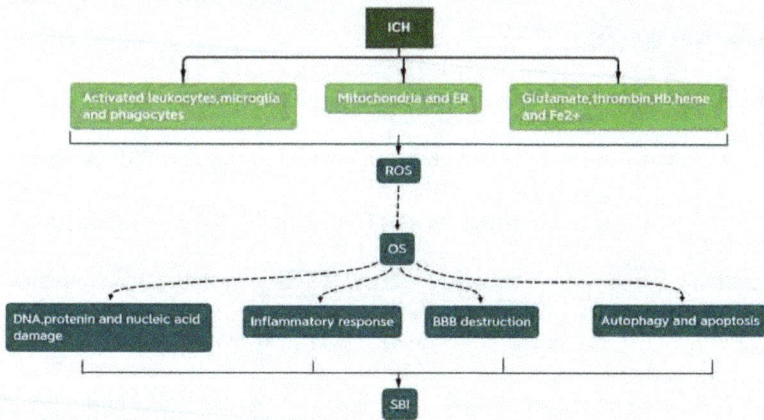

Figure 2: Summary of mechanisms by which OS aggravates SBI after ICH: after ICH, activated phagocytes, mitochondria, ER, and RBC lysates all cause excess release of ROS. This increase in OS exacerbates the inflammatory response, apoptosis, autophagy, and BBB disruption, with further SBI aggravation. BBB: blood-brain barrier; ICH: intracerebral hemorrhage; OS: oxidative stress; ROS: reactive oxygen species; SBI: secondary brain injury.

4. Markers for Detecting OS after ICH

4.1. Oxidative DNA Damage

4.1.1. 8-Oxo-7,8-Dihydro-2′Deoxyguanosine (8-OhdG) and 8-Oxo-7,8-Dihydro-Guanine (8-oxoGua). 8-OhdG and 8-oxoGua are sensitive markers for DNA oxidative damage that are produced through hydroxylation at the C-8 position of guanine. Various methods are used to measure 8-oxoGua and 8-oxodG concentrations in blood and urine samples, including gas chromatography-mass spectrometry (GCMS), high-performance liquid chromatography electrochemical detection (HPLC-ECD), immunohistochemistry, and enzyme-linked immunosorbent assay (ELISA). GC-MS and HPLC-ECD have higher specificity and are more accurate than ELISA [49]. At 24 h after ICH, 8-OhdG was detected at high levels at the borders of damaged and normal tissues, coinciding with an Increase In the number of apurinic/apyrimidinic sites; expression peaked in the first 3 days post-ICH and returned to baseline starting from day 7 [50]. The OS marker leukocyte 8-hydroxy-2′-deoxyguanosine was shown to be an independent predictor of 30-day outcome following ICH [51], while serum 8-OhdG and 8-oxoGua levels were related to 30-day mortality in ICH patients [52]. According to reports, the optimal cutoff of serum OGS levels in ICH patients is 4.94 ng/Ml (according to Youden's J index). When the OGS level of patients is higher than the cutoff value, the mortality rate is higher [52].

4.2. Lipid Peroxidation

4.2.1. Malondialdehyde (MDA). ICH leads to progressively higher levels of lipid peroxidation, as evidenced by increased diene conjugation and MDA levels [52]. MDA is the most commonly used biomarker of lipid peroxidation in clinical studies. Serum MDA levels were shown to increase rapidly at the early stage of ICH and were closely related to the severity of clinical symptoms [53]. MDA can be accurately detected by HPLC [53], whereas the detection of thiobarbituric acid-reactive substances by ultraviolet light (UV) spectrophotometry overestimated MDA levels in human plasma [43]. Serum MDA level at diagnosis of severe spontaneous ICH was shown to be associated with early mortality [54]. The study found that patients with spontaneous cerebral hemorrhage have a higher risk of death when the serum MDA is higher than 2.48 nmol/Ml [54]. It is common to use the thiobarbituric acid reactive substance (TBARS) method to determine the serum MDA of cerebral hemorrhage mouse models and patients with ICH [2, 52, 54–58].

4.2.2. 4-Hydroxynonenal (4-HNE).

4-HNE is a product of lipid peroxidation in the cell membrane that can be quantified by HPLC, GC-MS, LC-MS, and aldehyde-reactive probes [59]. 4-HNE levels in cerebrospinal fluid (CSF) and plasma samples of patients with Parkinson's disease have also been determined by GC-negative-ion chemical ionization mass spectrometry-based detection of

O-pentafluorobenzyl oxime [60]. Vasospasm in patients with SAH has been evaluated based on measurement of lipid peroxidation; the levels of polyunsaturated fatty acid cyclization products, F2-isoprostanes (F2-IsoPs), and neuroprostanes were highest on day 1 post-SAH and decreased over time, with similar trends observed in the levels of 4-HNE, 4-oxononenal, and MDA [61].

6. F2-IsoPs.

Another hallmark of lipid peroxidation is the production of F2-IsoPs, which can be detected by LC-MS and the gold standard method GC-MS, while ELISA is less effective [62]. 8-Iso-prostaglandin (8-iso-PG) F2α is an isomer derivative of F2-IsoP that serves as a biomarker for evaluating OS and lipid peroxidation. 8-Iso-PGF2α is present in a free form in tissue or in esterified form in lipids; levels in the blood were shown to be increased after ICH, which was positively correlated with the National Institute of Health Stroke Scale score and hematoma volume [60], and elevated plasma concentrations of 8-Iso-PGF2α were reported to be associated with the clinical severity and outcome of ICH.

The plasma level of 8-iso-PGF2α is an independent prognostic factor in ICH [63] and indicator of oxidation in analyses of F2-IsoP, isofuran, and F(4)-neuroprostane concentrations following aneurysmal SAH and traumatic brain injury. A higher level of F(4)-neuroprostanes in CSF more accurately reflects neural dysfunction than the elevated F2-IsoP level [64].

4.3. Enzyme Activity

4.3.1. SOD.

Studies have determined that the level of SOD in patients with cerebral hemorrhage (113:62 ± 9:14 U/Ml) is significantly lower than healthy (161:20 ± 21:12 U/Ml) [65].It is a common indicator for evaluating oxidative stress in mouse models of ICH [2, 6, 56, 58, 66, 67].

7. MPO.

The activity of MPO, a potent oxidizing enzyme, can be determined by quantifying the level of 3-Cl-Tyr and the conversion of hydroethidine to 2-chloroethidium. The MPO/H2O2/chloride system of leukocyte activation is responsible for the generation of 3-Cl-Tyr, which is a biomarker of neuroinflammation [68]. Moreover, serum MPO concentration was found to be increased in ICH patients, which was correlated with ICH severity and prognosis [69]. In ICH animal experiments, MPO can be measured with immunofluorescence assay [55].

4.4. Evaluation of Antioxidant Levels

4.4.1. Glutathione (GSH) and Oxidized Glutathione (GSSG).

The molar ratio of GSH to GSSG is a useful index of OS in ICH. Total GSH in cells is quantified by measuring the concentration of the glutathione-N-ethylmaleimide conjugate by UV/visible HPLC. However, under pathologic conditions, total GSH content is lower than that of GSSG. Spectrophotometry can be used to determine GSSG concentration by either the GSH recycling method or HPLC [70], while commercial GSH/GSSG detection kits are commonly used in studies involving ICH models [6, 57, 66].

7.4.2. Allantoin.

Allantoin is a physiologic antioxidant that can be detected in human plasma and serum samples by GC-MS [71]. It was also demonstrated that determination of urinary allantoin concentrations by GC-MS was useful for evaluating the efficacy of clinical interventions in preterm neonates diagnosed with germinal matrix IVH [64].

8. Thioredoxin (TRX).

TRX is an antioxidant that eliminates oxygen as well as OH− radicals. Serum concentrations of TRX can be determined by ELISA, with commercial kits widely available. Increased serum concentrations of TRX were shown to be related to hemorrhage severity and longterm mortality in patients with ICH [72].

Besides, the mouse ICH model can also use the ROS analysis kit to detect the level of oxidative stress. This kit uses the principle of the fluorescent probe 2′,7′-dichlorofluorescein diacetate to determine [6, 57, 67, 73].

9. Therapeutic Strategies Targeting OS.

Following ICH (Supplementary Table 1–2)

5.1. Regulation of Oxidant Signaling Pathways

5.1.1. Keap1/Nrf2/ARE Signaling (Supplementary Table 1).

The Keap1/Nrf2/ARE signaling pathway is one of the most important defense mechanisms against OS in ICH [74] as it promotes the expression of endogenous antioxidant enzymes including NQO1, CAT, SOD, HO-1, and GPX [75]. Nrf2 was upregulated following ICH, with peak level occurring at 24 h;

the time course of expression was shown to be correlated with the severity of brain edema and neurologic deficits. Heme oxygenase-1 is resistant to OS in the early stages of ICH but is thought to promote oxidation in subsequent stages of the disease process. Drugs targeting the Nrf2/ARE signaling pathway have therapeutic potential for reducing brain damage caused by OS and inflammation following ICH (Figure 3).

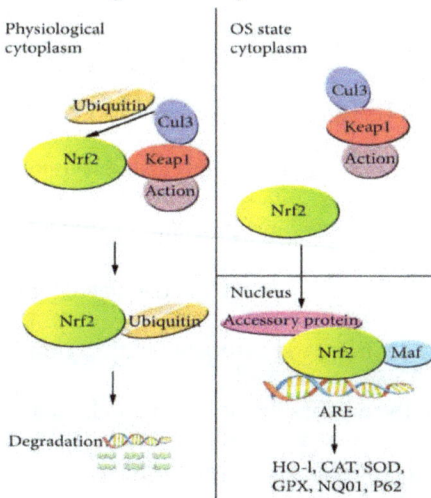

Figure 3: Description of antioxidant enzyme system regulation via the Keap1-Nrf2-ARE pathway.
(a) Under normal basal conditions, Keap1 binds Nrf2 and keeps its level low by ubiquitination and proteasomal degradation;
(b) under OS conditions, Keap1 is oxidized by OS, and dissociation of Nrf2 from Keap1 enables Nrf2 to translocate to the nucleus. Nrf2 combines with the small Maf protein to form a Nrf2-Maf

heterodimer, and Nrf2 binds to accessory protein and then ARE activates gene expression of HO- 1, NQO1, GPX, SOD, CAT, and the autophagy protein p62. ARE: antioxidant response element; CAT: catalase; Cul3: Cullin3; GPX: glutathione peroxidase; HO-1: heme oxygenase-1; ICH: intracerebral hemorrhage; Keap1: Kelch-like ECH-associated protein 1; Maf: musculoaponeurotic fibrosarcoma; NQO1: NAPDH quinone oxidoreductase 1; Nrf2: nuclear factor erythroid 2-related factor 2; OS: oxidative stress; SOD: superoxide dismutase.

The drugs used to treat ICH animal models by regulating the Nrf2-ARE signaling pathway include glycyrrhizin [6], simvastatin [76], methyl hydrogen fumarate [77], nicotinamide mononucleotide [56], astaxanthin [55], mangiferin [71], RS9 [78], silymarin [79], sulforaphane [80], Hb pretreatment [81], melatonin [82], and recombinant human erythropoietin [83], calycosin [84], (-)-epicatechin [67], luteolin [85], and ghrelin [86].

5.1.2. Peroxisome Proliferator-Activated Receptor (PPAR) γ Signaling.

PPARγ regulates CAT expression and is another antioxidant signaling pathway. CAT is ubiquitously expressed in all cell types including glia and neurons and is predominantly localized in peroxisomes. A PPAR response element is present in the CAT gene promoter, indicating a direct regulatory interaction. 15-Deoxy-Δ12,14-prostaglandin J2 (15d-PGJ2) is a nonenzymatic breakdown product of prostaglandin D2; unlike synthetic thiazolidinediones, 15d-PGJ2 acts as an endogenous ligand for PPARγ to promote the expression of CAT, which was shown to be associated with decreased inflammation, oxidative damage, and neuronal loss in a rat model of ICH [87]. It was noted in the cerebral hemorrhage model that telmisartan can induce the expression of receptor γ activated by endothelial nitric oxide synthase and peroxisome proliferators and reduce

oxidative stress, apoptosis signals, and tumor necrosis factor-α and

cyclooxygenase-2 expression [88].

5.2. Decreased ROS Production following ICH

5.2.1. NOX.

The inhibition of NOX reduces the generation of endogenous ROS. A

small ubiquitin-related modifier was shown to negatively regulate NOX5

in human neutrophils and vascular smooth muscle cells, thus limiting the

production of ROS. However, there is little known about the involvement

of small ubiquitin-related modifiers in ICH [89]. Melatonin was

previously found to inhibit ROS generation and OS after ICH [73].

Meanwhile, overexpression of the ubiquitin ligase ring finger (RNF) 34

exacerbated brain injury after ICH by promoting peroxisome proliferator-

activated receptor coactivator- (PGC-) 1α degradation while stimulating

the generation of mitochondrial ROS. Thus, genetic ablation of RNF34 is

a potential strategy for the treatment of ICH [90]. The NADPH oxidase

inhibitor apocynin improved the therapeutic efficacy of mesenchymal

stem cells in the acute stage of ICH by exerting neuroprotective effects

and enhancing the integrity of cerebral vasculature[12].

5.2.2. Mitochondria.

Sodium benzoate was reported to mitigate OS-induced secondary brain

injury, inhibit neuronal apoptosis, and suppress ROS production in mitochondria after ICH via DJ-1/protein kinase B (AKT)/IκB kinase

(IKK)/NF-Kb signaling [91]. The alleviation of neurologic deficits by

deferoxamine via inhibition of PGC-1α signaling was shown to reduce

OS caused by mitochondrial dysfunction[92]. Besides, drugs that can

reduce the oxidative stress induced by mitochondrial function damage in

ICH animal models include Dexmedetomidine (Dex) [92],

Pyrroloquinoline Quinone (PQQ) [93], and melatonin [73].

5.3. Elimination of ROS following ICH.

Intracerebroventricular injection of recombinant α1-microglobulin (A1M)

resulted in its coexistence with extracellular Hb, while injection of human

A1M mitigated the inflammatory response and mitochondrial damage in

a rabbit model of IVH [94]. As a radical scavenger, A1M eliminates both

heme and radicals, thus providing early protection to the immature brain

in preterm IVH [94]. The novel free radical scavenger NSP-116 was

found to alter cerebral blood flow and alleviate neurologic deficits in a

model of I/R injury caused by middle cerebral artery occlusion; it also

suppressed the expansion of hematomas and reduced neurologic deficits

[95].

Edaravone, a free radical scavenger, reduced cerebral edema, and lipid

peroxidation following IVH in rats and repeated administration improved

learning and memory performance [96]. Hydrogen gas was found to

reduce OS damage by eliminating OH− in a rat model of cerebral I/R

[97], and inhaled hydrogen diminishes OS and brain edema 24 h after

ICH, although it did not improve clinical outcome [98]. In addition,

Glibenclamide (GLI) [99] and tempol [100] are also free radical

scavengers for oxidative stress after ICH.

5.4. Effects of Antioxidants following ICH.

Melatonin (N-acetyl-5-methoxytryptamine) is an indolamine that is

primarily synthesized by the pineal gland and can easily pass through the

BBB. Melatonin improved severe ICH-induced brain injury by mitigating

OS, apoptosis, inflammation, DNA damage, brain edema, and BBB

damage and by inhibiting MPTP opening [73], and in a SAH model, it

mitigated cerebral OS by increasing the expression of HO-1, NQO1,

NADPH, and GST-α1, possibly via activation of the Nrf2/ARE signaling

pathway [82]. Baicalein treatment reduced OS in rats by increasing the

activity of SOD and GPX while downregulating the expression of MDA

in the brain. Thus, baicalein can potentially be used to treat ICH and

related brain injuries [101]. Danhong—a traditional Chinese medicine

extracted from 2 herbs (Salviae miltiorrhiza Bunge (Danshen, China) and

Carthamus tinctorius L (Honghua, China))—contains flavonoids and

phenolic compounds and was reported to increase the expression of

peroxiredoxin (Prx) 1 in astrocytes, thereby preventing severe brain

injury following ICH in aged rats [102]. In addition, carnosine [103],

COA-Cl (a novel synthesized nucleoside analog) [104], AE1-259-01 EP2 receptor agonists [105], green tea and red tea [57], protocatechuic acid (PCA) [106], nebivolol [107], 14Adiponectin (APN) [108], metformin [109], C1q/tumor necrosis factor-related protein 3 (CTRPs) [15], gastrodin [110], Naringin (NGN) [111], and Parthenolide (PN) [112] are all effective antioxidants in ICH animal models.

10. Summary and Outlook

The pathophysiologic processes that occur after ICH are complex, involving the neuroinflammatory response, OS, cytotoxicity caused by erythrocyte lysis, and the production of thrombin. Elucidating the causes of brain injury and the underlying molecular mechanisms and identifying novel markers of OS in the context of ICH will enable the development of effective interventions for the prevention and treatment of secondary brain injury following ICH.

REFERENCES:

[1] F. Siaw-Debrah, M. Nyanzu, H. Ni et al., "Preclinical studies and translational applications of intracerebral hemorrhage," BioMed Research International, vol. 2017, Article ID 5135429, 18 pages, 2017.

[2] J. F. Clark, M. Loftspring, W. L. Wurster et al., "Bilirubin oxidation products, oxidative stress, and intracerebral hemorrhage," Acta Neurochirurgica. Supplement, vol. 105, pp 7-12, 2008.

[3] J. W. Park, J. E. Kim, M. J. Kang et al., "Anti-oxidant activity of gallotannin-enriched extract of Galla Rhois can associate with the protection of the cognitive impairment through the regulation of BDNF signaling pathway and neuronal cell function in the scopolamine-treated ICR mice," Antioxidants, vol. 8, no. 10, p. 450, 2019.

[4] Y. Zhang, M. Xu, C. Hu et al., "Sargassum fusiforme fucoidan SP2 extends the lifespan of Drosophila melanogaster by upregulating the Nrf2-mediated antioxidant

signaling pathway," Oxidative Medicine and Cellular Longevity, vol. 2019, Article ID 8918914, 15 pages, 2019.

[5] D. P. Jones, "Radical-free biology of oxidative stress," American Journal of Physiology. Cell Physiology, vol. 295, no. 4,pp. C849–C868, 2008.

[6] J. Zeng, Y. Chen, R. Ding et al., "Isoliquiritigenin alleviates early brain injury after experimental intracerebral hemorrhage via suppressing ROS- and/or NF-κB-mediated NLRP3 inflammasome activation by promoting Nrf2 antioxidant pathway," Journal of Neuroinflammation, vol. 14, no. 1, p. 119, 2017.

[7] H. Shang, D. Yang, W. Zhang et al., "Time course of Keap1-Nrf2 pathway expression after experimental intracerebral haemorrhage: correlation with brain oedema and neurological deficit," Free Radical Research, vol. 47, no. 5, pp. 368–375, 2013.

[8] L. Zhang, J. Wu, X. Duan et al., "NADPH oxidase: a potential target for treatment of stroke," Oxidative Medicine and Cellular Longevity, vol. 2016, Article ID 5026984, 9 pages, 2016.

[9] A. Coyoy, A. Valencia, A. Guemez-Gamboa, and J. Morán, "Role of NADPH oxidase in the apoptotic death of cultured cerebellar granule neurons," Free Radical Biology & Medicine, vol. 45, no. 8, pp. 1056–1064, 2008.

[10] R. Reinehr, B. Görg, S. Becker et al., "Hypoosmotic swelling and ammonia increase oxidative stress by NADPH oxidase in cultured astrocytes and vital brain slices," Glia, vol. 55, no. 7, pp. 758–771, 2007.

[11] H. Sumimoto, K. Miyano, and R. Takeya, "Molecular composition and regulation of the Nox family NAD(P)H oxidases," Biochemical and Biophysical Research Communications, vol. 338, no. 1, pp. 677–686, 2005.

[12] S. Min, O. Kim, J. Bae, and T. Chung, "Effect of pretreatment with the NADPH oxidase inhibitor apocynin on the therapeutic efficacy of human placenta-derived mesenchymal stem cells in intracerebral hemorrhage," International Journal of Molecular Sciences, vol. 19, no. 11, p. 3679, 2018.

[13] M. T. Zia, A. Csiszar, N. Labinskyy et al., "Oxidative-nitrosative stress in a rabbit pup model of germinal matrix hemorrhage: role of NAD(P)H oxidase," Stroke, vol. 40, no. 6,pp. 2191–2198, 2009.

[14] J. Tang, J. Liu, C. Zhou et al., "Role of NADPH oxidase in the brain injury of intracerebral hemorrhage," Journal of Neurochemistry,vol. 94, no. 5, pp. 1342–1350, 2005.

[15] B. Yang, S. Wang, S. Yu et al., "C1q/tumor necrosis factor related protein 3 inhibits oxidative stress during intracerebral hemorrhage via PKA signaling," Brain Research, vol. 1657,pp. 176–184, 2017.

[16] L. Feng, Y. Chen, R. Ding et al., "P2X7R blockade prevents NLRP3 inflammasome activation and brain injury in a rat model of intracerebral hemorrhage: involvement of peroxynitrite," Journal of Neuroinflammation, vol. 12, no. 1, p. 190, 2015.

[17] R. Zhang, M. L. Brennan, Z. Shen et al., "Myeloperoxidase functions as a major enzymatic catalyst for initiation of lipid peroxidation at sites of inflammation*," The Journal of Biological Chemistry, vol. 277, no. 48, pp. 46116–46122, 2002.

[18] J. K. Y. Tse, "Gut microbiota, nitric oxide, and microglia as prerequisites for neurodegenerative disorders," ACS Chemical Neuroscience, vol. 8, no. 7, pp. 1438–1447, 2017.

[19] A. Sarniak, J. Lipińska, K. Tytman, and S. Lipińska, "Endogenous mechanisms of reactive oxygen species (ROS) generation," Postępy Higieny i Medycyny Doświadczalnej (Online), vol. 70, pp. 1150–1165, 2016.

[20] F. L. Muller, Y. Liu, and H. Van Remmen, "Complex III releases superoxide to both sides of the inner mitochondrial membrane*," The Journal of Biological Chemistry, vol. 279, no. 47, pp. 49064–49073, 2004.

[21] M. D. Brand, "The sites and topology of mitochondrial superoxide production," Experimental Gerontology, vol. 45, no. 7-8, pp. 466–472, 2010.

[22] J. Qu, W. Chen, R. Hu, and H. Feng, "The injury and therapy of reactive oxygen species in intracerebral hemorrhage looking at mitochondria," Oxidative Medicine and Cellular Longevity, vol. 2016, Article ID 2592935, 9 pages, 2016.

[23] Z. Z. Duan, F. Zhang, F. Y. Li et al., "Protease activated receptor 1 (PAR1) enhances Src-mediated tyrosine phosphorylation of NMDA receptor in intracerebral hemorrhage (ICH)," Scientific Reports, vol. 6, no. 1, p. 29246, 2016.

[24] Z. Jiao, X. Liu, Y. Ma et al., "Adipose-derived stem cells protect ischemia-reperfusion and partial hepatectomy by attenuating endoplasmic reticulum stress," Frontiers in Cell and Development Biology, vol. 8, p. 177, 2020.

[25] C. D. Ochoa, R. F. Wu, and L. S. Terada, "ROS signaling and ER stress in cardiovascular disease," Molecular Aspects of Medicine, vol. 63, pp. 18–29, 2018.

[26] S. S. Cao and R. J. Kaufman, "Endoplasmic reticulum stress and oxidative stress in cell fate decision and human disease," Antioxidants & Redox Signaling, vol. 21, no. 3, pp. 396–413, 2014.

[27] M. Niu, X. Dai, W. Zou et al., "Autophagy, endoplasmic reticulum stress and the unfolded protein response in intracerebral hemorrhage," Translational Neuroscience, vol. 8, pp. 37–48, 2017.

[28] J. Aronowski and X. Zhao, "Molecular pathophysiology of cerebral hemorrhage: secondary brain injury," Stroke, vol. 42, no. 6, pp. 1781–1786, 2011.

[29] M. Katsu, K. Niizuma, H. Yoshioka, N. Okami, H. Sakata, and P. H. Chan, "Hemoglobin-induced oxidative stress contributes to matrix metalloproteinase

activation and blood-brain barrier dysfunction in vivo," Journal of Cerebral Blood Flow
and Metabolism, vol. 30, no. 12, pp. 1939–1950, 2010.

[30] Y. Gu and S. Yang, "Effects of hemoglobin on the expression and distribution of inducible nitric oxide synthase after intracerebral hemorrhage," Zhonghua Yi Xue Za Zhi, vol. 94, no. 36, pp. 2857–2860, 2014.

[31] S. Yang, Y. Chen, X. Deng et al., "Hemoglobin-induced nitric oxide synthase overexpression and nitric oxide production contribute to blood-brain barrier disruption in the rat," Journal of Molecular Neuroscience, vol. 51, no. 2, pp. 352–363, 2013.

[32] J. M. Gutteridge and A. Smith, "Antioxidant protection by haemopexin of haem-stimulated lipid peroxidation," The Biochemical Journal, vol. 256, no. 3, pp. 861–865, 1988.

[33] R. F. Regan, J. Chen, and L. Benvenisti-Zarom, "Heme oxygenase-2 gene deletion attenuates oxidative stress in neurons exposed to extracellular hemin," BMC Neuroscience, vol. 5, no. 1, p. 34, 2004.

[34] K. A. Hanafy, J. A. Gomes, and M. Selim, "Rationale and current evidence for testing iron chelators for treating stroke," Current Cardiology Reports, vol. 21, no. 4, p. 20, 2019.

[35] J. Cadet, S. Loft, R. Olinski et al., "Biologically relevant oxidants and terminology, classification and nomenclature of oxidatively generated damage to nucleobases and 2-deoxyribose in nucleic acids," Free Radical Research, vol. 46, no. 4, pp. 367–381, 2012.

[36] C. L. Hawkins and M. J. Davies, "Detection, identification, and quantification of oxidative protein modifications," The Journal of Biological Chemistry, vol. 294, no. 51, pp. 19683–19708, 2019.

[37] A. Cipak Gasparovic, N. Zarkovic, K. Zarkovic et al., "Biomarkers of oxidative and nitro-oxidative stress: conventional and novel approaches," British Journal of Pharmacology,vol. 174, no. 12, pp. 1771–1783, 2017.

[38] T. Jiang, B. Harder, M. Rojo de la Vega, P. K. Wong, E. Chapman, and D. D. Zhang, "p62 links autophagy and Nrf2 signaling," Free Radical Biology and Medicine, vol. 88, no. Part B, pp. 199–204, 2015.

[39] R. Scherz-Shouval, E. Shvets, E. Fass, H. Shorer, L. Gil, and Z. Elazar, "Reactive oxygen species are essential for autophagy and specifically regulate the activity of Atg4," The EMBO Journal, vol. 38, no. 10, 2019.

[40] G. Filomeni, D. De Zio, and F. Cecconi, "Oxidative stress and autophagy: the clash between damage and metabolic needs," Cell Death and Differentiation, vol. 22, no. 3, pp. 377–388,2015.

[41] X. Shen, L. Ma, W. Dong et al., "Autophagy regulates intracerebral hemorrhage induced neural damage via apoptosis and NF-κB pathway," Neurochemistry International, vol. 96, pp. 100–112, 2016.

[42] Y. Fang, S. Chen, C. Reis, and J. Zhang, "The role of autophagy in subarachnoid hemorrhage: an update," Current Neuropharmacology, vol. 16, no. 9, pp. 1255–1266, 2018.

[43] G. Pistritto, D. Trisciuoglio, C. Ceci, A. Garufi, and G. D'Orazi, "Apoptosis as anticancer mechanism: function and dysfunction of its modulators and targeted therapeutic strategies," Aging (Albany NY), vol. 8, no. 4, pp. 603–619, 2016.

[44] C. Yang, K. E. Hawkins, S. Doré, and E. Candelario-Jalil, "Neuroinflammatory mechanisms of blood-brain barrier damage in ischemic stroke," American Journal of Physiology. Cell Physiology, vol. 316, no. 2, pp. C135–C153, 2019.

[45] W. Abdullahi, D. Tripathi, and P. T. Ronaldson, "Blood-brain barrier dysfunction in ischemic stroke: targeting tight junctions and transporters for vascular protection," American Journal of Physiology. Cell Physiology, vol. 315, no. 3, pp. C343–c356, 2018.

[46] J. Zheng, L. Shi, F. Liang et al., "Sirt3 ameliorates oxidative stress and mitochondrial dysfunction after intracerebral hemorrhage in diabetic rats," Frontiers in Neuroscience, vol. 12, p. 414, 2018.

[47] L. Fialkow, Y. Wang, and G. P. Downey, "Reactive oxygen and nitrogen species as signaling molecules regulating neutrophil function," Free Radical Biology & Medicine, vol. 42, no. 2, pp. 153–164, 2007.

[48] G. J. Maghzal, K. M. Cergol, S. R. Shengule et al., "Assessment of myeloperoxidase activity by the conversion of hydroethidine to 2-chloroethidium*," The Journal of Biological Chemistry, vol. 289, no. 9, pp. 5580–5595, 2014.

[49] J. Cadet, K. J. A. Davies, M. H. G. Medeiros, P. di Mascio, and J. R. Wagner, "Formation and repair of oxidatively generated damage in cellular DNA," Free Radical Biology & Medicine, vol. 107, pp. 13–34, 2017.

[50] T. Nakamura, R. F. Keep, Y. Hua, J. T. Hoff, and G. Xi, "Oxidative DNA injury after experimental intracerebral hemorrhage," Brain Research, vol. 1039, no. 1-2, pp. 30–36, 2005.

[51] Y. C. Chen, C. M. Chen, J. L. Liu, S. T. Chen, M. L. Cheng, and D. T. Y. Chiu, "Oxidative markers in spontaneous intracerebral hemorrhage: leukocyte 8-hydroxy-2′-deoxyguanosine as an independent predictor of the 30-day outcome," Journal of Neurosurgery, vol. 115, no. 6, pp. 1184–1190, 2011.

[52] L. Lorente, M. M. Martín, A. F. González-Rivero et al., "High serum DNA and RNA oxidative damage in non-surviving patients with spontaneous intracerebral hemorrhage," Neurocritical Care, vol. 33, no. 1, pp. 90–96, 2020.

[53] H. F. Moselhy, R. G. Reid, S. Yousef, and S. P. Boyle, "A specific, accurate, and sensitive measure of total plasma malondialdehyde by HPLC," Journal of Lipid Research, vol. 54, no. 3, pp. 852–858, 2013.

[54] L. Lorente, M. M. Martín, P. Abreu-González et al., "Serum malondialdehyde levels and mortality in patients with spontaneous intracerebral hemorrhage," World Neurosurgery, vol. 113, pp. e542–e547, 2018.

[55] Q. Wu, X. S. Zhang, H. D. Wang et al., "Astaxanthin activates nuclear factor erythroid-related factor 2 and the antioxidant responsive element (Nrf2-ARE) pathway in the brain after subarachnoid hemorrhage in rats and attenuates early brain injury," Marine Drugs, vol. 12, no. 12, pp. 6125–6141, 2014.

[56] C. C. Wei, Y. Y. Kong, G. Q. Li, Y. F. Guan, P. Wang, and C. Y. Miao, "Nicotinamide mononucleotide attenuates brain injury after intracerebral hemorrhage by activating Nrf2/HO-1 signaling pathway," Scientific Reports, vol. 7,no. 1, p. 717, 2017.

[57] P. M. Sosa, M. A. de Souza, and P. B. Mello-Carpes, "Green tea and red tea from Camellia sinensis partially prevented the motor deficits and striatal oxidative damage induced by hemorrhagic stroke in rats," Neural Plasticity, vol. 2018, Article ID 5158724, 8 pages, 2018.

[58] S. Duan, F. Wang, J. Cao, and C. Wang, "Exosomes derived from microRNA-146a-5p-enriched bone marrow mesenchymal stem cells alleviate intracerebral hemorrhage by inhibiting neuronal apoptosis and microglial M1 polarization," Drug Design, Development and Therapy, vol. Volume 14,pp. 3143–3158, 2020.

[59] C. M. Spickett, "The lipid peroxidation product 4-hydroxy-2- nonenal: advances in chemistry and analysis," Redox Biology, vol. 1, no. 1, pp. 145–152, 2013.

[60] M. L. Selley, "Determination of the lipid peroxidation product (E)-4-hydroxy-2-nonenal in clinical samples by gas chromatography–negative-ion chemical ionisation mass spectrometry of the O-pentafluorobenzyl oxime," Journal of Chromatography. B, Biomedical Sciences and Applications,vol. 691, no. 2, pp. 263–268, 1997.

[61] I. Jarocka-Karpowicz, A. Syta-Krzyżanowska, J. Kochanowicz, and Z. D. Mariak, "Clinical prognosis for SAH consistent with redox imbalance and lipid peroxidation," Molecules, vol. 25, no. 8, p. 1921, 2020.

[62] D. Il'yasova, J. D. Morrow, A. Ivanova, and L. E. Wagenknecht,

"Epidemiological marker for oxidant status: comparison of the ELISA and the gas

chromatography/mass
spectrometry assay for urine 2,3-dinor-5,6-dihydro-15-F2tisoprostane,"Annals of Epidemiology, vol. 14, no. 10, pp. 793–797, 2004.

[63] Q. du, W. H. Yu, X. Q. Dong et al., "Plasma 8-isoprostaglandin F2α concentrations and outcomes after acute intracerebral hemorrhage," Clinica Chimica Acta, vol. 437, pp. 141–146, 2014.

[64] T. B. Corcoran, E. Mas, A. E. Barden et al., "Are isofurans and neuroprostanes increased after subarachnoid hemorrhage and traumatic brain injury?," Antioxidants & Redox Signaling, vol. 15, no. 10, pp. 2663–2667, 2011.

[65] M. Zheng, X. Wang, J. Yang, S. Ma, Y. Wei, and S. Liu, "Changes of complement and oxidative stress parameters in patients with acute cerebral infarction or cerebral hemorrhage and the clinical significance," Experimental and Therapeutic Medicine, vol. 19, no. 1, pp. 703–709, 2020.

[66] Z. Wang, S. Guo, J. Wang, Y. Shen, J. Zhang, and Q. Wu, "Nrf2/HO-1 mediates the neuroprotective effect of mangiferin on early brain injury after subarachnoid hemorrhage by attenuating mitochondria-related apoptosis and neuroinflammation," Scientific Reports, vol. 7, no. 1, p. 11883, 2017.

[67] X. Lan, X. Han, Q. Li, and J. Wang, "(-)-Epicatechin, a natural flavonoid compound, protects astrocytes against hemoglobin toxicity via Nrf2 and AP-1 signaling pathways," Molecular Neurobiology, vol. 54, no. 10, pp. 7898–7907, 2017.

[68] T. Nybo, M. J. Davies, and A. Rogowska-Wrzesinska, "Analysis of protein chlorination by mass spectrometry," Redox Biology, vol. 26, p. 101236, 2019.

[69] G. R. Zheng, B. Chen, J. Shen et al., "Serum myeloperoxidase concentrations for outcome prediction in acute intracerebral hemorrhage," Clinica Chimica Acta, vol. 487, pp. 330–336, 2018.

[70] D. Giustarini, D. Tsikas, G. Colombo et al., "Pitfalls in the analysis of the physiological antioxidant glutathione (GSH) and its disulfide (GSSG) in biological samples: an elephant in the room," Journal of Chromatography. B, Analytical Technologies in the Biomedical and Life Sciences, vol. 1019, pp. 21–28, 2016.

[71] J. Gruber, S. Y. Tang, A. M. Jenner et al., "Allantoin in human plasma, serum, and nasal-lining fluids as a biomarker of oxidative stress: avoiding artifacts and establishing real in vivo concentrations," Antioxidants & Redox Signaling, vol. 11, no. 8, pp. 1767–1776, 2009.

[72] S. Q. Qian, X. C. Hu, S. R. He, B. B. Li, X. D. Zheng, and G. H. Pan, "Prognostic value of serum thioredoxin concentrations after intracerebral hemorrhage," Clinica Chimica Acta, vol. 455, pp. 15–19, 2016.

[73] Z. Wang, F. Zhou, Y. Dou et al., "Melatonin alleviates intracerebral hemorrhage-induced secondary brain injury in rats via suppressing apoptosis, inflammation, oxidative stress, DNA damage, and mitochondria injury," Translational Stroke Research, vol. 9, no. 1, pp. 74–91, 2018.

[74] X. Zhao, G. Sun, J. Zhang et al., "Transcription factor Nrf2 protects the brain from damage produced by intracerebral hemorrhage," Stroke, vol. 38, no. 12, pp. 3280–3286, 2007.

[75] S. Petri, S. Körner, and M. Kiaei, "Nrf2/ARE signaling pathway: key mediator in oxidative stress and potential therapeutic target in ALS," Neurology Research International,vol. 2012, Article ID 878030, 7 pages, 2012.

[76] C. Y. Zhang, X. M. Ren, H. B. Li et al., "Simvastatin alleviates inflammation and oxidative stress in rats with cerebral hemorrhage through Nrf2-ARE signaling pathway," European Review for Medical and Pharmacological Sciences, vol. 23, no. 14, pp. 6321–6329, 2019.

[77] Y. Y. Shi, H. F. Cui, and B. J. Qin, "Monomethyl fumarate protects cerebral hemorrhage injury in rats via activating microRNA-139/Nrf2 axis," European Review for Medical and Pharmacological Sciences, vol. 23, no. 11, pp. 5012–5019, 2019.

[78] T. Sugiyama, T. Imai, S. Nakamura et al., "A novel Nrf2 activator, RS9, attenuates secondary brain injury after intracerebral hemorrhage in sub-acute phase," Brain Research,vol. 1701, pp. 137–145, 2018.

[79] R. Yuan, H. Fan, S. Cheng et al., "Silymarin prevents NLRP3 inflammasome activation and protects against intracerebral hemorrhage," Biomedicine & Pharmacotherapy, vol. 93, pp. 308–315, 2017.

[80] G. Chen, Q. Fang, J. Zhang, D. Zhou, and Z. Wang, "Role of the Nrf2-ARE pathway in early brain injury after experimental subarachnoid hemorrhage," Journal of Neuroscience Research, vol. 89, no. 4, pp. 515–523, 2011.

[81] Y. Yang, Z. Xi, Y. Xue et al., "Hemoglobin pretreatment endows rat cortical astrocytes resistance to hemin- induced toxicity via Nrf2/HO-1 pathway," Experimental Cell Research, vol. 361, no. 2, pp. 217–224, 2017.

[82] Z. Wang, C. Ma, C. J. Meng et al., "Melatonin activates the Nrf2-ARE pathway when it protects against early brain injury in a subarachnoid hemorrhage model," Journal of Pineal Research, vol. 53, no. 2, pp. 129–137, 2012.

[83] J. Zhang, Y. Zhu, D. Zhou, Z. Wang, and G. Chen, "Recombinant human erythropoietin (rhEPO) alleviates early brain injury following subarachnoid hemorrhage in rats: possible involvement of Nrf2-ARE pathway," Cytokine, vol. 52, no. 3, pp. 252–257, 2010.

[84] C. Chen, J. Cui, X. Ji, and L. Yao, "Neuroprotective functions of calycosin against intracerebral hemorrhage-induced oxidative stress and neuroinflammation," Future Medicinal Chemistry, vol. 12, no. 7, pp. 583–592, 2020.

[85] X. Tan, Y. Yang, J. Xu et al., "Luteolin exerts neuroprotection via modulation of the p62/Keap1/Nrf2 pathway in intracerebral hemorrhage," Frontiers in Pharmacology, vol. 10, p. 1551,2020.

[86] Y. Cheng, B. Chen, W. Xie et al., "Ghrelin attenuates secondary brain injury following intracerebral hemorrhage by inhibiting NLRP3 inflammasome activation and promoting Nrf2/ARE signaling pathway in mice," International Immunopharmacology,
vol. 79, p. 106180, 2020.

[87] X. Zhao, Y. Zhang, R. Strong, J. C. Grotta, and J. Aronowski, "15d-

Prostaglandin J2Activates peroxisome proliferator activated Receptor-γ, promotes expression of catalase, and reduces inflammation, behavioral dysfunction, and neuronal loss after intracerebral hemorrhage in rats," Journal of Cerebral Blood Flow and Metabolism, vol. 26, no. 6, pp. 811– 820, 2005.

[88] K. H. Jung, K. Chu, S. T. Lee et al., "Blockade of AT1 receptor reduces apoptosis, inflammation, and oxidative stress in normotensive rats with intracerebral hemorrhage," The Journal of Pharmacology and Experimental Therapeutics, vol. 322, no. 3, pp. 1051–1058, 2007.

[89] D. Pandey, F. Chen, A. Patel et al., "SUMO1 negatively regulates reactive oxygen species production from NADPH oxidases,"Arteriosclerosis, Thrombosis, and Vascular Biology, vol. 31, no. 7, pp. 1634–1642, 2011.

[90] X. Qu, N. Wang, W. Chen, M. Qi, Y. Xue, and W. Cheng, "RNF34

overexpression exacerbates neurological deficits and brain injury in a mouse model of intracerebral hemorrhage by potentiating mitochondrial dysfunction-mediated oxidative stress," Scientific Reports, vol. 9, no. 1, p. 16296,2019.

[91] W. Xu, T. Li, L. Gao et al., "Sodium benzoate attenuates secondary brain injury by inhibiting neuronal apoptosis and reducing mitochondria-mediated oxidative stress in a rat model of intracerebral hemorrhage: possible involvement of DJ-1/Akt/IKK/NFκB pathway," Frontiers in Molecular Neuroscience, vol. 12, p. 105, 2019.

[92] J. Huang and Q. Jiang, "Dexmedetomidine protects against neurological dysfunction in a mouse intracerebral hemorrhage model by inhibiting mitochondrial dysfunction derived oxidative stress," Journal of Stroke and Cerebrovascular Diseases, vol. 28, no. 5, pp. 1281–1289, 2019.

[93] H. Lu, J. Shen, X. Song et al., "Protective effect of pyrroloquinoline quinone (PQQ) in rat model of intracerebral hemorrhage," Cellular and Molecular Neurobiology, vol. 35, no. 7, pp. 921–930, 2015.

[94] O. Romantsik, A. A. Agyemang, S. Sveinsdóttir et al., "The heme and radical scavenger α1-microglobulin (A1M) confers early protection of the immature brain following preterm intraventricular hemorrhage," Journal of Neuroinflammation, vol. 16, no. 1, p. 122, 2019.

[95] T. Imai, S. Iwata, D. Miyo, S. Nakamura, M. Shimazawa, and H. Hara, "A novel free radical scavenger, NSP-116, ameliorated the brain injury in both ischemic and hemorrhagic stroke models," Journal of Pharmacological Sciences, vol. 141, no. 3, pp. 119–126, 2019.

[96] Z. Chen, J. Zhang, Q. Chen, J. Guo, G. Zhu, and H. Feng, "Neuroprotective

effects of edaravone after intraventricular hemorrhage in rats," Neuroreport, vol. 25, no. 9, pp. 635–640, 2014.

[97] I. Ohsawa, M. Ishikawa, K. Takahashi et al., "Hydrogen acts as a therapeutic antioxidant by selectively reducing cytotoxic oxygen radicals," Nature Medicine, vol. 13, no. 6, pp. 688–694, 2007.

[98] A. Manaenko, T. Lekic, Q. Ma, R. P. Ostrowski, J. H. Zhang, and J. Tang, "Hydrogen inhalation is neuroprotective and improves functional outcomes in mice after intracerebral hemorrhage," Acta Neurochirurgica. Supplement, vol. 111, pp. 179–183, 2011.

[99] F. Zhou, Y. Liu, B. Yang, and Z. Hu, "Neuroprotective potential of glibenclamide is mediated by antioxidant and antiapoptotic pathways in intracerebral hemorrhage," Brain Research Bulletin, vol. 142, pp. 18–24, 2018.

[100] Y. Wanyong, T. Zefeng, X. Xiufeng et al., "Tempol alleviates intracerebral hemorrhage-induced brain injury possibly by attenuating nitrative stress," Neuroreport, vol. 26, no. 14, pp. 842–849, 2015.

[101] N. Wei, Y. Wei, B. Li, and L. Pang, "Baicalein promotes neuronal and behavioral recovery after Intracerebral hemorrhage via suppressing apoptosis, oxidative stress and neuroinflammation," Neurochemical Research, vol. 42, no. 5, pp. 1345–1353, 2017.

[102] S. Wang, L. Yu, G. Sun et al., "Danhong injection protects hemorrhagic brain by increasing peroxiredoxin 1 in aged rats," Frontiers in Pharmacology, vol. 11, p. 346, 2020.

[103] R. X. Xie, D. W. Li, X. C. Liu et al., "Carnosine attenuates brain oxidative stress and apoptosis after intracerebral hemorrhage in rats," Neurochemical Research, vol. 42, no. 2, pp. 541–551, 2017.

[104] F. Lu, T. Nakamura, N. Okabe et al., "COA-Cl, a novel synthesized nucleoside analog, exerts neuroprotective effects in the acute phase of intracerebral hemorrhage," Journal of Stroke and Cerebrovascular Diseases, vol. 25, no. 11, pp. 2637–2643, 2016.

[105] H. Wu, T. Wu, X. Han et al., "Cerebroprotection by the neuronal PGE2 receptor EP2 after intracerebral hemorrhage in middle-aged mice," Journal of Cerebral Blood Flow and Metabolism, vol. 37, no. 1, pp. 39–51, 2017.

[106] Z. Xi, X. Hu, X. Chen et al., "Protocatechuic acid exerts protective effects via suppression of the P38/JNK- NF-κB signaling pathway in an experimental mouse model of intracerebral haemorrhage," European Journal of Pharmacology,vol. 854, pp. 128–138, 2019.

[107] M. A. Aladag, Y. Turkoz, H. Parlakpinar, and M. Gul, "Nebivolol attenuates cerebral vasospasm both by increasing endothelial nitric oxide and by decreasing oxidative stress in an experimental subarachnoid haemorrhage," British Journal of Neurosurgery, vol. 31, no. 4, pp. 439–445, 2016.

[108] S. Wang, D. Li, C. Huang et al., "Overexpression of adiponectin alleviates intracerebral hemorrhage-induced brain injury in rats via suppression of oxidative stress," Neuroscience Letters, vol. 681, pp. 110–116, 2018.

[109] B. Qi, L. Hu, L. Zhu et al., "Metformin attenuates neurological deficit after intracerebral hemorrhage by inhibiting apoptosis, oxidative stress and neuroinflammation in rats," Neurochemical Research, vol. 42, no. 10, pp. 2912–2920, 2017.

[110] X. C. Liu, C. Z. Wu, X. F. Hu et al., "Gastrodin attenuates neuronal apoptosis and neurological deficits after experimental intracerebral hemorrhage," Journal of Stroke and Cerebrovascular Diseases, vol. 29, no. 1, p. 104483, 2020.

[111] N. Singh, Y. Bansal, R. Bhandari et al., "Naringin reverses neurobehavioral and biochemical alterations in intracerebroventricular collagenase-induced intracerebral hemorrhage in rats," Pharmacology, vol. 100, no. 3-4, pp. 172–187, 2017.

[112] J. A. Wang, M. L. Tong, B. Zhao, G. Zhu, D. H. Xi, and J. P. Yang, "Parthenolide ameliorates intracerebral hemorrhage induced brain injury in rats," Phytotherapy Research, vol. 34, no. 1, pp. 153–160, 2019.

CONFLICTS OF INTEREST

The authors declare no conflict of interest.

ACKNOWLEDGMENTS

This research was funded by the National Natural Science Foundation of China, grant number 81771294.

CHAPTER 5:

Ferroptosis, a regulated neuronal cell death type after intracerebral hemorrhage

ABSTRACT:

Ferroptosis is a term that describes one form of regulated non-apoptotic cell death. It's triggered by iron-dependent accumulation of lipid peroxides. Emerging evidence suggests a link between ferroptosis and the pathophysiological processes of neurological disorders, including stroke, degenerative diseases, neurotrauma, and cancer. Hemorrhagic stroke, also known as intracerebral hemorrhage (ICH), belongs to a devastating illness for its high level in morbidity and mortality. Currently, there are few established treatments and limited knowledge about the mechanisms of post-ICH neuronal death. The secondary brain damage after ICH is mainly attributed to oxidative stress and hemoglobin (Hb) lysate, including iron, which leads to irreversible damage to neurons. Therefore, ferroptosis is becoming a common trend in research of neuronal death after ICH. Accumulative data suggest the inhibition of ferroptosis may effectively prevent neuronal ferroptosis, thereby reducing secondary brain damage after ICH in animal models. Ferroptosis has a close relationship with oxidative damage and iron metabolism. In this review lies in revealing the pathological pathways and regulation mechanism of ferroptosis following ICH, then offer the potential intervention strategies to mitigate neuron death and dysfunction after ICH.

KEY WORDS: Ferroptosis, Intracerebral hemorrhage, Lipid peroxidation, antioxidation, Iron metabolism

1. INTRODUCTION

Ferroptosis, a regulated non-apoptotic cell death, is characterized by the overwhelming lipid peroxidation in an iron-dependent manner (1, 2). It was identified firstly in 2012 by handling tumour cells with the chemical probe erastin (1). As described below, the regulation of ferroptotic death is dramatically modulated by lipid peroxidation, antioxidant system, and iron metabolism. Emerging evidence suggests that a link between ferroptosis and the pathophysiological processes of neurological disorders, including stroke, degenerative diseases, neurotrauma, and cancer (3). Here, we will elaborate on the neuronal ferroptosis after ICH.

Intracerebral hemorrhage (ICH) is an acute subtype of cerebral stroke and accounts for 80% of hemorrhagic stroke and 10-15% of all types of strokes (4). Only six of ten patients can survive one month after the onset of ICH (5). And the poor outcomes after ICH result from complicated pathological processes that facilitate neuronal death. After ICH, Hb/heme/iron is recognized as one of the main contributors to delayed cerebral edema and irreversible damage to neurons and plays an essential role in lipid ROS production (6). It is discovered that ferroptosis, iron-dependent cell death, exactly occurs after ICH and makes a contribution to the death of neurons, so the manipulation of ferroptosis may preserve neuronal cells exposed to specific oxidative conditions (1, 7, 8). It has previously been observed that the inhibitor of ferroptosis reduced iron deposition and prevented neuronal death induced by Hb (7). However, the specific agencies of neuronal ferroptosis after ICH is unclear. This review seeks to investigate the regulatory mechanisms of ferroptosis and how ferroptosis works in neuronal death after ICH. Based on this, potential intervention strategies to mitigate neuronal cell death and dysfunction after ICH are also summarized.

2. THE MECHANISMS AND REGULATION OF FERROPTOSIS

Essentially, ferroptosis is a form of programmed cell death induced by iron-dependent lipid peroxidation. Dysregulation of iron handling, increased of the labile redox-active iron, and the increase of lipid peroxidation are viewed as a possible pathogenic mechanism of ferroptosis. So ferroptosis is related to the lipid peroxidation, antioxidant system, and iron metabolism. Here we will elaborate on the mechanisms underlying ferroptosis and its regulatory systems.

2.1. The Lipid Peroxidation Pathway in Ferroptosis

Lipid peroxidation refers to the process that oxygen combines with lipids to generate lipid hydroperoxides through the formation of peroxyl radicals, which is necessary for the execution of ferroptosis. It is confirmed that ferroptosis selective preferentially oxidizes specific polyunsaturated fatty acids (PUFAs) which contains phosphatidylethanolamine such as arachidonic acid (AA), leading to lipid peroxidation and ferroptosis (9). A recent study indicated that AA-OOH-PE induced ferroptosis (10). In this process, the formation of AA-CoA is catalyzed by the acyl-CoA synthetase long-chain family 4 (ACSL4) (11). Then lysophosphatidylcholine acyltransferase 3 (LPCAT3) esterify it to AA-PE (12), which is oxidized into AA-OOH-PE by lipoxygenases (LOXs) (13). When the content of AA-OOH-PE overwhelms the ability of the reduction system, ferroptosis will occur. And fatty acid desaturases can promote the formation of lipids containing PUFA, so it is a regulatory target for lipid peroxidation associated with ferroptosis.

2.2. The Antioxidant System of Ferroptosis

Lipid peroxidation is the outcome of ferroptosis, so the antioxidant system plays an essential role in preventing ferroptosis. We will describe the antioxidant system that induces ferroptosis in two aspects, GSH and FSP1-CoQ10- NAD(P)H Pathway.

2.2.1. GPX4 and GSH in Ferroptosis

Glutathione peroxidase 4 (GPX4), a selenium-dependent endogenous antioxidant enzyme, can complete the conversion of lipid peroxides to non-toxic lipids which will resist lipid peroxidation (14), then prevent ferroptotic death. Glutathione (GSH) is the synthetic substrate for GPX4 and is a cofactor for GPX4 to exert its antioxidant function (15). So it is currently regarded as the critical regulator of ferroptosis. The study suggests GSH and selenium are necessary to maintain the operation of GPX4 and resist ferroptosis (16). GSH is synthesized by glycine, glutamate, and cysteine. Cysteine is transformed by intracellular cystine with a quick reduction reaction. And the transfer of cystine into the cell is promoted by System xc−, accompanied by glutamate out of the cell. System xc−, a heterodimeric cystine/glutamate antiporter, is made up of catalytic subunit solute carrier family 7 member 11 (SLC7A11) and solute carrier family 3 member 2 (SLC3A2). In cells that cysteine is obtained with the supply of cystine from system xc−, glutathione depletion is caused by the inhibition of the system xc− (17), so it is the most critical event of ferroptosis. (Figure1)

The inhibition of system xc− can result in cysteine reduction and the lack of GSH synthetic, then reduced the antioxidant function of GPX4, which finally caused lipid peroxidation, leading to ferroptosis. The inhibitors of system xc leading to ferroptosis should rely entirely on inhibition of cystine uptake. Erastin, piperazine erastin(PE), and Imidazole ketone erastin(IKE) induce ferroptosis by the inhibition of system xc–, but PE and IKE have substantially improved potency (1, 18). DPI2 and RSL5 may also be system xc– inhibitors because of the similar effects to erastin, although the potential mechanism has not yet been reported (18). Besides, the multi-targeted kinase inhibitor sorafenib inhibits system xc– function and can trigger ferroptosis, while a necrotic death can be induced when it comes to slightly higher concentrations (17). Sulfasalazine is another kind of system xc– inhibitor (19), but there is no reliable evidence that sulfasalazine can lead to ferroptosis currently. Furthermore, it is proved that the glutamate and amino acid can inhibit system xc– and promote ferroptosis in specific cellular contexts (20). Lipid peroxidation occurs when the activity of GPX4 is inhibited. It suggested that GPX4 can be covalently inhibited by another inhibitor, named RSL3, which blocks the antioxidant system of GPX4 (21) and leads to ferroptosis. The transcription factor nuclear factor erythroid 2-related factor 2 (Nrf2) increases the resistance to ferroptosis by upregulating xCT, glutathione, and GPX4 (22). Selenium is proven to be an indispensable micronutrient for the function of GPX4. So when it was replaced by sulfur in GPX4, GPX4 fails in the activity of resisting overoxidation and inhibiting ferroptosis (9, 23).

2.2.2. FSP1- CoQ10- NAD(P)H Pathway in Ferroptosis

A recent study indicated the ferroptosis suppressor protein 1 (FSP1)-coenzyme Q10 (CoQ10) -nicotinamide adenine dinucleotide phosphate (NAD(P)H) pathway existed as a stand-alone parallel system independent of GPX4 and GSH, which could also play an antioxidant role and inhibit ferroptosis (24). FSP1 is transferred to the plasma membrane through myristoylation, where it mediates the reduction of CoQ10 to ubiquinol using the reducing equivalents of NAD(P)H (24-26). And ubiquinol is a lipophilic radical-trapping antioxidant (RTA) that exerts an antioxidant effect to inhibit lipid peroxides (25). Vitamin E, a lipid-soluble antioxidant localized in the cell membrane, is also a RTA, that can restrain lipid peroxidation through its radical-trapping activities (26, 27). (Figure1)

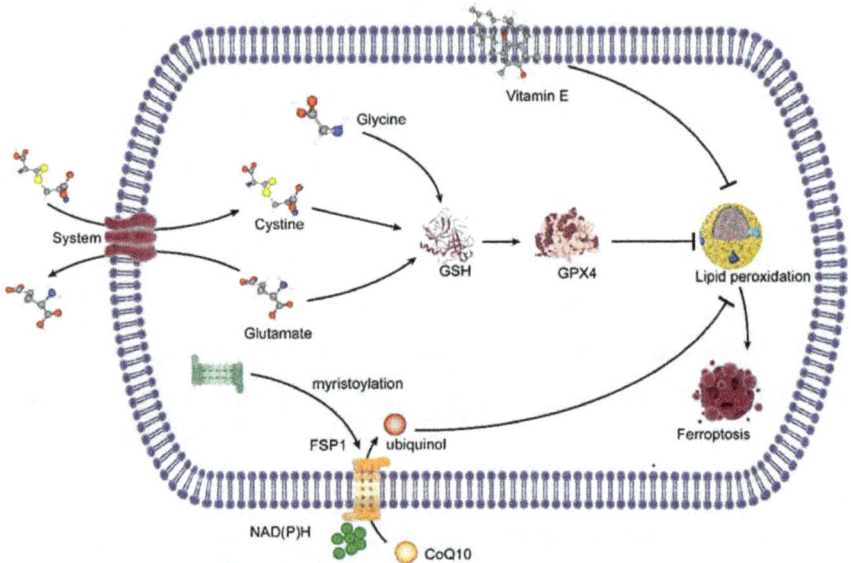

Figure1. The Lipid Peroxidation Pathway and Antioxidant System of Ferroptosis

2.3. The Iron Metabolism-Related Pathway in Ferroptosis

Ferroptosis is iron-depended cell death. Iron is a metal with redox activity and participates in the formation of free radicals and lipid peroxidation. Therefore, the increase of iron may promote ferroptotic death. Hydroperoxy lipids (L-OOH), the mainly enzymatic products of lipid peroxidation, is catalyzed by the iron centres of LOXs, and its decomposition products, oxidatively truncated electrophilic products, is yielded by Fe(II) from the labile iron pool (LIP), which triggers lipid peroxidation (28, 29), eventually leading to ferroptosis. Therefore, iron metabolism can regulate ferroptosis.

Under physiological conditions, Fe(II) can catalyze the transformation of hydrogen peroxide into highly reactive intermediate substance, which attacks and oxidatively damages multiple cellular components, especially lipids containing PUFAs (29). Almost all iron in the plasma is Fe (III) and combine with circulating transferrin(TF) to form transferrin bound iron (TBI). Then TBI is transported into cell through endocytosis after combining with transferrin receptor 1 (TfR1) on the cell surface. Also, Fe (III) can be transported directly into cells without binding to Tf. Iron is liberated from TF and reduced to Fe(II) by the ferric reductases in the Steap family when the endosomal environment is acidified, and Fe(II) is transported into cytosol across the membrane through ZRT/IRT-like Protein (ZIP) 14 or 8, or Divalent Metal Transporter 1 (DMT1) (28, 30). And the Poly rC Binding-Protein (PCBP) family, PCBP2 can combine iron and promote its transport into the cytosol by interacting with DMT1 (31). Ferritin transporter (Fpn), the only iron transmembrane export, can export Fe(II) out of the cells. (32). PCBP2 modulates the export of iron in the cells by delivering cytosolic iron to Fpn (33). Moreover, PCBP1 can bind iron and promote it loading onto client proteins like ferritin, which can be affected by PCBP2 (28). Once Fe(II) is transported out of the cell, it is quickly oxidized to Fe(III) to be loaded onto TF. Under conditions of iron deficiency, Nuclear Co-Activator 4(NCOA4) can directly deliver ferritin to autophagosome and facilitates its autophagic degradation (34), which transferred back to the cytosol or the mitochondria for heme synthesis (Figure2).

Heme oxygenase (HO)-1 has the dual effect of promoting and inhibiting ferroptosis by regulating iron. HO-1 mainly catalyzes the decomposition of heme into Fe (II). And the accumulation of Fe (II) has pro-oxidant activity and helps induce ferroptosis (35). However, the free Fe (II) produced by HO-1 alone does not facilitate ferroptosis (36). And the early study has shown that the expression of HO-1 can be upregulated by oxidative stress through the p62-Keap1-NRF2 pathway, thereby inducing ferroptosis (37). Moreover, the increase of HO-1 will also affect the intracellular iron distribution through the enhanced heme degradation and ferritin synthesis (38). Study suggests that the activation of the medium level of HO-1 plays a role in cell protection, while the excessive activation of HO-1 plays a role in cytotoxic because of the over-regulation of unstable Fe(II) (35).

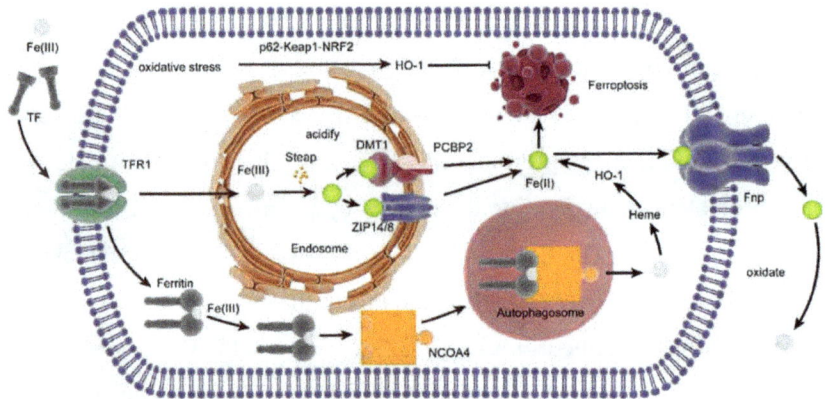

Figure2. The Iron Metabolism-Related Pathway in Ferroptosis

3. THE UNDERLYING MECHANISMS OF NEURONAL FERROPTOSIS AFTER ICH

ICH is a fatal subtype of stroke with high mortality and morbidity because there are few established treatments and limited understanding of the type and related mechanisms of neuronal death after ICH. It is observed various types of neuronal death after ICH, including apoptosis, pyroptosis, necrosis, ferroptosis, and autophagy (5, 39). Ferroptotic cells show shrunken mitochondria and increased membrane density in transmission electron microscopy (TEM), which is the difference between ferroptosis and other types of cell death (1, 40). In the ICH cell model and ICH-affected human brain tissue, the expression of iron death-related genes is up-regulated (42). It has been shown that ferroptosis is present in the acute phase of ICH, and it also happens in neurons far from the centre of the hematoma (42). After ICH, the iron released from Hb in the blood can produce a large number of reactive oxygen species (ROS), which leads to oxidative stress in neuronal cells and secondary brain injury. Pharmacologic inhibition of ferroptosis is beneficial in animal models of ICH, revealing that ferroptotic inhibitors can be used as new agents for the treatment of ICH (43). After ICH, mice treated with ferrostatin-1, a specific inhibitor of ferroptosis, could prevent the death of neurons by inhibiting lipid ROS production and reduce iron deposition induced by Hb, thereby exerted a long-term neuroprotective effect and improved neurological function (7, 42, 44). Here, we explore the underlying regulatory mechanism of ferroptosis following ICH. (Figure3)

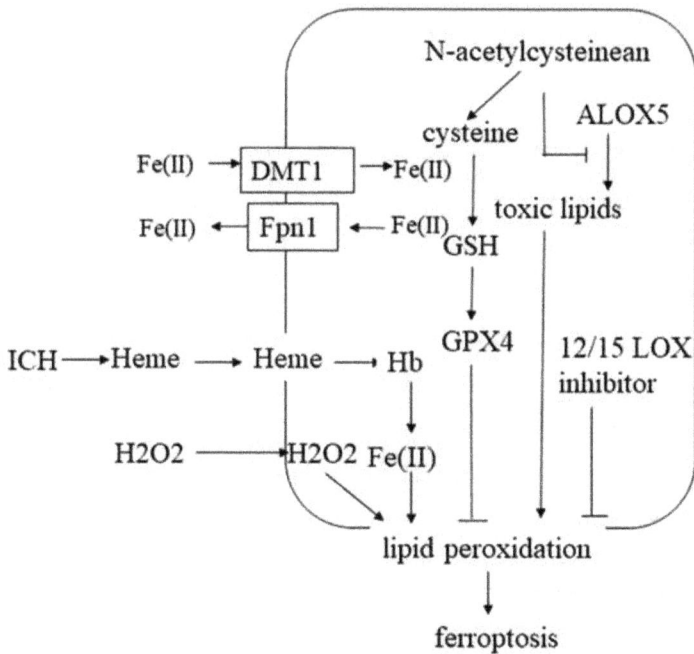

Figure3. The regulatory mechanism of ferroptosis following ICH

3.1. The Lipid Peroxidation in Ferroptosis after ICH

A large amount of ROS can promote cell damage in the way of lipid peroxidation, due to the disruption of the dynamic balance between the antioxidant system and ROS. Hb is the main component in blood, and Hb/heme/iron plays an indispensable role in the production of ROS and lipid ROS after ICH, which leads to secondary brain damage. After ICH, the heme can incorporate into the plasma membrane, and facilitate lipid peroxidation by increasing the sensitivity to the exogenous H2O2 (45, 46). ICH-induced ROS can lead to cell damage through lipid peroxidation, including apoptosis and another parallel pathway, maybe ferroptosis (47). Oxygen free radicals can enhance lipid peroxidation, which can cause the foundation of ferroptosis (48). Edaravone, a scavenger for oxygen free radicals, decreased cerebral oedema and inhibited lipid peroxidation after intraventricular hemorrhage in rats (49). 12/15 LOX inhibitor, a lipid peroxidation inhibitor, reduces hemorrhagic transformation in warfarin-treated mice after experimental stroke, and there is a contribution of this inhibitor to intracerebral bleeding (50, 51). Ferroptosis selective preferentially oxidizes PUFAs. The content of PUFA glycerophospholipids is high in the brain, especially in neuronal membranes, so neurons are easily oxidized (16). However, there is no research on the connection between neuronal PUFA and ferroptosis after ICH, which requires further investigation. N-acetylcysteinean can neutralize toxic lipids produced by arachidonate-dependent arachidonate 5-lipoxygenase (ALOX5) to prevent lipid peroxidation and heme-induced neuronal ferroptosis after ICH(52). Therefore, the inhibition of lipid peroxidation can prevent neurons from ferroptosis, which provides a therapeutic target for ICH.

3.2. The Antioxidant System for Ferroptosis after ICH

Redox balance is vital for the maintenance of brain health, so that excessive oxidative reactions can result in neuronal death in central nervous system. Oxidative stress and lipid peroxidation in neurons is critical for the occurrence of the secondary brain injury after ICH, and essentially, ferroptosis is a lipid peroxidation damage in cells. So the ferroptosis-related antioxidant system can inhibit neuronal ferroptosis after ICH.

After ICH, ferroptosis is caused by a defect in the synthesis of GSH and the reduce of GPX4. It was reported that systemic administration of N-acetylcysteinean, an approved cysteine prodrug, increased levels of cellular cysteine and synthesis of GSH to inhibit neuronal ferroptosis after ICH (52). After ICH, GSH was significantly decreased (53), and GSH treatment in ICH mice could decrease brain oedema and attenuate neural injury (54). It was showed that GPX4 protein levels were markedly reduced in neurons after ICH, the inhibition of GPX4 could exacerbate brain injury after ICH, and the upregulation of GPX4 could protect neurons from ferroptosis and ameliorate ICH-induced neuronal dysfunction in rats (55). In addition, selenium delivered into the brain could promote the expression of antioxidant GPX4, inhibit neuronal ferroptotic death, and improve function in a hemorrhagic stroke model (56). The cystine/glutamate antiporter, system xc−, is the foundation of GSH production. The study indicated the glutaminolysis could contribute to the death of neurons after ICH in vivo, But it does not affect the toxicity induced by Hb in vitro (7). Moreover, it has been shown that inhibiting the activation of the oxide-metabolic driver activating transcription factor 4 can eliminates ferroptosis induced by glutamate analogue and promote the recovery of brain function after ICH (57). Therefore, upregulation of GSH and GPX4 or increase the functionality of the system xc− may be a potential proposal to reduce the brain damage caused by ICH.

3.3. Iron Metabolism in Ferroptosis after ICH

Iron, one of the essential elements, is vital for the function of many enzymes and the average survival of cells. However, iron can also result in cell damage due to its ability to catalyze the production of ROS (58). And ferroptosis, the iron-dependent cell death, may occur through this process. The absence of iron response element binding protein 2 (IREB2) in neurons can lead to resistance the toxicity of Hb, and it was shown that the expression of IREB2 mRNA was upregulated after ICH (7). Our previous study showed that DMT1 and Fpn1 increase in ICH rats, and there is a positive correlation between Fe (II) and them (59). And Fpn1 upregulation is neuroprotective by facilitating Fe (II) export, but DMT1 has an adverse effect on through enhancing iron import (60). The study indicated that the iron-handling proteins, including ferritin, TF, and TfR levels and HO-1, were significantly increased in the brain after ICH(61) (Figure4). Excessive iron is generated, causing brain damage after ICH. After ICH, the microglia and macrophages were activated in the damaged area, which engulfs Hb released from lysed red blood cells, degrade it, and release Fe(II) (8). And heme, the degradation product of Hb, can also act as a Fenton reagent, producing Fe(II) (45). Then, Fe(II) is transported out of them and accumulates in neurons via the Tf–TfR system, which produces highly toxic hydroxyl radical, resulting in oxidative stress and the occurrence of lipid peroxidation (8). And ferroptosis, the iron-dependent cell death, may occur through this process. After ICH, HO catalyzes the oxidation of heme to Fe (II). And two types of HO were found in the brain: HO-1 and HO-2. HO-1 is mainly expressed in astrocytes and microglia, while HO-2 is highly expressed by neurons (45). A study suggests ICH induces mostly the expression of HO-1 and HO-1 knockout mice exhibit smaller infarct volumes after ICH than wild-type mice (62), which shows HO-1 is harmful to ICH. However, another study states (-)-Epicatechin (EC), a brain-permeable flavanol, could reduce lesion volume, ameliorate neurologic deficits, and neuronal degeneration via Nrf2 signaling, HO-1 induction, and brain iron deposition after ICH (63). And after subarachnoid hemorrhage, microglial HO-1 is essential for virtually eliminating heme and attenuating neuronal cell death (64). So, HO-1 plays a dual role after ICH, which is similar to the effect of HO-1 on ferroptosis.

The efficacy of iron chelation therapy has been shown in the preclinical studies of ICH. Research showed the decrease of iron accumulation with iron Chelators, including minocycline and VK-28, reduced ICH-related perihematomal iron accumulation and improved neurological outcomes after experimental ICH (65, 66). Still, it is not clear whether or not it inhibits ferroptosis.

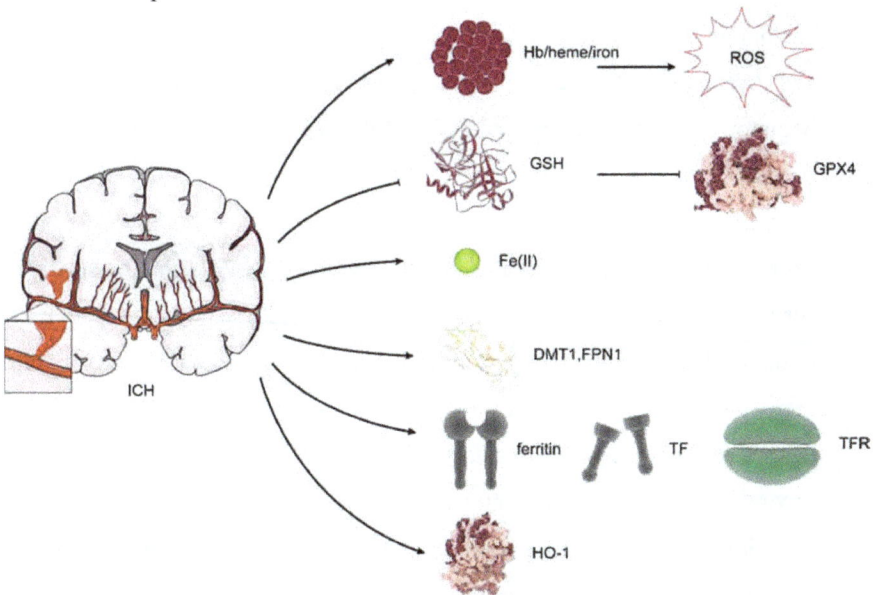

Figure4. Changes of ferroptosis regulators after ICH

4. SUMMARY

Ferroptosis is a regulated nonapoptotic cell death caused by lipid peroxidation depending on the excessive production of ROS and the accumulation of intracellular iron, but its physiological mechanism has not been determined. When ferroptosis occurs, the morphological changes of mitochondria are most apparent, such as the contraction of mitochondria, the evolution of membrane potential, the reduction of the mitochondrial cristae, electron-dense mass formation under ultrastructure, and rupture of mitochondria outer membrane (9). We find it is mediated and regulated by lipid peroxidation, antioxidant system (including GPX4, GSH, system xc– and FSP1- CoQ10- NAD(P)H Pathway) and iron metabolism. Essentially, ferroptosis results from an imbalance between oxidation and antioxidant systems.

ICH, a stroke subtype, is a disease that seriously affects the quality of life. It is characterized by a sudden rupture of cerebral blood vessels into surrounding brain tissue, which causes primary and secondary brain injury and irreversible damage to neurons. The physical compression of the hematoma causes primary damage. While the secondary damage mainly caused by the lysis of red blood cells, and the degradation of Hb, which then results in the accumulation of iron and the formation of ROS (67, 68). More than one-third of patients with ICH will not survive, and most of the surviving patients have permanent disabilities (69). The therapy for ICH remains elusive. Some patients undergo surgical hematoma evacuation, but there is no noticeable effect compared with conservative treatment (69, 70). So the therapeutic strategies for ICH remain elusive, and the study of secondary damage is of intense interest. After ICH, neuronal lipid peroxidation increases, the antioxidant GPX4 expression decreases, while DMT1, Fpn1, iron-treated protein and HO-1 increase. And neuronal lipid peroxidation, the disorder of the antioxidant system, and iron metabolism are essential for secondary brain injury. The preclinical research suggests that the inhibition of ferroptosis can prevent neuronal ferroptosis after ICH. However, the detailed mechanism still needs further exploration to provide better treatment for patients with ICH.

In this review, we explained the underlying mechanism of neuronal ferroptosis. The generalisability of these results is subject to certain limitations, including the ferroptosis of astrocytes, oligodendrocytes, microglia and their crosstalk. Study shows that ERK1/2, the vital marker of ferroptosis, is increased in astrocytes treated by heme (71). And the reduced GSH in astrocytes was depleted through Inflammatory reaction induced by heme (72). Therefore, the ferroptosis of astrocytes may occur after ICH, which affects the function of neurons. GPX4 is localized to the nucleus of oligodendrocytes in vivo, and the inhibition of GPX4 induces ferroptosis in oligodendrocytes (73). Moreover, the up-regulation of OH-1 in astrocytes and microglia affects the death of neurons. Therefore, there is a close connection between glia cell and neurons after ICH. The study indicated that the combined use of the inhibitors of different cell death has a better effect than only using one (7). In addition to ferroptosis, lipid peroxidation and increased ROS by oxidative stress after ICH can induce apoptosis via protein kinase C (PKC)/protein kinase (CK2) pathway, NF-κB pathway and cytochrome c (74). And superoxide generated by excessive oxidative stress resulting in the switch from apoptosis to necrosis (48). The inhibitors of necroptosis and ferroptosis each decrease neuronal death by greater than 80% and have similar windows for treatment in vitro (44). However, it remains to be studied how to induce different modes of cell death in a cell after ICH and what crosstalk occurs between them. Moreover, the temporal and spatial characteristics of various cell deaths caused by ICH still require to be further explored. Solving the above problems may clarify the time window for therapy targeting different ways of cell death, which provides us with research directions and new targets for exploring the treatment of ICH.

In conclusion, neuronal ferroptosis may occur after ICH, and the inhibition of ferroptosis may prevent ferroptotic death of neurons. Our review may bring insight a possible option for ferroptosis-based ICH treatment in the future.

REFERENCES:

1. Dixon SJ, Lemberg KM, Lamprecht MR, Skouta R, Zaitsev EM, Gleason CE, et al. Ferroptosis: An Iron-Dependent Form of Non-Apoptotic Cell Death. Cell (2012) 149(5):1060-72. doi: 10.1016/j.cell.2012.03.042.

2. Stockwell BR, Friedmann Angeli JP, Bayir H, Bush AI, Conrad M, Dixon SJ, et al. Ferroptosis: A Regulated Cell Death Nexus Linking Metabolism, Redox Biology, and Disease. Cell (2017) 171(2):273-85. Epub 2017/10/07. doi: 10.1016/j.cell.2017.09.021.

3. Li J, Cao F, Yin HL, Huang ZJ, Lin ZT, Mao N, et al. Ferroptosis: past, present and future. Cell death & disease (2020) 11(2):88. Epub 2020/02/06. doi: 10.1038/s41419-020-2298-2.

4. Donkor ES. Stroke in the 21(st) Century: A Snapshot of the Burden, Epidemiology, and Quality of Life. Stroke Res Treat (2018) 2018:3238165. Epub 2019/01/02. doi: 10.1155/2018/3238165.

5. Li Q, Weiland A, Chen X, Lan X, Han X, Durham F, et al. Ultrastructural Characteristics of Neuronal Death and White Matter Injury in Mouse Brain Tissues After Intracerebral Hemorrhage: Coexistence of Ferroptosis, Autophagy, and Necrosis. Frontiers in neurology (2018) 9:581. Epub 2018/08/02. doi: 10.3389/fneur.2018.00581.

6. Xiong XY, Wang J, Qian ZM, Yang QW. Iron and intracerebral hemorrhage: from mechanism to translation. Transl Stroke Res (2014) 5(4):429-41. Epub 2013/12/24. doi: 10.1007/s12975-013-0317-7.

7. Li Q, Han X, Lan X, Gao Y, Wan J, Durham F, et al. Inhibition of neuronal ferroptosis protects hemorrhagic brain. JCI insight (2017) 2(7):e90777. Epub 2017/04/14. doi: 10.1172/jci.insight.90777.

8. Wan J, Ren H, Wang J. Iron toxicity, lipid peroxidation and ferroptosis after intracerebral haemorrhage. Stroke and vascular neurology (2019) 4(2):93-5. Epub 2019/07/25. doi: 10.1136/svn-2018-000205.

9. Song X, Long D. Nrf2 and Ferroptosis: A New Research Direction for Neurodegenerative Diseases. Frontiers in neuroscience (2020) 14:267. Epub 2020/05/07. doi: 10.3389/fnins.2020.00267.

10. Kagan VE, Mao G, Qu F, Angeli JP, Doll S, Croix CS, et al. Oxidized arachidonic and adrenic PEs navigate cells to ferroptosis. Nat Chem Biol (2017) 13(1):81-90. Epub 2016/11/15. doi: 10.1038/nchembio.2238.

11. Doll S, Proneth B, Tyurina YY, Panzilius E, Kobayashi S, Ingold I, et al. ACSL4 dictates ferroptosis sensitivity by shaping cellular lipid composition. Nat Chem Biol (2017) 13(1):91-8. Epub 2016/11/15. doi: 10.1038/nchembio.2239.

12. Dixon SJ, Winter GE, Musavi LS, Lee ED, Snijder B, Rebsamen M, et al. Human Haploid Cell Genetics Reveals Roles for Lipid Metabolism Genes in Nonapoptotic Cell Death. ACS Chem Biol (2015) 10(7):1604-9. Epub 2015/05/13. doi: 10.1021/acschembio.5b00245.

13. Yang WS, Kim KJ, Gaschler MM, Patel M, Shchepinov MS, Stockwell BR. Peroxidation of polyunsaturated fatty acids by lipoxygenases drives ferroptosis. Proceedings of the National Academy of Sciences of the United States of America (2016) 113(34):E4966-75. Epub 2016/08/11. doi: 10.1073/pnas.1603244113.

14. Ursini F, Maiorino M, Gregolin C. The selenoenzyme phospholipid hydroperoxide glutathione peroxidase. Biochim Biophys Acta (1985) 839(1):62-70. Epub 1985/03/29. doi: 10.1016/0304-4165(85)90182-5.

15. Feng H, Stockwell BR. Unsolved mysteries: How does lipid peroxidation cause ferroptosis? PLoS Biol (2018) 16(5):e2006203. Epub 2018/05/26. doi: 10.1371/journal.pbio.2006203.

16. Yan HF, Tuo QZ, Yin QZ, Lei P. The pathological role of ferroptosis in ischemia/reperfusion-related injury. Zool Res (2020) 41(3):220-30. Epub 2020/04/22. doi: 10.24272/j.issn.2095-8137.2020.042.

17. Dixon SJ, Patel DN, Welsch M, Skouta R, Lee ED, Hayano M, et al. Pharmacological inhibition of cystine-glutamate exchange induces endoplasmic reticulum stress and ferroptosis. Elife (2014) 3:e02523. Epub 2014/05/23. doi: 10.7554/eLife.02523.

18. Stockwell BR, Jiang X. The Chemistry and Biology of Ferroptosis. Cell Chem Biol (2020) 27(4):365-75. Epub 2020/04/16. doi: 10.1016/j.chembiol.2020.03.013.

19. Gout PW, Buckley AR, Simms CR, Bruchovsky N. Sulfasalazine, a potent suppressor of lymphoma growth by inhibition of the x(c)- cystine transporter: a new action for an old drug. Leukemia (2001) 15(10):1633-40. Epub 2001/10/06. doi: 10.1038/sj.leu.2402238.

20. Murphy TH, Miyamoto M, Sastre A, Schnaar RL, Coyle JT. Glutamate toxicity in a neuronal cell line involves inhibition of cystine transport leading to oxidative stress. Neuron (1989) 2(6):1547-58. Epub 1989/06/01. doi: 10.1016/0896-6273(89)90043-3.

21. Yang WS, SriRamaratnam R, Welsch ME, Shimada K, Skouta R, Viswanathan VS, et al. Regulation of ferroptotic cancer cell death by GPX4. Cell (2014) 156(1-2):317-31. Epub 2014/01/21. doi: 10.1016/j.cell.2013.12.010.

22. Chen J, Wang Y, Wu J, Yang J, Li M, Chen Q. The Potential Value of Targeting Ferroptosis in Early Brain Injury After Acute CNS Disease. Front Mol Neurosci (2020) 13:110. Epub 2020/07/07. doi: 10.3389/fnmol.2020.00110.

23. Ingold I, Berndt C, Schmitt S, Doll S, Poschmann G, Buday K, et al. Selenium Utilization by GPX4 Is Required to Prevent Hydroperoxide-Induced Ferroptosis. Cell (2018) 172(3):409-22.e21. Epub 2018/01/02. doi: 10.1016/j.cell.2017.11.048.

24. Doll S, Freitas FP, Shah R, Aldrovandi M, da Silva MC, Ingold I, et al. FSP1 is a glutathione-independent ferroptosis suppressor. Nature (2019) 575(7784):693-8. Epub 2019/10/22. doi: 10.1038/s41586-019-1707-0.

25. Li D, Li Y. The interaction between ferroptosis and lipid metabolism in cancer. Signal transduction and targeted therapy (2020) 5(1):108. Epub 2020/07/02. doi: 10.1038/s41392-020-00216-5.

26. Bersuker K, Hendricks JM, Li Z, Magtanong L, Ford B, Tang PH, et al. The CoQ oxidoreductase FSP1 acts parallel to GPX4 to inhibit ferroptosis. Nature (2019) 575(7784):688-92. Epub 2019/10/22. doi: 10.1038/s41586-019-1705-2.

27. Matsushita M, Freigang S, Schneider C, Conrad M, Bornkamm GW, Kopf M. T cell lipid peroxidation induces ferroptosis and prevents immunity to infection. J Exp Med (2015) 212(4):555-68. Epub 2015/04/01. doi: 10.1084/jem.20140857.

28. Stoyanovsky DA, Tyurina YY, Shrivastava I, Bahar I, Tyurin VA, Protchenko O, et al. Iron catalysis of lipid peroxidation in ferroptosis: Regulated enzymatic or random free radical reaction? Free radical biology & medicine (2019) 133:153-61. Epub 2018/09/16. doi: 10.1016/j.freeradbiomed.2018.09.008.

29. Bayir H, Anthonymuthu TS, Tyurina YY, Patel SJ, Amoscato AA, Lamade AM, et al. Achieving Life through Death: Redox Biology of Lipid Peroxidation in Ferroptosis. Cell Chem Biol (2020) 27(4):387-408. Epub 2020/04/11. doi: 10.1016/j.chembiol.2020.03.014.

30. Ohgami RS, Campagna DR, McDonald A, Fleming MD. The Steap proteins are metalloreductases. Blood (2006) 108(4):1388-94. Epub 2006/04/13. doi: 10.1182/blood-2006-02-003681.

31. Yanatori I, Yasui Y, Tabuchi M, Kishi F. Chaperone protein involved in transmembrane transport of iron. Biochem J (2014) 462(1):25-37. Epub 2014/05/24. doi: 10.1042/BJ20140225.

32. Drakesmith H, Nemeth E, Ganz T. Ironing out Ferroportin. Cell Metab (2015) 22(5):777-87. Epub 2015/10/07. doi: 10.1016/j.cmet.2015.09.006.

33. Yanatori I, Richardson DR, Imada K, Kishi F. Iron Export through the Transporter Ferroportin 1 Is Modulated by the Iron Chaperone PCBP2. J Biol Chem (2016) 291(33):17303-18. Epub 2016/06/16. doi: 10.1074/jbc.M116.721936.

34. Mancias JD, Wang X, Gygi SP, Harper JW, Kimmelman AC. Quantitative proteomics identifies NCOA4 as the cargo receptor mediating ferritinophagy. Nature (2014) 509(7498):105-9. Epub 2014/04/04. doi: 10.1038/nature13148.

35. Chiang SK, Chen SE, Chang LC. A Dual Role of Heme Oxygenase-1 in Cancer Cells. International journal of molecular sciences (2018) 20(1). Epub 2018/12/26. doi: 10.3390/ijms20010039.

36. Adedoyin O, Boddu R, Traylor A, Lever JM, Bolisetty S, George JF, et al. Heme oxygenase-1 mitigates ferroptosis in renal proximal tubule cells. Am J Physiol Renal

Physiol (2018) 314(5):F702-F14. Epub 2017/05/19. doi: 10.1152/ajprenal.00044.2017.

37. Sun X, Ou Z, Chen R, Niu X, Chen D, Kang R, et al. Activation of the p62-Keap1-NRF2 pathway protects against ferroptosis in hepatocellular carcinoma cells. Hepatology (2016) 63(1):173-84. Epub 2015/09/26. doi: 10.1002/hep.28251.

38. Lanceta L, Li C, Choi AM, Eaton JW. Haem oxygenase-1 overexpression alters intracellular iron distribution. Biochem J (2013) 449(1):189-94. Epub 2012/09/20. doi: 10.1042/BJ20120936.

39. Zhao H, Chen Y, Feng H. P2X7 Receptor-Associated Programmed Cell Death in the Pathophysiology of Hemorrhagic Stroke. Curr Neuropharmacol (2018) 16(9):1282-95. Epub 2018/05/17. doi: 10.2174/1570159X16666180516094500.

40. Xie Y, Hou W, Song X, Yu Y, Huang J, Sun X, et al. Ferroptosis: process and function. Cell Death Differ (2016) 23(3):369-79. Epub 2016/01/23. doi: 10.1038/cdd.2015.158.

41. Dixon SJ, Lemberg KM, Lamprecht MR, Skouta R, Zaitsev EM, Gleason CE, et al. Ferroptosis: an iron-dependent form of nonapoptotic cell death. Cell (2012) 149(5):1060-72. Epub 2012/05/29. doi: 10.1016/j.cell.2012.03.042.

42. Chen B, Chen Z, Liu M, Gao X, Cheng Y, Wei Y, et al. Inhibition of neuronal ferroptosis in the acute phase of intracerebral hemorrhage shows long-term cerebroprotective effects. Brain Res Bull (2019) 153:122-32. Epub 2019/08/24. doi: 10.1016/j.brainresbull.2019.08.013.

43. Bartnikas TB, Steinbicker AU, Enns CA. Insights into basic science: what basic science can teach us about iron homeostasis in trauma patients. Current opinion in anaesthesiology (2020) 33(2):240-5. Epub 2019/12/27. doi: 10.1097/aco.0000000000000825.

44. Zille M, Karuppagounder SS, Chen Y, Gough PJ, Bertin J, Finger J, et al. Neuronal Death After Hemorrhagic Stroke In Vitro and In Vivo Shares Features of Ferroptosis and Necroptosis. Stroke (2017) 48(4):1033-43. Epub 2017/03/03. doi: 10.1161/STROKEAHA.116.015609.

45. Robinson SR, Dang TN, Dringen R, Bishop GM. Hemin toxicity: a preventable source of brain damage following hemorrhagic stroke. Redox Rep (2009) 14(6):228-35. Epub 2009/12/17. doi: 10.1179/ 135100009 X12525712409931

46. Chen-Roetling J, Cai Y, Lu X, Regan RF. Hemin uptake and release by neurons and glia. Free Radic Res (2014) 48(2):200-5. Epub 2013/10/30. doi: 10.3109/10715762.2013.859386.

47. Qu J, Chen W, Hu R, Feng H. The Injury and Therapy of Reactive Oxygen Species in Intracerebral Hemorrhage Looking at Mitochondria. Oxid Med Cell Longev (2016) 2016:2592935. Epub 2016/06/14. doi: 10.1155/2016/2592935.

48. Duan X, Wen Z, Shen H, Shen M, Chen G. Intracerebral Hemorrhage, Oxidative Stress, and Antioxidant Therapy. Oxid Med Cell Longev (2016) 2016:1203285. Epub

2016/05/18. doi: 10.1155/2016/1203285.

49. Chen Z, Zhang J, Chen Q, Guo J, Zhu G, Feng H. Neuroprotective effects of edaravone after intraventricular hemorrhage in rats. Neuroreport (2014) 25(9):635-40. Epub 2013/10/31. doi: 10.1097/WNR. 0000000000000050.

50. Zheng Y, Liu Y, Karatas H, Yigitkanli K, Holman TR, van Leyen K. Contributions of 12/15-Lipoxygenase to Bleeding in the Brain Following Ischemic Stroke. Adv Exp Med Biol (2019) 1161:125-31. Epub 2019/09/29. doi: 10.1007/978-3-030-21735-8_12.

51. Liu Y, Zheng Y, Karatas H, Wang X, Foerch C, Lo EH, et al. 12/15-Lipoxygenase Inhibition or Knockout Reduces Warfarin-Associated Hemorrhagic Transformation After Experimental Stroke. Stroke (2017) 48(2):445-51. Epub 2017/01/07. doi: 10.1161/STROKEAHA.116.014790.

52. Zille M, Karuppagounder SS, Chen Y, Gough PJ, Bertin J, Finger J, et al. Neuronal Death After Hemorrhagic Stroke In Vitro and In Vivo Shares Features of Ferroptosis and Necroptosis. Stroke (2017) 48(4):1033-43. Epub 2017/03/03. doi: 10.1161/STROKEAHA.116.015609.

53. Wang S, Li D, Huang C, Wan Y, Wang J, Zan X, et al. Overexpression of adiponectin alleviates intracerebral hemorrhage-induced brain injury in rats via suppression of oxidative stress. Neurosci Lett (2018) 681:110-6. Epub 2018/06/06. doi: 10.1016/j.neulet.2018.05.050.

54. Diao X, Zhou Z, Xiang W, Jiang Y, Tian N, Tang X, et al. Glutathione alleviates acute intracerebral hemorrhage injury via reversing mitochondrial dysfunction. Brain Res (2020) 1727:146514. Epub 2019/10/20. doi: 10.1016/j.brainres.2019.146514.

55. Zhang Z, Wu Y, Yuan S, Zhang P, Zhang J, Li H, et al. Glutathione peroxidase 4 participates in secondary brain injury through mediating ferroptosis in a rat model of intracerebral hemorrhage. Brain Res (2018) 1701:112-25. Epub 2018/09/12. doi: 10.1016/j.brainres.2018.09.012.

56. Alim I, Caulfield JT, Chen Y, Swarup V, Geschwind DH, Ivanova E, et al. Selenium Drives a Transcriptional Adaptive Program to Block Ferroptosis and Treat Stroke. Cell (2019) 177(5):1262-79 e25. Epub 2019/05/06. doi: 10.1016/j.cell.2019.03.032.

57. Zille M, Kumar A, Kundu N, Bourassa MW, Wong VSC, Willis D, et al. Ferroptosis in Neurons and Cancer Cells Is Similar But Differentially Regulated by Histone Deacetylase Inhibitors. eNeuro (2019) 6(1). Epub 2019/02/21. doi: 10.1523/eneuro.0263-18.2019.

58. Wang W, Di X, D'Agostino RB, Jr., Torti SV, Torti FM. Excess capacity of the iron regulatory protein system. J Biol Chem (2007) 282(34):24650-9. Epub 2007/07/03. doi: 10.1074/jbc.M703167200.

59. Wang G, Shao A, Hu W, Xue F, Zhao H, Jin X, et al. Changes of ferrous iron and its transporters after intracerebral hemorrhage in rats. Int J Clin Exp Pathol (2015) 8(9):10671-9. Epub 2015/12/01. PubMed PMID: 26617777.

60. Wang G, Hu W, Tang Q, Wang L, Sun XG, Chen Y, et al. Effect Comparison of Both Iron Chelators on Outcomes, Iron Deposit, and Iron Transporters After Intracerebral Hemorrhage in Rats. Molecular neurobiology (2016) 53(6):3576-85. Epub 2015/06/24. doi: 10.1007/s12035-015-9302-3.

61. Wu J, Hua Y, Keep RF, Nakamura T, Hoff JT, Xi G. Iron and iron-handling proteins in the brain after intracerebral hemorrhage. Stroke (2003) 34(12):2964-9. Epub 2003/11/15. doi: 10.1161/01.STR.0000103140. 52838. 45.

62. Wang J, Dore S. Inflammation after intracerebral hemorrhage. Journal of cerebral blood flow and metabolism : official journal of the International Society of Cerebral Blood Flow and Metabolism (2007) 27(5):894-908. Epub 2006/10/13. doi: 10.1038/sj.jcbfm.9600403.

63. Chang CF, Cho S, Wang J. (-)-Epicatechin protects hemorrhagic brain via synergistic Nrf2 pathways. Ann Clin Transl Neurol (2014) 1(4):258-71. Epub 2014/04/18. doi: 10.1002/acn3.54.

64. Schallner N, Pandit R, LeBlanc R, 3rd, Thomas AJ, Ogilvy CS, Zuckerbraun BS, et al. Microglia regulate blood clearance in subarachnoid hemorrhage by heme oxygenase-1. J Clin Invest (2015) 125(7):2609-25. Epub 2015/05/27. doi: 10.1172/JCI78443.

65. Li Q, Wan J, Lan X, Han X, Wang Z, Wang J. Neuroprotection of brain-permeable iron chelator VK-28 against intracerebral hemorrhage in mice. Journal of cerebral blood flow and metabolism: official journal of the International Society of Cerebral Blood Flow and Metabolism (2017) 37(9):3110-23. Epub 2017/05/24. doi: 10.1177/0271678x17709186.

66. Dai S, Hua Y, Keep RF, Novakovic N, Fei Z, Xi G. Minocycline attenuates brain injury and iron overload after intracerebral hemorrhage in aged female rats. Neurobiology of disease (2019) 126:76-84. Epub 2018/06/08. doi: 10.1016/j.nbd.2018.06.001.

67. Wagner KR, Sharp FR, Ardizzone TD, Lu A, Clark JF. Heme and iron metabolism: role in cerebral hemorrhage. Journal of cerebral blood flow and metabolism: official journal of the International Society of Cerebral Blood Flow and Metabolism (2003) 23(6):629-52. Epub 2003/06/11. doi: 10.1097/01.WCB.0000073905.87928.6D.

68. Aronowski J, Zhao X. Molecular pathophysiology of cerebral hemorrhage: secondary brain injury. Stroke (2011) 42(6):1781-6. Epub 2011/04/30. doi: 10.1161/STROKEAHA.110.596718.

69. Bamford J, Sandercock P, Dennis M, Burn J, Warlow C. A prospective study of acute cerebrovascular disease in the community: the Oxfordshire Community Stroke Project--1981-86. 2. Incidence, case fatality rates and overall outcome at one year of cerebral infarction, primary intracerebral and subarachnoid haemorrhage. J Neurol Neurosurg Psychiatry (1990) 53(1):16-22. Epub 1990/01/01. doi: 10.1136/jnnp.53.1.16.

70. Kuramatsu JB, Biffi A, Gerner ST, Sembill JA, Sprugel MI, Leasure A, et al.

Association of Surgical Hematoma Evacuation vs Conservative Treatment With Functional Outcome in Patients With Cerebellar Intracerebral Hemorrhage. JAMA (2019) 322(14):1392-403. Epub 2019/10/09. doi: 10.1001/jama.2019.13014.

71. Regan RF, Wang Y, Ma X, Chong A, Guo Y. Activation of extracellular signal-regulated kinases potentiates hemin toxicity in astrocyte cultures. J Neurochem (2001) 79(3):545-55. Epub 2001/11/10. doi: 10.1046/j.1471-4159.2001.00590.x.

72. Laird MD, Wakade C, Alleyne CH, Jr., Dhandapani KM. Hemin-induced necroptosis involves glutathione depletion in mouse astrocytes. Free radical biology & medicine (2008) 45(8):1103-14. Epub 2008/08/19. doi: 10.1016/j.freeradbiomed.2008.07.003.

73. Fan BY, Pang YL, Li WX, Zhao CX, Zhang Y, Wang X, et al. Liproxstatin-1 is an effective inhibitor of oligodendrocyte ferroptosis induced by inhibition of glutathione peroxidase 4. Neural regeneration research (2021) 16(3):561-6. Epub 2020/09/29. doi: 10.4103/1673-5374.293157.

74. Hu X, Tao C, Gan Q, Zheng J, Li H, You C. Oxidative Stress in Intracerebral Hemorrhage: Sources, Mechanisms, and Therapeutic Targets. Oxid Med Cell Longev (2016) 2016:3215391. Epub 2016/02/05. doi: 10.1155/2016/3215391.

ACKNOWLEDGEMENT:

This work was supported by a grant from National Natural Science Foundation of China (81771294).

DECLARATION: This chapter was authored by Qinqin Bai, Jiachen Liu and Gaiqing Wang published as "Ferroptosis, a regulated neuronal cell death type after intracerebral hemorrhage" in "Frontiers in Cellular Neuroscience", 2020; 14:591874

CHAPTER 6:

Microglia: A double-edged sword in intracerebral hemorrhage from basic mechanisms to clinical research

ABSTRACT:

Microglia are the resident immune cells of the central nervous system (CNS). It is well established that microglia are activated and polarized to acquire different inflammatory phenotypes, either pro-inflammatory or anti-inflammatory phenotypes, which act as a critical component in the neuroinflammation following intracerebral hemorrhage (ICH). Microglia produce pro-inflammatory mediators at the early stages after ICH onset, anti-inflammatory microglia with neuroprotective effects appear to be suppressed. Previous research found that driving microglia towards an anti-inflammatory phenotype could restrict inflammation and engulf cellular debris. The principal objective of this review is to analyze the phenotypes and dynamic profiles of microglia as well as their shift in functional response following ICH. The results may further the understanding of the body's self-regulatory functions involving microglia following ICH. On this basis, suggestions for future clinical development and research are provided.

KEY WORDS: Intracerebral hemorrhage, Microglia, Phenotype switch, Neuroimmunology, Neuroinflammation

1. INTRODUCTION

Microglia constitute 5-10% of adult brain cells and form the largest group of immune cells in the CNS (1). The primary source of microglia is yolk sac erythromyeloid precursors (EMPs) that migrate into the brain rudiment during embryo development (2). Under physiological conditions, microglia self-renew for the entire lifespan of the organism and interact with numerous other cells in the brain, such as astrocytes, neurons, and oligodendrocytes (3). Mounting evidence suggests that microglia, as brain resident immune cells, play an essential role in maintaining normal brain function. When pathologic changes disrupt homeostasis in the brain, microglia are activated to exert regulatory effects (4). Microglia are highly diverse, and their phenotype depends on the context and type of stressor or pathology (5). Specifically, during the different periods after intracerebral hemorrhage (ICH), microglia may polarize to produce pro-inflammatory mediators or acquire a more anti-inflammatory phenotype, which has a decisive influence on ICH progression (Figure 1) (6).

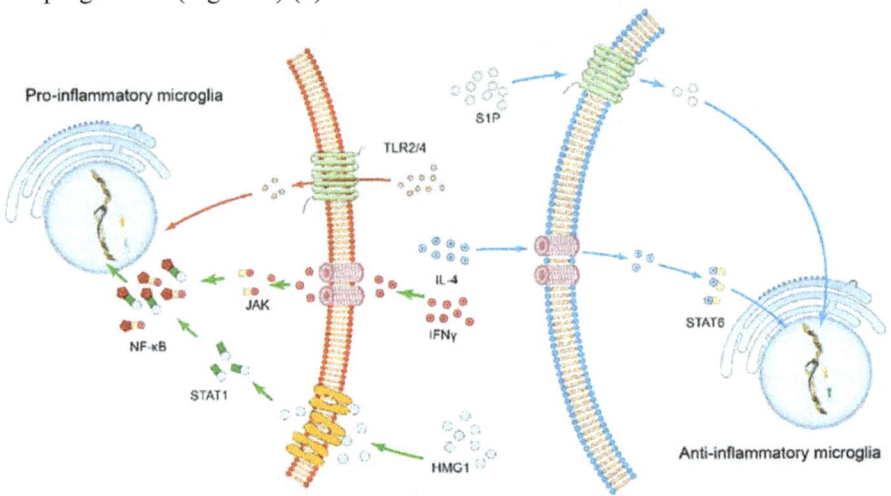

Figure 1. The induction of microglial polarization by several transcription factors. Activation of high mobility histone 1 (HMG1) and Toll-like receptor (TLR) 2 or TLR4 promotes the pro-inflammatory phenotypic polarization of microglia. Interferon-gamma (IFN-γ) promotes the pro-inflammatory phenotypic polarization of microglia through the signaling sensors signal transducer and activator of transcription (STAT) 1 and Janus kinase (JAK). This series of processes involves the nuclear factor kappa B (NF-κB) signaling pathway. On the other hand, STAT6 accumulates under the action of IL-4 and is responsible for the transcription of M2 phenotype-related genes. The sphingosine-1-phosphate (S1P) receptor signaling pathway downregulates the expression of pro-inflammatory cytokines and enhances anti-inflammatory responses following intracerebral hemorrhage.

Pathological analysis of microglial activity during ICH has revealed that microglia induce potent immune responses after extravasation of blood into the brain (7). The strong inflammatory response in microglia is caused by the rapid accumulation of blood-derived products (e.g., hemoglobin, heme, and iron) after ICH (8), which can directly damage the brain parenchyma, and a sustained microglia-mediated inflammatory response results in neurologic deterioration (9). Interestingly, Chang et al. (10) have experimentally proven that as early as 1-1.5 hours after ICH, microglia respond to hemorrhagic injury and exhibit a protective alternative activation phenotype.

The role of microglia following ICH is complex, and the entirely different action of different phenotypes of microglia plays an essential role in the development of cerebral inflammatory injury and recovery of the brain after ICH (Figure 2). Besides, the neuroprotective effect of microglia may serve as promising targets for ICH treatment. For example, the primary role of activated microglia is to phagocytose the hematoma, thereby reducing ICH-induced brain swelling and neuronal loss and improving neurological deficits (11). Microglial depletion can lead to more severe brain swelling, neuronal loss, and functional defects following ICH (12).

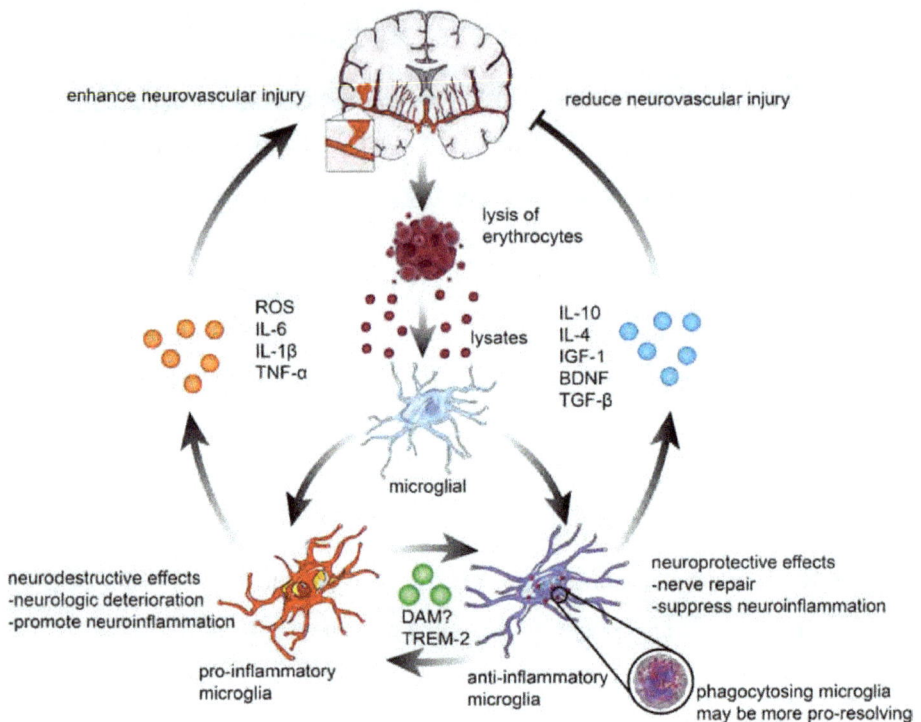

Figure 2. Microglial activation and polarization following ICH.

The polarization of microglia in response to stimulation with erythrocyte lysates after ICH can be broadly classified into two categories. 1) pro-inflammatory microglia elevate the levels of ROS, interleukin-6 (IL-6), interleukin-1β (IL-1β) and tumor necrosis factor-α (TNF-α), hence enhancing the pro-inflammatory and destructive effects of ICH on the brain. 2) anti-inflammatory microglia, on the contrary, mainly exert neuroprotective effects, including actions related to nerve repair and anti-inflammatory effects, through phagocytosis of lysates, which are always associated with higher expression of IL-10, IL-4, insulin-like growth factor-1 (IGF-1), brain-derived neurotrophic factor (BDNF) and transforming growth factor-β (TGF-β). In recent years, an increasing number of studies have revealed that microglia can also be polarized into neuroprotective and neurodestructive phenotypes, such as disease-associated microglia (DAM) and triggering receptor expressed on myeloid cells 2 (TREM2) phenotypes, which remain to be further investigated.

2. The dual role of microglia after ICH

2.1. The effects of microglia on the blood-brain barrier following ICH

Destruction of the blood-brain barrier (BBB) and consequent brain edema is the most common secondary causes of life-threatening events after ICH

(13). One recent study by Chen et al. showed that microglia-derived TNF-α mediates endothelial necroptosis contributing to blood-brain-barrier disruption (14). Besides, activated microglia cause an imbalance between endogenous vasodilators and vasoconstrictors, further leading to edema formation after ICH (15).

Anti-inflammatory actions of microglia may mediate BBB protection and neural repair by producing anti-inflammatory cytokines, extracellular matrix proteins, glucocorticoids, and other substances (16). As signaling via IL-4 and IL-10 can induce an anti-inflammatory phenotype of microglia, it can be targeted for ICH treatment through modulating BBB physiology (17).

2.2 The functions of microglia in secondary brain damage following ICH

Intracranial hematoma is a crucial factor contributing to brain injury after ICH. Mechanical damage is induced in adjacent tissues due to compression and dissection. Simultaneously, iron, heme, and cytotoxic hemoglobin can be passively released due to the lysis of erythrocytes adjacent to the hematoma (18). Microglial phagocytosis of hematoma occurs before erythrocytes lysis to protect the brain (19, 20). This process can be regulated by alternative activation of microglia via activating the CCR4/ERK/Nrf2 pathway and peroxisome proliferator-activated receptor γ (PPAR-γ) (21-23). (Figure 3)

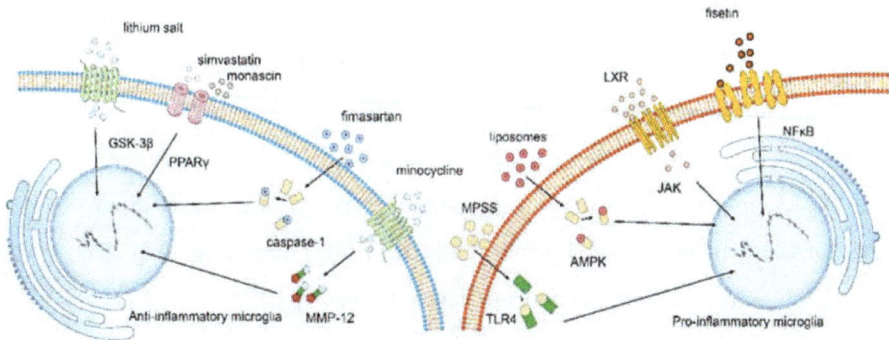

Figure 3. Potential intervention strategies targeting the microglial phenotypic shift following ICH. Interventions that induce the polarization of pro-inflammatory microglia towards the anti-inflammatory phenotype exert beneficial effects following ICH. For example, fisetin mediates the NFκB pathway, and liver X receptor (LXR)-mediated JAK, liposome-mediated adenosine monophosphate-activated protein kinase (AMPK), and methylprednisolone sodium succinate (MPSS)-mediated TLR4 inhibit M1 microglia. While lithium salt mediates glycogen synthase kinase-3beta (GSK-3β) expression, simvastatin and monascin mediate peroxisome proliferator-activated receptor gamma (PPARγ) levels, fimasartan mediates caspase-1 levels, and minocycline upregulates matrix metalloproteinase 12 (MMP-12) expression.

There is ample evidence that microglial activation is essential for secondary damage to the brain after ICH (24). For example, microglia also produce pro-inflammatory factors (TNF-α, IL-1β, IL-6) and chemokines (CXCL2), which promote neuroinflammation (25, 26). Besides, the absorption of hematoma may also trigger a series of inflammatory reactions leading to primary and secondary brain damage (27).

3 Microglial polarization following ICH

Although the terminology of "microglia polarization" is still widely used in the literature, most commonly in the M1 and M2 phenotypes. Complex high-content experiment and multi-omics technologies, including transcriptomic, epigenomic, and proteomics, have found novel microglia polarization states beyond the standard M1/M2 dichotomy, which leads to a fierce debate in microglial M1/M2 polarization in recent years (28).

As early as 2013, Chiu and colleagues utilized flow cytometry and deep RNA sequencing of acutely isolated spinal cord microglia. The study aimed to prove that microglial reactions must be interpreted in light of the tissue in which the activating stimulus is present (29). However, the M1/M2 model is not a pure phenomenon in vivo, as previously proven by Butovsky, by profiling CNS cells with an MG400 microglial chip (30), which ignores the crucial concept demonstrated by Chiu et al.(30).

Besides, transcriptionally distinguishable subpopulations of microglia that appear to be a transcriptional continuum of the local population of microglia can be detected during homeostasis (31, 32), representing a transcriptional basis for the microglia phenotype diversity (33).

Single-cell RNA-sequence analysis of microglia suggested converged expression of M1 and M2 markers due to the influence of disease-related inflammatory processes (34). Furthermore, precise categorization of different microglia or monocyte subtypes based on specific types and stages of pathology or their relation to specific tissue injury types is also possible (35). In conclusion, a precise definition of microglial polarization has proven elusive, and the description of M1 or M2 phenotypes is an oversimplification of the complex biology of microglia.

In a recent transcriptional single-cell study, Keren-Shaul et al. found that microglial phenotypes other than the M1/M2 phenotypes exist. For example, a new subpopulation named disease-associated microglia (DAM) has been discovered through genome-wide transcriptomic analyses of microglia under different disease conditions. Although the gene profile of DAM and M1 microglia partially overlapped, the molecular signatures have shown apparent differences (36). Interestingly, DAM also exhibits anti-inflammatory/phagocytic and pro-inflammatory profiles (37). Activation of DAM depends on triggering receptors expressed on myeloid cells 2 (TREM2), a receptor located mainly on the surface of microglia. TREM2 promotes the phagocytosis of apoptotic neurons producing tiny quantities of pro-inflammatory cytokines (38). Research has also shown that TREM2 is activated in perihematomal areas, which improved attenuated neuroinflammation and neuronal apoptosis after ICH (39). Besides, according to a study done by Gao et al. in 2019, CEBPα, IRF1, and LXRβ are likely regulators of pro-inflammatory and anti-inflammatory DAM states. Based on emerging findings, it is possible to conclude that DAM represents a switch that substantially alters microglial function (40). While the DAM concept has been widely used in neurodegenerative diseases such as Alzheimer's disease rather than ICH, it is clear that microglia is in a constant flux state and exquisitely sensitive to their environment.

Many studies have investigated the spatially and temporally restricted subsets of microglia during development and disease, further identifying the distinct molecular hallmarks and diverse cellular kinetics using massively parallel single-cell analysis and computational modeling (32, 41). For example, using single-cell RNA sequencing from human cerebral cortex samples, Olah et al. confirm the presence of four microglial subsets and elucidate the significance of subsets, such as the association with Alzheimer's disease (AD) (42). More recently, Ochocka et al. demonstrate cellular and functional heterogeneity of microglia using flow cytometry and scRNAseq. In this experiment, multiple microglial clusters were obtained, and gene expression profiles underlying a specific cluster could reflect different functions. Hom-MG and activated microglia (Act-MG) were identified, which shows the distinct spatial distribution in experimental gliomas (43). Furthermore, an environment-dependent transcriptional network specifying microglia-specific programs have been developed, which identified substantial subsets of microglia associate with neurodegenerative and behavioral diseases (44).

In summary, microglia are activated by various pathologic events or changes in brain homeostasis, which are highly diverse and depend on the context and type of stressor or pathology. The complicated functional roles of microglia support the existence of distinct pro-inflammatory and anti-inflammatory functional states following ICH. The significance of defining microglial subtypes is to identify novel microglial functional conditions; determine the impact of molecules on microglia types, and discover ways to mediate functions in healthy physiology or disease (45). During the ICH progress, most investigators continue to use the expression of M1/M2 markers and microglia polarization as a surrogate for a genuine mechanistic understanding of how microglial function changes (46). Therefore, it would be interesting to identify the regulators and influencing factors that contribute to the polarization of microglia towards a neuroprotective or neurodestructive phenotype, which may shed new light on the pathogenetic role of microglia following ICH.

3.1 Endogenous mechanisms of microglia

Much of the literature has emphasized the autoregulation of microglia during ICH progress. For example, studies by Wu et al. showed that soluble epoxide hydrolase expression is upregulated in microglia after ICH, which causes neuroinflammatory responses by degrading anti-inflammatory epoxyeicosatrienoic acid (47). Other studies have provided further evidence that microglial recruitment is associated with TWIK-related K+ channel 1 (TREK-1), which also triggers the secretion of pro-inflammatory factors such as IL-1β and TNF-α as well as cell adhesion molecules following ICH (48). Besides, low-density LRP1 in the neurovascular unit interacts with Mac-1 expressed by microglia to promote tPA-mediated activation of platelet-derived growth factor-cc (PDGF-cc). Activation of potential PDGF-cc and PDGF receptor-α signals can increase the permeability of the blood-brain barrier and deterioration following ICH (13).

Microglia have similarly been shown to be involved in anti-inflammatory and phagocytic effects on the hematoma, contributing to neurologic recovery after ICH. The correlation between regulatory T lymphocytes

(Tregs) and neuroinflammatory response after ICH has been defined. In vitro experiments have demonstrated that Tregs modulate microglia polarization toward the anti-inflammation phenotype through the IL-10/GSK3β/PTEN axis in this regulatory process (49, 50).

3.1.1 The regulatory effect of miRNAs

As gene expression is regulated through genetic and epigenetic regulatory networks, there is growing evidence that miRNAs play essential roles in the microglial effects after ICH (51). For example, miRNA-7 (miR-7) can inhibit the expression of Toll-like receptor 4 (TLR4) and provoke a secondary microglia-mediated inflammatory response after ICH (52). Further studies have confirmed that agents that target TLR4 and miR-7, such as ligustilide (LIG) and senkyunolide H (SH), can exert neuroprotective effects against ICH by inhibiting Prx1/TLR4/NF-κB signaling via activation of microglia and astrocytes (53).

Recent studies have found that inhibition of miRNA-222 suppresses microglia-mediated inflammatory responses and improves neurological functions in a preclinical mouse model of ICH. Integrin subunit β8 (ITGB8) was identified as a directly negatively regulated target of miR-222 in microglial cells, leading to the attenuation of inflammation and apoptosis (54). Besides, miR-132 enhances the cholinergic blockade of the inflammatory response by targeting acetylcholinesterase (AChE), which also inhibits the activation of pro-inflammatory microglia and provides protection against neuronal death caused by ischemia (55).

Furthermore, as the critical factors in autophagy, miRNAs negatively regulate gene expression and autophagic activity of microglia. For example, miRNA-144 targets mTOR by directly interacting with 3' untranslated regions (UTRs), which are involved in hemoglobin-mediated activation of microglial autophagy and inflammatory responses (56). The specific function of autophagy is dualistic and has been difficult to assess whether it has harmful or beneficial effects following ICH thus far. Despite many studies demonstrated that autophagy could enhance the protection of endoplasmic reticulum stress and reducing oxidative damage after ICH via clearing up the cell rubbish and oxidative-stress products (57, 58), recent studies showed autophagy positively regulates inflammation following ICH (59, 60).

3.1.2 Regulation of microglia function by intracellular signaling following ICH

Anti-inflammatory microglia functions are accomplished by combining various signaling pathways that compose a complex network involved in multiple biological processes. Exploring the network of biological signaling pathways and its molecular basis contributes to novel interventions targeting signaling pathways that block the pathological progression of ICH. (Figure 3)

The roles of the AMPK pathway and AdipoR1 in microglia function following ICH

It has been demonstrated that adenosine monophosphate-activated protein kinase (AMPK) can drive the phenotypic shift from a pro-inflammatory state to an anti-inflammatory state (61). The expression of endogenous C1q/TNF-related protein 9 (CTRP9), an upstream trigger of the AMPK signaling pathway and an agonist of AdipoR1, is increased after ICH in animal models of long-term neurobehavior, peaking at 24 hours after ICH. Further experiments have confirmed that the expression of AdipoR1 and p-AMPK can reduce the expression of inflammatory cytokines after ICH (62). Besides, the activation of MC4R also alleviates neurological deficits through the AMPK pathway following ICH, and interventions targeting MC4R, such as RO27-3225 administration, have been proven to be effective in animal experiments (63).

The roles of the JNK pathway in microglia function following ICH

As mentioned above, Treg cells inhibit microglia-mediated inflammatory responses and improve neurological function in vivo, mainly by activate NF-κB through the JNK pathway (49, 64). There are controversies regarding the role of the JNK signaling pathway following ICH, which has received increased attention in the clinic in recent years. For example, the synthesis of the liver X receptor (LXR) agonist TO901317 was shown to exert specific effects in an ICH model by inhibiting JNK signaling. The hyperbaric oxygen preconditioning (HBOP) model of ICH has demonstrated the potential relevance between JNK phosphorylation and the immunological activity of anti-inflammatory microglia (65). As current practical limitations include drug side effects, uncertainties regarding efficacy, surgical injuries, and complications, there are no standardized clinical interventions for ICH except intracranial pressure-lowering therapies. Therefore, hyperbaric oxygen therapy provides a feasible alternative intervention with mild adverse effects against ICH, and the mechanism of HBOP in ICH needs further exploration and verification.

The impact of the Toll-like receptor 4 (TLR-4) pathway on microglia function

Toll-like receptor 4 (TLR4) plays a crucial role in the innate immune response. It can be concluded that loss of TLR4 reduces the recruitment of pro-inflammatory microglia and markedly alleviates inflammation around the hematoma in the animal model (66). Further studies have shown that TLR4 also inhibits the phagocytosis of microglia on the surface of red blood cells, resulting in hematoma absorption delay and severe neurological deficits in ICH patients (67). TLR4-mediated autophagy of microglial activation contributes to secondary brain injury and brain recovery and inflammatory damage following ICH (68).

The role of TLR4 in secondary brain damage following ICH has been elaborated in detail, and therapeutic strategies targeting TLR4 are relatively well-developed. Therefore, TLR4 remains a promising target for inhibiting undesired microglial responses, and interventions targeting TLR4-related pathways may represent future candidates for ICH therapy.

3.2 Regulation of microglia function by extracellular signals following ICH

As the regulatory effects of intracellular signaling pathways on microglia after ICH have been discussed, the final section of this paper addresses how extracellular signaling regulators influence microglial morphology and function. Compared with intracellular signals, extracellular signals are more complicated and vulnerable to disruption, which means they have the potential to be translated into clinically effective targeted therapies for ICH.

3.2.1 Interventions targeting microglia functions for ICH

Interleukins

The interleukins (ILs) level is intimately associated with the development and progression of ICH, which may be achieved by modulation of microglia functions. For example, activation of the IL-4/transcription 6 (STAT6) axis improved long-term functional recovery in a mouse model of ICH (69). Conversely, expression of IL-15 exacerbates brain injury following ICH by mediate the crosstalk between microglia and astrocytes (70).

Besides, antibodies against IL-17A can prevent ICH-induced expression of TNF-α, IL-1β and IL-6 and inhibit microglial activation (71). Further examination revealed that IL-17A promotes autophagy in pro-inflammatory microglia, thus maintaining the body's normal immune response and alleviating brain edema after ICH (60). Notably, recent studies have found that intraventricular infusion of IL-33 can alleviate neurological deficits following ICH by promoting the transformation of pro-inflammatory microglia (72). Deferoxamine (DFA) can also inhibit the activation of pro-inflammatory microglia by downregulating IL-1β and TNF expression, reducing secondary brain insult following ICH.

Nuclear factor-κB

Evidence has suggested that NF-κB translocates to the nucleus, and pro-inflammatory mediators (NO, TNF-a, and IL-6) are produced following inflammatory response after ICH. These results suggest that combined targeting of NF-κB signaling pathway inhibition may be a more effective anti-neuroinflammatory strategy following ICH (53).

Regulation of NF-κB activity may also have promising clinical benefits following ICH. Analysis of thrombin toxicity in vitro shows that has thrombin release after ICH led to the increased expression of NF-κB in microglia (73, 74). Treatment modalities disrupting this harmful process, such as miR-181c mimic therapy, are expected to regulate thrombin-driven inflammation after cerebral hemorrhage (75).

Glycogen synthase kinase-3β

It is widely acknowledged that glycogen synthase kinase-3beta (GSK-3β) exerts a potent pro-inflammatory effect following ICH (76). Studies have shown that the hematoma volume is significantly decreased by GSK-3β inhibition after ICH due to enhanced microglia-mediated phagocytosis (77). Consistently, the GSK-3β inhibitor 6-bromoindirubin-3'-oxime (BIO) has been shown to relieve inflammation by blocking GSK-3β

Tyr216 phosphorylation/activation following ICH. BIO may exert a protective effect against ICH by increasing the number of anti-inflammatory microglia through inactivating GSK-3β (78).

It is interesting to note that the molecular mechanism by which lithium salt can treat ICH in clinical practice has already been elucidated. Recently, it has been shown that LiCl treatment decreased the death of mature oligodendrocytes (OLGs) in ICH mice, which may be regulated by the LiCl-induced inhibition of glycogen synthase kinase-3β (GSK-3β) (79).

Peroxisome proliferator-activated receptor gamma (PPAR-γ)

The phagocytic activity of microglia is required to remove the hematoma after ICH; however, the pro-inflammatory mediators and free radicals released as a result of microglial activation and phagocytosis are toxic to neighboring cells and lead to secondary brain damage following ICH (80). ICH mouse model demonstrated that peroxisome proliferator-activated receptor gamma (PPAR-γ) prevents LPS-induced pro-inflammatory microglial activation while facilitating microglial polarization towards the anti-inflammatory phenotype (81). Besides, PPAR-γ promotes phagocytosis in a timely and effective manner, limiting the toxic effects of hemolysis by facilitating hematoma clearance following ICH (82).

Studies have demonstrated that PPAR-γ activation is imperative for enhancing the phagocytic ability of anti-inflammatory microglia by CD36 (18). Furthermore, 15(S)-hydroxyeicosatetraenoic acid, an exogenous PPAR-γ agonist, improves functional recovery following ICH and exerts neuroprotective effects (83).

Based on in-depth basic research, PPAR-γ agonists have been widely used in clinical treatment. For example, the neuroprotective effects of statins following ICH through PPAR-γ activation and enhancement of microglia-induced erythrocyte phagocytosis have been established (84). Besides, monascin, as a novel dual agonist of PPAR-γ and Nrf2, facilitates microglial phagocytosis of the hematoma and exerts neuroprotective effects following ICH (85, 86).

Caspase family

Caspase-mediated cascades play an essential role in mediating anti-inflammatory microglial death (87). For example, AC-YVAD-CMK can alleviate brain edema by inhibiting the activation of pro-caspase-1 and downregulating the expression of inflammation-related factors, which is accompanied by decreasing activated microglia at 24 h post-ICH (88).

Clinical studies have found that fimasartan (an angiotensin II receptor blocker) significantly reduces the activation of the caspase-1 pathway after ICH (89), suggesting that it is effective in ICH by regulating caspase-1-mediated microglial autophagy.

Matrix metalloproteinases (MMPs)

The first serious discussions of MMP-12, which is harmful and contributes to secondary damage after ICH, emerged in 2005 (90). Subsequent studies found that MMP-9 binds to injured neurons in culture, activates pro-inflammatory microglia, and exerts neurotoxic effects after ICH (91). Based on this, further research proposed that inhibition of MMP-9 improves prognosis following ICH (92).

MMP-mediated microglial activation has become a potential therapeutic target for ICH. For example, minocycline, a widely available drug that alleviates brain damage, effectively reduces early upregulation of MMP-12 expression (93, 94) and induces anti-inflammation microglial polarization, which reduces the levels of inflammatory cytokines and the number of microglia surrounding the hematoma after ICH (86). It should be noted that although the molecular mechanism is unclear, MMP-12 expression and microglial infiltration around the hematoma are significantly reduced after stem cell transplantation following ICH (95, 96).

Iron chelators

Iron overload is a significant cause of brain damage because iron toxicity contributes to pro-inflammatory microglial activation following collagenase-induced ICH. Therefore, reducing the accumulation of iron can moderately improve the outcomes after ICH (97). As an iron chelator, minocycline can reduce free iron and iron handling protein levels, thus prevent neuronal death (98). Besides, VK-28, a brain-permeable iron chelator, is superior to and less toxic than DFA following ICH (99, 100).

The evidence from observational studies shows that microglia function is controlled by complex regulatory networks (Table 1), an understanding of which is critical for elucidating phenotypic and genotypic variations in microglia and developing therapeutic interventions for ICH (Figure 4).

Phenotype	Activating signals (events)	Markers (events)	Result	Purpose
Pro-inflammatory microglia	JNK (TO901317, HBOP -) GSK-3β (Lithium, BIO -) miR-222 (Fisetin -) TLR4 (Ligustilide, Senkyunolide H, MPSS, Eupatilin -) miR-124 TREK-1	MMP (Minocycline, sinomenine -) Caspase-1 (AC-YVAD-CMK, Fimasartan -) TNF-α IL-1β NF-κB (ITGB8, Andrographolide -) IL-6 IL-1	Pro-inflammation	Neurological deficit

Anti-inflammatory microglia	Tregs AMPK (CTRP9, AdipoR1 +) IL-33	TGF-β IL-10 (Atorvastatin +) Tregs MC4R (RO27-3225 +)	Phagocytosis Anti-inflammation	Neurological recovery

Table1. Potential interventions for microglia polarization after intracerebral hemorrhage.

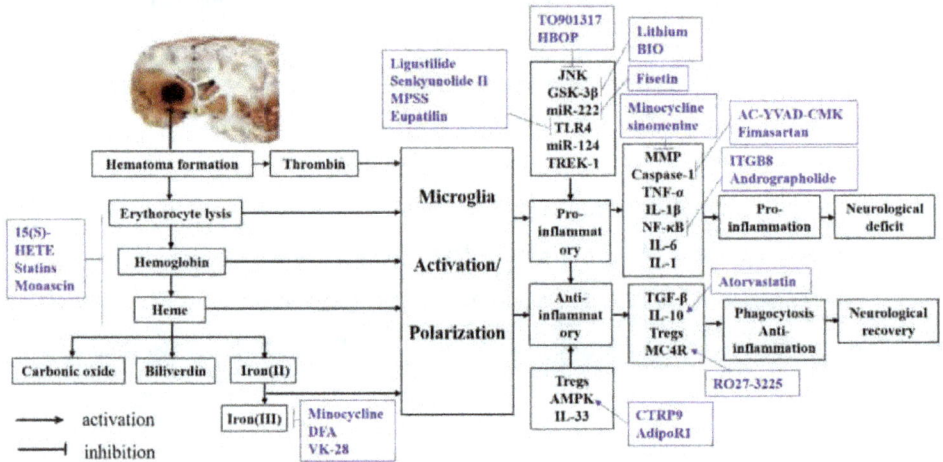

FIGURE 4 | Summary of interventions for ICH targeting microglial polarization. Available intervention strategies are labeled blue.

4 Potential therapeutic strategies targeting microglia function after ICH

Exploring the regulatory mechanism of microglial immunophenotype changes may help identify the hematoma scavenging mechanism and a precise therapeutic target for ICH. The multi-omics technologies have made significant achievements in the research of microglial activation (101). The application of systematic multi-omics approaches to precision medicine and systems biology has great potential to improve the care of patients with ICH. Notably, the target gene identified by multi-omics studies can potentially be used for drug repositioning in ICH, which is approved to be cheaper, quicker, and effective (102).

5 Conclusion

This review aimed to objectively discuss and assess the role of microglia in regulating neuronal injury after ICH. The findings indicate that pro-inflammatory or anti-inflammatory microglia have divergent effects, which have significant implications for understanding microglia function via intracellular and extracellular signal-regulated pathways. Besides, this review provides the first comprehensive assessment of cellular and molecular mechanisms and pathways responsible for regulating microglia, including an in-depth analysis of signaling pathways strongly associated with microglia following ICH. Notwithstanding the relatively limited number of reliable clinical trials and the lack of molecular genetic studies on the phenotypic change of microglia, this work offers valuable insights into a novel therapeutic strategy for ICH that targets microglia. Further research on interventions associated with microglial physiology is an essential next step in confirming a framework for assessing the feasibility of the novel therapy mentioned above.

REFERENCES:

1. Ajami, B., Samusik, N., Wieghofer, P., Ho, P. P., Crotti, A., Bjornson, Z., Prinz, M., Fantl, W. J., Nolan, G. P. and Steinman, L. (2018) 'Single-cell mass cytometry reveals distinct populations of brain myeloid cells in mouse neuroinflammation and neurodegeneration models', Nat Neurosci, 21(4), 541-551.

2. Apolloni, S., Amadio, S., Fabbrizio, P., Morello, G., Spampinato, A. G., Latagliata, E. C., Salvatori, I., Proietti, D., Ferri, A., Madaro, L., Puglisi-Allegra, S., Cavallaro, S. and Volonté, C. (2019) 'Histaminergic transmission slows progression of amyotrophic lateral sclerosis', J Cachexia Sarcopenia Muscle, 10(4), 872-893.

3. Arcuri, C., Mecca, C., Bianchi, R., Giambanco, I. and Donato, R. (2017) 'The Pathophysiological Role of Microglia in Dynamic Surveillance, Phagocytosis and Structural Remodeling of the Developing CNS', Front Mol Neurosci, 10, 191.

4. Armando, R. G., Mengual Gómez, D. L. and Gomez, D. E. 'New drugs are not enough-drug repositioning in oncology: An update', (1791-2423 (Electronic)).

5. Bai, Y. Y. and Niu, J. Z. (2020) 'miR222 regulates brain injury and inflammation following intracerebral hemorrhage by targeting ITGB8', Mol Med Rep, 21(3), 1145-1153.

6. Bian, Z., Gong, Y., Huang, T., Lee, C. Z. W., Bian, L., Bai, Z., Shi, H., Zeng, Y., Liu, C., He, J., Zhou, J., Li, X., Li, Z., Ni, Y., Ma, C., Cui, L., Zhang, R., Chan, J. K.

Y., Ng, L. G., Lan, Y., Ginhoux, F. and Liu, B. (2020) 'Deciphering human macrophage development at single-cell resolution', Nature, 582(7813), 571-576.

7.   Brown, G. C. and St George-Hyslop, P. H. (2017) 'Deciphering microglial diversity in Alzheimer's disease', Science, 356(6343), 1123-1124.

8.   Carson, M. J., Doose, J. M., Melchior, B., Schmid, C. D. and Ploix, C. C. (2006) 'CNS immune privilege: hiding in plain sight', Immunol Rev, 213, 48-65.

9.   Chang, C. F., Goods, B. A., Askenase, M. H., Hammond, M. D., Renfroe, S. C., Steinschneider, A. F., Landreneau, M. J., Ai, Y., Beatty, H. E., da Costa, L. H. A., Mack, M., Sheth, K. N., Greer, D. M., Huttner, A., Coman, D., Hyder, F., Ghosh, S., Rothlin, C. V., Love, J. C. and Sansing, L. H. (2018) 'Erythrocyte efferocytosis modulates macrophages towards recovery after intracerebral hemorrhage', J Clin Invest, 128(2), 607-624.

10.   Chang, C. F., Wan, J., Li, Q., Renfroe, S. C., Heller, N. M. and Wang, J. (2017) 'Alternative activation-skewed microglia/macrophages promote hematoma resolution in experimental intracerebral hemorrhage', Neurobiol Dis, 103, 54-69.

11.   Chen, A. Q., Fang, Z., Chen, X. L., Yang, S., Zhou, Y. F., Mao, L., Xia, Y. P., Jin, H. J., Li, Y. N., You, M. F., Wang, X. X., Lei, H., He, Q. W. and Hu, B. (2019) 'Microglia-derived TNF-alpha mediates endothelial necroptosis aggravating blood brain-barrier disruption after ischemic stroke', Cell Death Dis, 10(7), 487.

12.   Chen, M., Li, X., Zhang, X., He, X., Lai, L., Liu, Y., Zhu, G., Li, W., Li, H., Fang, Q., Wang, Z. and Duan, C. (2015) 'The inhibitory effect of mesenchymal stem cell on blood-brain barrier disruption following intracerebral hemorrhage in rats: contribution of TSG-6', J Neuroinflammation, 12, 61.

13.   Chen, S., Peng, J., Sherchan, P., Ma, Y., Xiang, S., Yan, F., Zhao, H., Jiang, Y., Wang, N., Zhang, J. H. and Zhang, H. (2020) 'TREM2 activation attenuates neuroinflammation and neuronal apoptosis via PI3K/Akt pathway after intracerebral hemorrhage in mice', J Neuroinflammation, 17(1), 168.

14.   Chen, S., Zhao, L., Sherchan, P., Ding, Y., Yu, J., Nowrangi, D., Tang, J., Xia, Y. and Zhang, J. H. (2018) 'Activation of melanocortin receptor 4 with RO27-3225 attenuates neuroinflammation through AMPK/JNK/p38 MAPK pathway after intracerebral hemorrhage in mice', J Neuroinflammation, 15(1), 106.

15.   Chen, Z., Xu, N., Dai, X., Zhao, C., Wu, X., Shankar, S., Huang, H. and Wang, Z. (2019) 'Interleukin-33 reduces neuronal damage and white matter injury via selective microglia M2 polarization after intracerebral hemorrhage in rats', Brain Res Bull, 150, 127-135.

16.   Chiu, I. M., Morimoto, E. T., Goodarzi, H., Liao, J. T., O'Keeffe, S., Phatnani, H. P., Muratet, M., Carroll, M. C., Levy, S., Tavazoie, S., Myers, R. M. and Maniatis, T. (2013) 'A neurodegeneration-specific gene-expression signature of acutely isolated microglia from an amyotrophic lateral sclerosis mouse model', Cell Rep, 4(2), 385-401.

17. Dai, S., Hua, Y., Keep, R. F., Novakovic, N., Fei, Z. and Xi, G. (2019) 'Minocycline attenuates brain injury and iron overload after intracerebral hemorrhage in aged female rats', Neurobiol Dis, 126, 76-84.

18. Davis, M. J., Tsang, T. M., Qiu, Y., Dayrit, J. K., Freij, J. B., Huffnagle, G. B. and Olszewski, M. A. (2013) 'Macrophage M1/M2 polarization dynamically adapts to changes in cytokine microenvironments in Cryptococcus neoformans infection', mBio, 4(3), e00264-13.

19. Deng, S., Sherchan, P., Jin, P., Huang, L., Travis, Z., Zhang, J. H., Gong, Y. and Tang, J. (2020) 'Recombinant CCL17 Enhances Hematoma Resolution and Activation of CCR4/ERK/Nrf2/CD163 Signaling Pathway After Intracerebral Hemorrhage in Mice', Neurotherapeutics, 17(4), 1940-1953.

20. Desale, S. E. and Chinnathambi, S. (2020) 'Role of dietary fatty acids in microglial polarization in Alzheimer's disease', J Neuroinflammation, 17(1), 93.

21. Duan, X. C., Wang, W., Feng, D. X., Yin, J., Zuo, G., Chen, D. D., Chen, Z. Q., Li, H. Y., Wang, Z. and Chen, G. (2017) 'Roles of autophagy and endoplasmic reticulum stress in intracerebral hemorrhage-induced secondary brain injury in rats', CNS Neurosci Ther, 23(7), 554-566.

22. Eldahshan, W., Fagan, S. C. and Ergul, A. (2019) 'Inflammation within the neurovascular unit: Focus on microglia for stroke injury and recovery', Pharmacol Res, 147, 104349.

23. Fang, H., Chen, J., Lin, S., Wang, P., Wang, Y., Xiong, X. and Yang, Q. (2014) 'CD36-mediated hematoma absorption following intracerebral hemorrhage: negative regulation by TLR4 signaling', J Immunol, 192(12), 5984-92.

24. Fang, Y., Tian, Y., Huang, Q., Wan, Y., Xu, L., Wang, W., Pan, D., Zhu, S. and Xie, M. (2019) 'Deficiency of TREK-1 potassium channel exacerbates blood-brain barrier damage and neuroinflammation after intracerebral hemorrhage in mice', J Neuroinflammation, 16(1), 96.

25. Friedman, B. A., Srinivasan, K., Ayalon, G., Meilandt, W. J., Lin, H., Huntley, M. A., Cao, Y., Lee, S. H., Haddick, P. C. G., Ngu, H., Modrusan, Z., Larson, J. L., Kaminker, J. S., van der Brug, M. P. and Hansen, D. V. (2018) 'Diverse Brain Myeloid Expression Profiles Reveal Distinct Microglial Activation States and Aspects of Alzheimer's Disease Not Evident in Mouse Models', Cell Rep, 22(3), 832-847.

26. García-Revilla, J., Alonso-Bellido, I. M., Burguillos, M. A., Herrera, A. J., Espinosa-Oliva, A. M., Ruiz, R., Cruz-Hernández, L., García-Domínguez, I., Roca-Ceballos, M. A., Santiago, M., Rodríguez-Gómez, J. A., Soto, M. S., de Pablos, R. M. and Venero, J. L. (2019) 'Reformulating Pro-Oxidant Microglia in Neurodegeneration', J Clin Med, 8(10).

27. Geraghty, J. R., Davis, J. L. and Testai, F. D. (2019) 'Neuroinflammation and Microvascular Dysfunction After Experimental Subarachnoid Hemorrhage: Emerging Components of Early Brain Injury Related to Outcome', Neurocrit Care, 31(2), 373-

389.

28. Gosselin, D., Skola, D., Coufal, N. G., Holtman, I. R., Schlachetzki, J. C. M., Sajti, E., Jaeger, B. N., O'Connor, C., Fitzpatrick, C., Pasillas, M. P., Pena, M., Adair, A., Gonda, D. D., Levy, M. L., Ransohoff, R. M., Gage, F. H. and Glass, C. K. (2017) 'An environment-dependent transcriptional network specifies human microglia identity', Science, 356(6344).

29. Jing, C., Bian, L., Wang, M., Keep, R. F., Xi, G. and Hua, Y. (2019) 'Enhancement of Hematoma Clearance With CD47 Blocking Antibody in Experimental Intracerebral Hemorrhage', Stroke, 50(6), 1539-1547.

30. Jung, K. H., Chu, K., Lee, S. T., Kim, S. J., Song, E. C., Kim, E. H., Park, D. K., Sinn, D. I., Kim, J. M., Kim, M. and Roh, J. K. (2007) 'Blockade of AT1 receptor reduces apoptosis, inflammation, and oxidative stress in normotensive rats with intracerebral hemorrhage', J Pharmacol Exp Ther, 322(3), 1051-8.

31. Lan, X., Han, X., Li, Q., Yang, Q. W. and Wang, J. (2017) 'Modulators of microglial activation and polarization after intracerebral haemorrhage', Nat Rev Neurol, 13(7), 420-433.

32. Lassmann, H. (2020) 'Pathology of inflammatory diseases of the nervous system: Human disease versus animal models', Glia, 68(4), 830-844.

33. Li, M., Xia, M., Chen, W., Wang, J., Yin, Y., Guo, C., Li, C., Tang, X., Zhao, H., Tan, Q., Chen, Y., Jia, Z., Liu, X. and Feng, H. (2020) 'Lithium treatment mitigates white matter injury after intracerebral hemorrhage through brain-derived neurotrophic factor signaling in mice', Transl Res, 217, 61-74.

34. Li, Q., Wan, J., Lan, X., Han, X., Wang, Z. and Wang, J. (2017) 'Neuroprotection of brain-permeable iron chelator VK-28 against intracerebral hemorrhage in mice', J Cereb Blood Flow Metab, 37(9), 3110-3123.

35. Li, R., Liu, Z., Wu, X., Yu, Z., Zhao, S. and Tang, X. (2019) 'Lithium chloride promoted hematoma resolution after intracerebral hemorrhage through GSK-3beta-mediated pathways-dependent microglia phagocytosis and M2-phenotype differentiation, angiogenesis and neurogenesis in a rat model', Brain Res Bull, 152, 117-127.

36. Li, Y., Zhu, Z. Y., Lu, B. W., Huang, T. T., Zhang, Y. M., Zhou, N. Y., Xuan, W., Chen, Z. A., Wen, D. X., Yu, W. F. and Li, P. Y. (2019) 'Rosiglitazone ameliorates tissue plasminogen activator-induced brain hemorrhage after stroke', CNS Neurosci Ther, 25(12), 1343-1352.

37. Liang, H., Guan, D., Gao, A., Yin, Y., Jing, M., Yang, L., Ma, W., Hu, E. and Zhang, X. (2014) 'Human amniotic epithelial stem cells inhibit microglia activation through downregulation of tumor necrosis factor-alpha, interleukin-1beta and matrix metalloproteinase-12 in vitro and in a rat model of intracerebral hemorrhage', Cytotherapy, 16(4), 523-34.

38. Liang, H., Sun, Y., Gao, A., Zhang, N., Jia, Y., Yang, S., Na, M., Liu, H., Cheng, X., Fang, X., Ma, W., Zhang, X. and Wang, F. (2019) 'Ac-YVAD-cmk improves neurological function by inhibiting caspase-1-mediated inflammatory response in the intracerebral hemorrhage of rats', Int Immunopharmacol, 75, 105771.

39. Liu, D. L., Zhao, L. X., Zhang, S. and Du, J. R. (2016) 'Peroxiredoxin 1-mediated activation of TLR4/NF-kappaB pathway contributes to neuroinflammatory injury in intracerebral hemorrhage', Int Immunopharmacol, 41, 82-89.

40. Martinez, F. O. and Gordon, S. (2014) 'The M1 and M2 paradigm of macrophage activation: time for reassessment', F1000Prime Rep, 6, 13.

41. Masuda, T., Sankowski, R., Staszewski, O., Böttcher, C., Amann, L., Sagar, Scheiwe, C., Nessler, S., Kunz, P., van Loo, G., Coenen, V. A., Reinacher, P. C., Michel, A., Sure, U., Gold, R., Grün, D., Priller, J., Stadelmann, C. and Prinz, M. (2019) 'Spatial and temporal heterogeneity of mouse and human microglia at single-cell resolution', Nature, 566(7744), 388-392.

42. Miao, H., Li, R., Han, C., Lu, X. and Zhang, H. (2018) 'Minocycline promotes posthemorrhagic neurogenesis via M2 microglia polarization via upregulation of the TrkB/BDNF pathway in rats', J Neurophysiol, 120(3), 1307-1317.

43. Ochocka, N., Segit, P., Walentynowicz, K. A., Wojnicki, K., Cyranowski, S., Swatler, J., Mieczkowski, J. and Kaminska, B. (2021) 'Single-cell RNA sequencing reveals functional heterogeneity of glioma-associated brain macrophages', Nat Commun, 12(1), 1151.

44. Ohnishi, M., Katsuki, H., Fujimoto, S., Takagi, M., Kume, T. and Akaike, A. (2007) 'Involvement of thrombin and mitogen-activated protein kinase pathways in hemorrhagic brain injury', Exp Neurol, 206(1), 43-52.

45. Olah, M., Menon, V., Habib, N., Taga, M. F., Ma, Y., Yung, C. J., Cimpean, M., Khairallah, A., Coronas-Samano, G., Sankowski, R., Grün, D., Kroshilina, A. A., Dionne, D., Sarkis, R. A., Cosgrove, G. R., Helgager, J., Golden, J. A., Pennell, P. B., Prinz, M., Vonsattel, J. P. G., Teich, A. F., Schneider, J. A., Bennett, D. A., Regev, A., Elyaman, W., Bradshaw, E. M. and De Jager, P. L. (2020) 'Single cell RNA sequencing of human microglia uncovers a subset associated with Alzheimer's disease', Nat Commun, 11(1), 6129.

46. Prinz, M., Erny, D. and Hagemeyer, N. (2017) 'Ontogeny and homeostasis of CNS myeloid cells', Nat Immunol, 18(4), 385-392.

47. Prinz, M., Jung, S. and Priller, J. (2019) 'Microglia Biology: One Century of Evolving Concepts', Cell, 179(2), 292-311.

48. Rangaraju, S., Dammer, E. B., Raza, S. A., Rathakrishnan, P., Xiao, H., Gao, T., Duong, D. M., Pennington, M. W., Lah, J. J., Seyfried, N. T. and Levey, A. I. (2018) 'Identification and therapeutic modulation of a pro-inflammatory subset of disease-associated-microglia in Alzheimer's disease', Mol Neurodegener, 13(1), 24.

49. Ransohoff, R. M. (2016) 'A polarizing question: do M1 and M2 microglia exist?', Nat Neurosci, 19(8), 987-91.

50. Ronaldson, P. T. and Davis, T. P. (2020) 'Regulation of blood-brain barrier integrity by microglia in health and disease: A therapeutic opportunity', J Cereb Blood Flow Metab, 40(1_suppl), S6-s24.

51. Ryu, J., Pyo, H., Jou, I. and Joe, E. (2000) 'Thrombin induces NO release from cultured rat microglia via protein kinase C, mitogen-activated protein kinase, and NF-kappa B', J Biol Chem, 275(39), 29955-9.

52. Sansing, L. H., Harris, T. H., Welsh, F. A., Kasner, S. E., Hunter, C. A. and Kariko, K. (2011) 'Toll-like receptor 4 contributes to poor outcome after intracerebral hemorrhage', Ann Neurol, 70(4), 646-56.

53. Sekerdag, E., Solaroglu, I. and Gursoy-Ozdemir, Y. (2018) 'Cell Death Mechanisms in Stroke and Novel Molecular and Cellular Treatment Options', Curr Neuropharmacol, 16(9), 1396-1415.

54. Shi, H., Wang, J., Wang, J., Huang, Z. and Yang, Z. (2018) 'IL-17A induces autophagy and promotes microglial neuroinflammation through ATG5 and ATG7 in intracerebral hemorrhage', J Neuroimmunol, 323, 143-151.

55. Shi, S. X., Li, Y. J., Shi, K., Wood, K., Ducruet, A. F. and Liu, Q. (2020) 'IL (Interleukin)-15 Bridges Astrocyte-Microglia Crosstalk and Exacerbates Brain Injury Following Intracerebral Hemorrhage', Stroke, 51(3), 967-974.

56. Su, E. J., Cao, C., Fredriksson, L., Nilsson, I., Stefanitsch, C., Stevenson, T. K., Zhao, J., Ragsdale, M., Sun, Y. Y., Yepes, M., Kuan, C. Y., Eriksson, U., Strickland, D. K., Lawrence, D. A. and Zhang, L. (2017) 'Microglial-mediated PDGF-CC activation increases cerebrovascular permeability during ischemic stroke', Acta Neuropathol, 134(4), 585-604.

57. Tan, X., Yang, Y., Xu, J., Zhang, P., Deng, R., Mao, Y., He, J., Chen, Y., Zhang, Y., Ding, J., Li, H., Shen, H., Li, X., Dong, W. and Chen, G. (2019) 'Luteolin Exerts Neuroprotection via Modulation of the p62/Keap1/Nrf2 Pathway in Intracerebral Hemorrhage', Front Pharmacol, 10, 1551.

58. Taylor, R. A., Chang, C. F., Goods, B. A., Hammond, M. D., Mac Grory, B., Ai, Y., Steinschneider, A. F., Renfroe, S. C., Askenase, M. H., McCullough, L. D., Kasner, S. E., Mullen, M. T., Hafler, D. A., Love, J. C. and Sansing, L. H. (2017) 'TGF-beta1 modulates microglial phenotype and promotes recovery after intracerebral hemorrhage', J Clin Invest, 127(1), 280-292.

59. Tschoe, C., Bushnell, C. D., Duncan, P. W., Alexander-Miller, M. A. and Wolfe, S. Q. (2020) 'Neuroinflammation after Intracerebral Hemorrhage and Potential Therapeutic Targets', J Stroke, 22(1), 29-46.

60. Vainchtein, I. D. and Molofsky, A. V. (2020) 'Astrocytes and Microglia: In Sickness and in Health', Trends Neurosci, 43(3), 144-154.

61. Vinukonda, G., Liao, Y., Hu, F., Ivanova, L., Purohit, D., Finkel, D. A., Giri, P., Bapatla, L., Shah, S., Zia, M. T., Hussein, K., Cairo, M. S. and La Gamma, E. F. (2019) 'Human Cord Blood-Derived Unrestricted Somatic Stem Cell Infusion Improves Neurobehavioral Outcome in a Rabbit Model of Intraventricular Hemorrhage', Stem Cells Transl Med, 8(11), 1157-1169.

62. Wan, S., Cheng, Y., Jin, H., Guo, D., Hua, Y., Keep, R. F. and Xi, G. (2016) 'Microglia Activation and Polarization After Intracerebral Hemorrhage in Mice: the Role of Protease-Activated Receptor-1', Transl Stroke Res, 7(6), 478-487.

63. Wang, G., Li, T., Duan, S. N., Dong, L., Sun, X. G. and Xue, F. (2018a) 'PPAR-gamma Promotes Hematoma Clearance through Haptoglobin-Hemoglobin-CD163 in a Rat Model of Intracerebral Hemorrhage', Behav Neurol, 2018, 7646104.

64. Wang, G., Li, Z., Li, S., Ren, J., Suresh, V., Xu, D., Zang, W., Liu, X., Li, W., Wang, H. and Guo, F. (2019) 'Minocycline Preserves the Integrity and Permeability of BBB by Altering the Activity of DKK1-Wnt Signaling in ICH Model', Neuroscience, 415, 135-146.

65. Wang, G., Wang, L., Sun, X. G. and Tang, J. (2018b) 'Haematoma scavenging in intracerebral haemorrhage: from mechanisms to the clinic', J Cell Mol Med, 22(2), 768-777.

66. Wang, J. (2010) 'Preclinical and clinical research on inflammation after intracerebral hemorrhage', Prog Neurobiol, 92(4), 463-77.

67. Wang, M., Cheng, L., Chen, Z. L., Mungur, R., Xu, S. H., Wu, J., Liu, X. L. and Wan, S. (2019a) 'Hyperbaric oxygen preconditioning attenuates brain injury after intracerebral hemorrhage by regulating microglia polarization in rats', CNS Neurosci Ther, 25(10), 1126-1133.

68. Wang, M., Hua, Y., Keep, R. F., Wan, S., Novakovic, N. and Xi, G. (2019b) 'Complement Inhibition Attenuates Early Erythrolysis in the Hematoma and Brain Injury in Aged Rats', Stroke, 50(7), 1859-1868.

69. Wang, Y., Chen, Q., Tan, Q., Feng, Z., He, Z., Tang, J., Feng, H., Zhu, G. and Chen, Z. (2018) 'Simvastatin accelerates hematoma resolution after intracerebral hemorrhage in a PPARgamma-dependent manner', Neuropharmacology, 128, 244-254.

70. Wang, Z., Yuan, B., Fu, F., Huang, S. and Yang, Z. (2017) 'Hemoglobin enhances miRNA-144 expression and autophagic activation mediated inflammation of microglia via mTOR pathway', Sci Rep, 7(1), 11861.

71. Wasserman, J. K. and Schlichter, L. C. (2007) 'Minocycline protects the blood-brain barrier and reduces edema following intracerebral hemorrhage in the rat', Exp Neurol, 207(2), 227-37.

72. Wasserman, J. K., Zhu, X. and Schlichter, L. C. (2007) 'Evolution of the inflammatory response in the brain following intracerebral hemorrhage and effects of

delayed minocycline treatment', Brain Res, 1180, 140-54.

73. Wells, J. E., Biernaskie, J., Szymanska, A., Larsen, P. H., Yong, V. W. and Corbett, D. (2005) 'Matrix metalloproteinase (MMP)-12 expression has a negative impact on sensorimotor function following intracerebral haemorrhage in mice', Eur J Neurosci, 21(1), 187-96.

74. Wolf, S. A., Boddeke, H. W. and Kettenmann, H. (2017) 'Microglia in Physiology and Disease', Annu Rev Physiol, 79, 619-643.

75. Wu, C. H., Shyue, S. K., Hung, T. H., Wen, S., Lin, C. C., Chang, C. F. and Chen, S. F. (2017) 'Genetic deletion or pharmacological inhibition of soluble epoxide hydrolase reduces brain damage and attenuates neuroinflammation after intracerebral hemorrhage', J Neuroinflammation, 14(1), 230.

76. Wu, H., Wu, T., Xu, X., Wang, J. and Wang, J. (2011) 'Iron toxicity in mice with collagenase-induced intracerebral hemorrhage', J Cereb Blood Flow Metab, 31(5), 1243-50.

77. Xiao, H., Chen, H., Jiang, R., Zhang, L., Wang, L., Gan, H., Jiang, N., Zhao, J., Zhai, X. and Liang, P. (2020) 'NLRP6 contributes to inflammation and brain injury following intracerebral haemorrhage by activating autophagy', J Mol Med (Berl), 98(9), 1319-1331.

78. Xu, J., Chen, Z., Yu, F., Liu, H., Ma, C., Xie, D., Hu, X., Leak, R. K., Chou, S. H. Y., Stetler, R. A., Shi, Y., Chen, J., Bennett, M. V. L. and Chen, G. (2020) 'IL-4/STAT6 signaling facilitates innate hematoma resolution and neurological recovery after hemorrhagic stroke in mice', Proc Natl Acad Sci U S A, 117(51), 32679-32690.

79. Xu, R., Wang, S., Li, W., Liu, Z., Tang, J. and Tang, X. (2017) 'Activation of peroxisome proliferator-activated receptor-gamma by a 12/15-lipoxygenase product of arachidonic acid: a possible neuroprotective effect in the brain after experimental intracerebral hemorrhage', J Neurosurg, 127(3), 522-531.

80. Xue, M., Hollenberg, M. D. and Yong, V. W. (2006) 'Combination of thrombin and matrix metalloproteinase-9 exacerbates neurotoxicity in cell culture and intracerebral hemorrhage in mice', J Neurosci, 26(40), 10281-91.

81. Yang, X., Sun, J., Kim, T. J., Kim, Y. J., Ko, S. B., Kim, C. K., Jia, X. and Yoon, B. W. (2018) 'Pretreatment with low-dose fimasartan ameliorates NLRP3 inflammasome-mediated neuroinflammation and brain injury after intracerebral hemorrhage', Exp Neurol, 310, 22-32.

82. Yang, Z., Jiang, X., Zhang, J., Huang, X., Zhang, X., Wang, J., Shi, H. and Yu, A. (2018) 'Let-7a promotes microglia M2 polarization by targeting CKIP-1 following ICH', Immunol Lett, 202, 1-7.

83. Yang, Z., Liu, B., Zhong, L., Shen, H., Lin, C., Lin, L., Zhang, N. and Yuan, B. (2015) 'Toll-like receptor-4-mediated autophagy contributes to microglial activation and inflammatory injury in mouse models of intracerebral haemorrhage', Neuropathol

Appl Neurobiol, 41(4), e95-106.

84. Yang, Z., Yu, A., Liu, Y., Shen, H., Lin, C., Lin, L., Wang, S. and Yuan, B. (2014a) 'Regulatory T cells inhibit microglia activation and protect against inflammatory injury in intracerebral hemorrhage', Int Immunopharmacol, 22(2), 522-5.

85. Yang, Z., Zhao, T., Zou, Y., Zhang, J. H. and Feng, H. (2014b) 'Curcumin inhibits microglia inflammation and confers neuroprotection in intracerebral hemorrhage', Immunol Lett, 160(1), 89-95.

86. Yao, S. T., Cao, F., Chen, J. L., Chen, W., Fan, R. M., Li, G., Zeng, Y. C., Jiao, S., Xia, X. P., Han, C. and Ran, Q. S. (2017) 'NLRP3 is Required for Complement-Mediated Caspase-1 and IL-1beta Activation in ICH', J Mol Neurosci, 61(3), 385-395.

87. Yin, M., Chen, Z., Ouyang, Y., Zhang, H., Wan, Z., Wang, H., Wu, W. and Yin, X. (2017a) 'Thrombin-induced, TNFR-dependent miR-181c downregulation promotes MLL1 and NF-kappaB target gene expression in human microglia', J Neuroinflammation, 14(1), 132.

88. Yin, M., Chen, Z., Ouyang, Y., Zhang, H., Wan, Z., Wang, H., Wu, W. and Yin, X. (2017b) 'Thrombin-induced, TNFR-dependent miR-181c downregulation promotes MLL1 and NF-κB target gene expression in human microglia', J Neuroinflammation, 14(1), 132.

89. Yu, A., Duan, H., Zhang, T., Pan, Y., Kou, Z., Zhang, X., Lu, Y., Wang, S. and Yang, Z. (2016) 'IL-17A promotes microglial activation and neuroinflammation in mouse models of intracerebral haemorrhage', Mol Immunol, 73, 151-7.

90. Zhang, X. D., Fan, Q. Y., Qiu, Z. and Chen, S. (2018) 'MiR-7 alleviates secondary inflammatory response of microglia caused by cerebral hemorrhage through inhibiting TLR4 expression', Eur Rev Med Pharmacol Sci, 22(17), 5597-5604.

91. Zhang, Y., Han, B., He, Y., Li, D., Ma, X., Liu, Q. and Hao, J. (2017) 'MicroRNA-132 attenuates neurobehavioral and neuropathological changes associated with intracerebral hemorrhage in mice', Neurochem Int, 107, 182-190.

92. Zhang, Z., Zhang, Z., Lu, H., Yang, Q., Wu, H. and Wang, J. (2017) 'Microglial Polarization and Inflammatory Mediators After Intracerebral Hemorrhage', Mol Neurobiol, 54(3), 1874-1886.

93. Zhao, F., Hua, Y., He, Y., Keep, R. F. and Xi, G. (2011) 'Minocycline-induced attenuation of iron overload and brain injury after experimental intracerebral hemorrhage', Stroke, 42(12), 3587-93.

94. Zhao, L., Chen, S., Sherchan, P., Ding, Y., Zhao, W., Guo, Z., Yu, J., Tang, J. and Zhang, J. H. (2018) 'Recombinant CTRP9 administration attenuates neuroinflammation via activating adiponectin receptor 1 after intracerebral hemorrhage in mice', J Neuroinflammation, 15(1), 215.

95. Zhao, S., Liu, Z., Yu, Z., Wu, X., Li, R. and Tang, X. (2019) 'BIO alleviates

inflammation through inhibition of GSK-3beta in a rat model of intracerebral hemorrhage', J Neurosurg, 1-9.

96. Zhao, X., Grotta, J., Gonzales, N. and Aronowski, J. (2009) 'Hematoma resolution as a therapeutic target: the role of microglia/macrophages', Stroke, 40(3 Suppl), S92-4.

97. Zhao, X., Sun, G., Zhang, J., Strong, R., Song, W., Gonzales, N., Grotta, J. C. and Aronowski, J. (2007) 'Hematoma resolution as a target for intracerebral hemorrhage treatment: role for peroxisome proliferator-activated receptor gamma in microglia/macrophages', Ann Neurol, 61(4), 352-62.

98. Zheng, J., Liu, Z., Li, W., Tang, J., Zhang, D. and Tang, X. (2017) 'Lithium posttreatment confers neuroprotection through glycogen synthase kinase-3beta inhibition in intracerebral hemorrhage rats', J Neurosurg, 127(4), 716-724.

99. Zhou, K., Zhong, Q., Wang, Y. C., Xiong, X. Y., Meng, Z. Y., Zhao, T., Zhu, W. Y., Liao, M. F., Wu, L. R., Yang, Y. R., Liu, J., Duan, C. M., Li, J., Gong, Q. W., Liu, L., Yang, M. H., Xiong, A., Wang, J. and Yang, Q. W. (2017) 'Regulatory T cells ameliorate intracerebral hemorrhage-induced inflammatory injury by modulating microglia/macrophage polarization through the IL-10/GSK3beta/PTEN axis', J Cereb Blood Flow Metab, 37(3), 967-979.

100. Zhou, Y., Wang, Y., Wang, J., Anne Stetler, R. and Yang, Q. W. (2014) 'Inflammation in intracerebral hemorrhage: from mechanisms to clinical translation', Prog Neurobiol, 115, 25-44.

101. Zhuang, J., Peng, Y., Gu, C., Chen, H., Lin, Z., Zhou, H., Wu, X., Li, J., Yu, X., Cao, Y., Zeng, H., Fu, X., Xu, C., Huang, P., Cao, S., Wang, C., Yan, F. and Chen, G. (2020) 'Wogonin Accelerates Hematoma Clearance and Improves Neurological Outcome via the PPAR-γ Pathway After Intracerebral Hemorrhage', Transl Stroke Res.

102. Zlokovic, B. V. (2008) 'The blood-brain barrier in health and chronic neurodegenerative disorders', Neuron, 57(2), 178-201.

CONFLICT OF INTEREST

The authors declare that the research was conducted in the absence of any commercial or financial relationships that could be construed as a potential conflict of interest.

ACKNOWLEDGEMENT

This work was supported by a grant from National Natural Science Foundation of China (81771294)

DECLARATION: This chapter was authored by Jiachen Liu, Lirong Liu, Xiaoyu Wang, Rundong Jiang, Qinqin Bai and Gaiqing Wang published as "Microglia: A double-edged sword in intracerebral hemorrhage from basic mechanisms to clinical research" in "Frontiers in Immunology", 2021;675660

CHAPTER 7:

Interaction of microglia and astrocytes in the neurovascular unit

ABSTRACT:

The interaction between microglia and astrocytes significantly influences neuroinflammation. Microglia/astrocytes, part of the neurovascular unit (NVU), are activated by various brain insults. The local extracellular and intracellular signals determine their characteristics and switch of phenotypes. Microglia and astrocytes are activated into two polarization states: the pro-inflammatory phenotype (M1 and A1) and the anti-inflammatory phenotype (M2 and A2). During neuroinflammation, induced by stroke or lipopolysaccharides, microglia are more sensitive to pathogens, or damage; they are thus initially activated into the M1 phenotype and produce common inflammatory signals such as IL-1 and TNF-α to trigger reactive astrocytes into the A1 phenotype. These inflammatory signals can be amplified not only by the self-feedback loop of microglial activation but also by the unique anatomy structure of astrocytes. As the pathology further progresses, resulting in local environmental changes, M1-like microglia switch to the M2 phenotype, and M2 crosstalk with A2. While astrocytes communicate simultaneously with neurons and blood vessels to maintain the function of neurons and the blood–brain barrier (BBB), their subtle changes may be identified and responded by astrocytes, and possibly transferred to microglia. Although both microglia and astrocytes have different functional characteristics, they can achieve immune "optimization" through their mutual communication and cooperation in the NVU and build a cascaded immune network of amplification.

KEY WORDS: Microglia; Astrocyte; Neuroinflammation; Stroke; Polarization phenotype; Neurovascular unit;

INTRODUCTION

Neuroinflammation often runs through the entire process of pathological development. There is a dynamic change over time with the regulation of pro and anti-inflammatory signals (1, 2). Microglia/astrocytes, part of the neurovascular unit (NVU), are activated by various brain insults. The local extracellular and intracellular signals determine their characteristics and switch of phenotypes. Generally, microglia and astrocytes are activated into two states: the pro-inflammatory phenotype (M1/A1) and the anti-inflammatory phenotype (M2/A2), corresponding to either the destructive or reparative functions in the NVU, respectively (3–5). The activated microglia and astrocytes have dynamic phenotypic changes (6–9). The crosstalk between microglia and astrocytes occurs through a variety of molecule signals such as adenosine triphosphate (ATP), cytokines, etc (10).

Liddelow et al (9) showed that reactive astrocytes (A1) can be induced by the cytokines secreted from activated microglia(M1), which are induced by lipopolysaccharides (LPS) in vitro and in vivo (11). Microglia appear to be more sensitive to pathogens or damage, which stimulate them and promote secretion of "molecular signals" to trigger reactive astrocytes. Neuroinflammation, such as in stroke, may exhibit a similar mechanism and interaction between microglia, and astrocytes may share the common molecular language in various diseases. It has been previously shown that neuroinflammation between the microglia and astrocytes has a cascade of amplification (12–14), but its mechanism needs further elucidation. As the pathology progresses, thus causing environmental changes, it promotes the switch from M1 to M2, which is also closely associated with A2. While astrocytes, an essential component of the NVU, communicate simultaneously with both neurons and blood vessels as versatile cells to maintain the function of neurons and the blood–brain barrier (BBB), there seems to be a difference in the communication of astrocytes from microglia. This review is concerned with the origin, anatomy, and physiological function of microglia and astrocytes, particularly their communication and cooperation in pathological conditions. The activated microglia and astrocytes may achieve immune "optimization" through their interaction in the NVU.

MICROGLIA AND ASTROCYTES IN THE NVU

The NVU, a structural and functional unit, is composed of microglia, neurons, the BBB, and the extracellular matrix (15). Its primary function is to meet the brain's dynamic metabolic needs by regulating the cerebral blood flow (CBF) in response to physiological or pathological stimuli in the CNS (16, 17). The BBB consists of vascular endothelial cells (ECs), tight junctions, and basement membranes, pericytes, or smooth muscle cells, and astrocytes. It separates parenchyma of the central nervous system (CNS) from blood, and it thus maintains a stable micro-environmental homeostasis of CNS (18, 19). The BBB maintains the low permeability through the tight-junction between endothelial cells with membrane-bound transporters, and perivascular cells, such as pericytes, astrocytes, and the extracellular matrix, also contribute to this (17, 20). Astrocytes promote the maintenance of the BBB via sonic hedgehog and b-catenin, which strengthen the tight junction and integrity (21). Meanwhile, reactive astrocytes disrupt the local BBB by the release of vascular endothelial growth factor (VEGF), increase permeability, and allow entry of peripheral immune cells (22, 23). Astrocytes are considered an indispensable element of the NVU or extended BBB. In the context of the NVU, astrocytes are located in the center between neurons and ECs. The strategic position of astrocytes enable them to regulate CBF to adapt to dynamic changes in neuronal metabolism and synaptic activity (18, 24). Astrocytes co-originate with neurons and oligodendrocytes and are produced in the final stages of neurogenesis (25, 26). They are the most abundant and heterogeneous glia cell type, tiling throughout the brain in a non-overlapping manner in the CNS (27).

Astrocytes are closely associated with neurons and blood vessels as versatile cells (28, 29) and communicate with neuronal pre- and post-synaptic terminals to help modulate synaptic transmission by the release of glutamate, D-serine, and ATP. It has been reported that one astrocyte can supervise over 100,000 synapses (30–33). Astrocytes can be extensively coupled into syncytial structures of up to 100 units by gap junctions, composed of connexin (CX) proteins such as CX-43 and CX−30 subtypes, allowing for the rapid facilitation of long- range signaling through calcium waves (34–37). Astrocytes extend end-feet processes to cover the surface of cerebral blood vessels with a ratio of ~99% to modulate CBF or the BBB(24). Furthermore, the end-feet with high levels of aquaporin-4 water channel proteins promote perivascular clearance by the newly characterized "glymphatic system" (CNS waste clearance system) (38, 39).

Astrocytes were, in the past, considered simply as a supportive or "glue-" like function in the CNS; now, their essential functions are increasingly being elucidated (28). Besides the abovementioned effects of "glymphatic system" (39, 40), astrocytes also have neurotrophic support, promote formation, and maintenance of synaptic activity, and transmission, regulate CBF, and determine some functions, and properties of the BBB, or NVU (27). In physiological conditions, astrocytes restrict the entry of peripheral immune cells passing through the BBB (41). While in pathological conditions, astrocytes participate in innate immune reactions (42) and the adaptive immune responses by their strategic position (43, 44).

Microglia, an important partner of the NVU, are the primary immune cells and account for ~5–15% of all cells in the human brain (45, 46). Early in development, microglia derive from the yolk sac, and seed in the brain as the first glial cells,

and they develop concurrently with neurons into highly plastic cells with mobility (47–49). Under physiological or pathological conditions, microglia continuously survey their surrounding environment and always firstly respond to any insult in the CNS (50-52).

There is a local network of immune cells via communication and collaboration in the CNS against pathogenic insults, injury, or stress (44). Microglia, scattered throughout the brain, wander more observantly and detect modifications of their environment as sentinels (42, 53). Whether as the first glial cells seeded in the brain early in embryonic development or as the first to respond to insults in CNS, microglia are always the "pioneers" in the NVU. On the other hand, astrocytes with a more dominant quantity may be "reserve forces" and amplify the neuroinflammation, owing to syncytium of the structure and function and strategic position to mobilize peripheral immunity (54).

ASSOCIATION OF MICROGLIA, ASTROCYTES, AND NEUROINFLAMMATION

Neuroinflammation is constantly present at every different pathological state in CNS diseases. Neuroinflammation is induced when the NVU responds to specific stimuli involved in the activation of microglia and astrocytes, breakdown of the BBB, infiltration of peripheral leukocytes, and inflammation factors, etc. (55). Activated microglia and reactive astrocytes play a crucial role in neuroinflammation. The dynamic phenotypic changes of microglia and astrocytes determine their detrimental or beneficial character at particular stages (7, 9). Microglia and astrocytes in NVU is illustrated in Figure 1.

Microglia

Microglia, the first activated innate immune cells, can be activated within minutes of tissue damage (56). Activated microglia, with changes from the ramified morphology into an amoeboid shape, upregulate the secretion of numerous inflammation factors, and microglial phagocytosis (57).

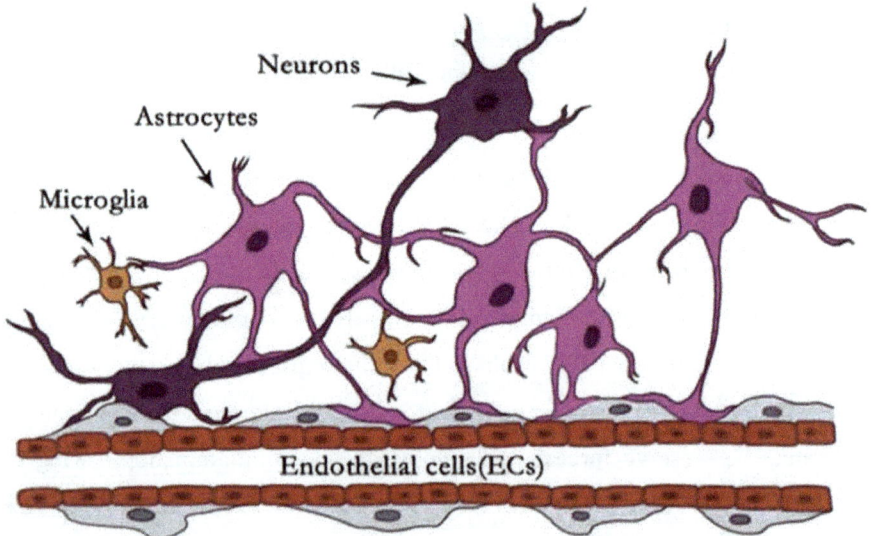

FIGURE 1 | Illustration of microglia and astrocytes in NVU. In the context of the NVU, astrocytes are located in the center between neurons and endothelial cells (ECs). Astrocytes are closely associated with neurons and blood vessels as versatile cells. Astrocytes communicate with neuronal pre- and postsynaptic terminals to help modulate synaptic transmission. It has been reported that one astrocyte can supervise over 100,000 synapses. Astrocytes extend end-feet processes to cover the surface of cerebral blood vessels with a ratio of ~99% to modulate CBF or the BBB. Astrocytes can be organized into syncytial structures of up to 100 units by gap junctions to facilitate long-range signaling. Microglia account for about 5–15% of all cells in the human brain. Under physiological or pathological conditions, they scan their environment through scavenging functions. Microglia firstly react to brain insults like "pioneers," monitoring and transmitting "danger." Astrocytes with dominant quantity may be "reserve forces" and amplify the neuroinflammation, owing to their syncytium of the structure, and function, and strategic position to mobilize peripheral immunity.

The local extracellular and intracellular signals determine their characteristics and switch of phenotypes, which range from "M1-like" phenotypes characterized by increase of inflammatory mediators, such as tumor necrosis factor (TNF), interleukin 1 beta (IL-1β), and reactive oxygen species (ROS) (58), to "M2-like" phenotypes characterized by upregulation of anti-inflammatory mediators, such as Interleukin IL-10, transforming growth factor beta (TGFβ), and glucocorticoids (59). The M1-like phenotype is considered to be destructive to NVU (60), while the M2- like phenotype is interpreted to be nerve repair cells in CNS diseases (61). Moreover, microglia display intermediate phenotypes with diverse combination of polarization markers ranging from M1 to M2, representing the crossroads of diverse pro- and anti- inflammatory (62–64). Although the supposed dichotomy of M1/M2 phenotypes hardly reflect a wide range of microglial phenotypes, this facilitates understanding of the activated state of microglia in various CNS disorders (3).

Astrocytes

Astrocytes are another type of glial cells that actively participate in regulation of neuroinflammation, depending on the timing and context (65). Following diverse brain injuries, astrocytes undergo a significant transformation called "reactive astrocytosis," whereby they upregulate many genes, increase the size of cytoskeleton, process extension, increase expression and immunoreactivity of glial fibrillary acidic protein (GFAP), and form a glial scar (5, 66, 67). Reactive astrocytes were purified and genetically analyzed in mice about neuroinflammation induced by systemic injection of LPS or cerebral ischemia induced by middle cerebral artery occlusion (MCAO). Neuroinflammation and ischemia induced two different types of reactive astrocytes, which correspond to "A1" pro-inflammatory and "A2" anti- inflammatory, respectively. This nomenclature is similar to the "M1" and "M2" of microglia (9). Different polarizations of astrocytes are marked by different biochemical and functional characteristics (68–70). A1 reactive astrocytes elevate levels of many genes of the classic complement cascade, such as C1r, C1s, C3, and C4, which are harmful for the NVU. Meanwhile, A2 reactive astrocytes upregulate beneficial inflammatory factors, such as CLCF1 (cardiotrophin-like cytokine factor 1), LIF (hypoxia induce factor), IL-6, IL-10, and thrombospondins, to promote the NVU remodeling (5, 9). Reactive astrocytosis also represents a spectrum of alterations reflecting the specific insults in the CNS (9, 54).

The association of microglia, astrocytes, and neuroinflammation is illustrated in Figure 2.

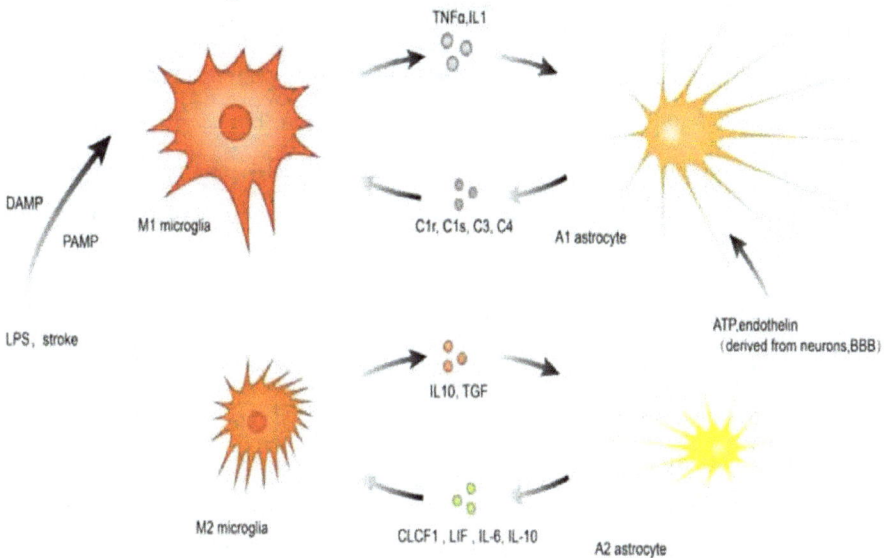

FIGURE 2 | Illustration of microglia, astrocytes, and neuroinflammation. Microglia are more sensitive to pathogens/damage such as LPS or stroke, firstly activated into M1-like phenotypes via PAMP/DAMP and promote the secretion of inflammatory factors such as TNF-a, IL-1, etc. to trigger reactive astrocyte (A1). As the insult limited and the NVU is remodeling, the local environmental factors change and determine M2-like phenotype to upregulate microglial phagocytosis and secretion of IL10, TGF, etc. Simultaneously, the local environmental factors may promote the switch to A2. Astrocytes communicate simultaneously with both neurons and blood vessels as versatile cells to maintain the function of neurons and the blood–brain barrier, and their subtle changes may be captured and responded by astrocytes and even transferred to microglia. A variety of molecular signals such as ATP, endothelin, etc. trigger reactive astrocytes (A1) and A1 upregulates many genes of the classic complement cascade such as C1r, C1s, C3, and C4, which communicate with microglia via some corresponding complement receptors; A2 elevates the levels of neurotrophic factors and cytokines such as CLCF1, LIF, IL-6, IL-10, and thrombospondins to promote neuronal survival and repair; the local environmental factors promote the switch to M2-like phenotype.

INTERACTION OF MICROGLIA AND ASTROCYTES IN THE NVU

The Common Molecular Signals of Interaction

Reactive astrocytes are induced by LPS-activated microglia (11, 56, 71). Liddelow et al. (9) showed that reactive astrocytes (A1) can be induced by cytokines, such as interleukin-1 alpha (IL-1α), TNF-α, and the complement component subunit 1q(C1q), which secreted by activated microglia (M1) both in vitro and in vivo. (11). Microglia appear to be more sensitive to pathogens; they activate and secrete "molecular signals" to trigger reactive astrocytes. Interaction between activated microglia and astrocytes plays a crucial role in the process of neuroinflammation. Neuroinflammation of diverse CNS diseases such as stroke may share the common "molecular signals" to trigger astrocytes reaction, and these inflammation signals may be amplified (72).

The activation of microglia occurs early in the timeline of neuroinflammation following stroke besides LPS-induced inflammation. Microglial activation within the perihematomal region, by immunofluorescence staining, was seen within 1 h of intracerebral hemorrhage (ICH) in a model of ICH (73, 74). In a clinical study of perihematomal brain tissue, TNF and IL-1β levels increased within 1 day of ICH (75, 76). After collagenase- induced or autologous blood-induced ICH, IL-1β, TNF, IL-6 (77, 78), and inducible nitric oxide synthase (iNOS) (25), mRNA levels were generally upregulated in the acute phase, starting to rise in the first 3 h after ICH and peaking at 3 days (79, 80). Changes in the protein levels corresponded to the timeline (25, 80, 81). Similarly, in the acute phase of ischemic stroke, microglia were activated first and invaded the peri-infarct and infarct core to orchestrate the post-stroke neuroinflammatory response and communicated with astrocytes through soluble and membrane-bound signaling molecules (82–84), including the cytokines IL-1β, TNF, and IL-1 receptor antagonist (IL- 1Ra) (82, 83, 85). These studies imply that microglia in stroke are more sensitive to pathogens/damage; which are activated and produce then produce the common "molecular signals," such as IL- 1 and TNF, to trigger reactive astrocytes (11, 86).

Meanwhile, another study showed highly enriched astrocyte cultures produced only a very few inflammatory factors, such as TNF-α, reactive oxygen species (ROS), and nitric oxide (NO), in response to LPS stimulation. Astrocytes seem to be sluggish in response to pathogens stimulation and fail to be completely activated in the absence of microglia (87). TNF-α is a multi-effect cytokine mostly released from microglia/macrophages (88) and neutrophils (89). The IL-1 cytokine family has a large number of members, and the most important are IL-1α, IL-1β, and the natural receptor antagonist IL-Ra (90). Further, IL-1β ismainly derived from microglia/macrophages (91). Both TNF-α and IL-1 primarily produced by microglia/macrophages are overexpressed within the first 2 h after experimental ICH (92–94) and as early as 24 h after ischemic stroke in mice (82).

Microglia are firstly activated via TLR4 by the pathogens or damage and release the inflammation mediators TNF-α (95). Sansing et al. (96) showed that activated microglia express high levels of TLR4, which result in neuroinflammation after ICH. Meanwhile, astrocytes respond through activation of TLR2, TLR3, and TLR4, almost depending on the presence of microglia (97). In the case of TLR4 activation in response to LPS, microglia directly trigger or promote astrocytic responses by upregulating the expression levels of soluble mediators. The results indicate that microglia play a critical role in astrocytic activation via TLR4 in response to insults, injury, or inflammation in CNS disorders (14, 97).

It is observed that human astrocytes are highly sensitive to IL-1β but unresponsive to LPS stimulation, and reactive astrogliosis is also induced by IL-1β alone (98). Within 24 h of IL- 1β induction, large numbers of reactive astrocytes are observed, and elevate the matrixmetalloprotease

(MMP)-9 expression (98-100). Although astrocytes produce certain pro-inflammatory factors, microglia are the main source of cytokines (101). Primary mediators, such as TNF, IL-1β, and IFNγ, promote the produce of secondary mediators, such as MMP, nitric oxide (NO), and arachidonic acid (72).

These evidences suggest that, in the process of neuroinflammation induced by stroke or LPS, microglia are more sensitive to pathogens/damage and activated via PAMP/DAMP and release the common "molecular signals" or primary mediators, such as IL- 1 and TNF-α, to trigger reactive astrocytes, while astrocytes are unresponsive to pathogens/damage in the absence of microglial cells.

HMGB1

High-mobility group protein box-1(HMGB1), a highly conserved non-histone DNA-binding protein, is involved in pro-inflammatory cytokine gene transcription in diverse inflammatory diseases (56, 102–104). In a rabbit subarachnoid hemorrhage (SAH) model, the Murakami group found that the HMGB1 protein are located in microglia and macrophages with a ratio >90% (105). In a collagenase-induced mode of ICH in rats, the release of HMGB1 into the cytoplasm in the brain was detected within 1 h, and express levels of HMG1 protein was substantially elevated at 24 h after ICH (106–108). These suggest that HMGB1 also primarily arise from microglia/macrophages and seem to be produced concurrently with cytokines such as IL- 1 and TNF-α.

In vitro, microglia stimulated by TNF-α release large amounts of HMGB1 (109), and recombinant human HMGB1 (rhHMGB1) can activate microglia, increase NF-κB activity, and promote inflammation factors including TNF-α, IL-1β, cyclooxygenase (COX)–2, and NO (110). However, these effects disappeared in TLR4–/– microglia treated with rhHMGB1(110). These observations indicate that not only pathogens /damage but also HMGB1 can ignite microglial activation via TLR4 and promotes the produce of TNF-α, which in turn stimulates microglia to release large amounts of HMGB1 to active more microglia. There seems to be self-feedback loop in the process of microglial activation.

Signal Can be Amplified

Molecular languages, such as TNF-α and IL-1 is not only the proinflammatory factors of M1-like phenotypes, but more like "signals" to trigger reactivity astrocytes, and these inflammatory signals may be amplified by the unique physiological structure of astrocytes. A rat model experiment indicated that primary microglia are more sensitive to lead (Pb) exposure; compared to astrocytes, Pb is more likely to reduce microglial viability, while astrocytes have greater uptake of Pb (111). Similarly, the Kirkley group found that microglia can amplify the inflammatory activation of astrocytes by the release of cytokines and chemokines (12).

ATP and analogs interact with G protein-coupled P2Y receptors to promote astrocyte proliferation and the growth of long, branched processes (101). It has also been shown that microglial cells quickly released small amounts of ATP, and astrocytes in turn amplified this release, increasing the frequency of excitatory postsynaptic currents through P2Y1 (14). This response can be blocked by inhibitors of connexin channels. In the case of connexin channel inhibitors, microglial movement is also significantly impeded (112). These results reveal that microglia as upstream partners ignite the response and astrocytes with the syncytium coupled by connexin channels magnify this.

In conclusion, microglia firstly react like "pioneers" in the NVU, initiate immune cascades, release inflammatory mediators, and form network regulation. Meanwhile, astrocytes with dominant quantity may be "reserve forces" and amplify the neuroinflammation, owing to their syncytium of structure and function. In addition, the amplification of neuroinflammation may be also related to astrocytic strategic position to mobilize peripheral immunity.

Communication Between M2 and A2

As mentioned above, the M1-like microglia secrete some pro-inflammatory mediators to induce A1 astrocytes, which amplify the cascaded neuroinflammation. With the process of the insults limited and the NVU remodeling, the local environmental factors change and determine the switch of microglial and astrocytic phenotypes. Activated microglia-Derived Cytokines (TNF-α, IL- 1β and IL-6) induced the switch of astrocyte phenotype after brain trauma (113). The interaction of microglia and astrocytes plays a vital role in the switch of phenotypes. In addition, activated M2-like microglia produce the anti-inflammatory cytokine IL-10, which matches the IL-10 receptor (IL-10R) primarily expressed in A2 astrocytes, and this allows astrocytes to secrete TGF-β, which reduces microglial activation (114). The communication between M2 and A2 significantly promotes neuronal survival and repair and is even amplified by the unique anatomy structure of astrocytes.

Astrocytic Dialogue to Microglia

In physiological conditions, astrocytes communicate simultaneously with both neurons and blood vessels as versatile cells to maintain the function of neurons and the blood–brain barrier (27). In pathological conditions, reactive astrogliosis, and astrocytic proliferation become dominant, and the process is triggered by diverse molecular signals, such as cytokines, ATP, endothelin, sonic hedgehog, fibroblast growth factor2 (FGF2), thrombin, and bone morphogenic proteins (BMP) (27, 115). The communications among neurons, BBB and microglia/macrophage mostly rely on these molecular signals (11, 13, 21, 116). Early triggers contain nucleotides released from damaged cells and pro-inflammatory cytokines as well as purines/pyrimidines such as ATP and elevated excitotoxic transmission, as ATP is co-released with neurotransmitters (101). In physiological or pathological conditions, astrocytes seem to primarily sense the signals derived from neurons and blood–brain barrier components including microglia in the NVU.

During development, astrocytes can sense subtle changes in neurons to induce the production of C1q in neuronal synapses, which interacts with the microglial C3a receptor (C3aR) to prune the neuronal synapses through the classic cascade complement pathway (117). In the context of Alzheimer's disease (AD) pathology, overproduction of AD promote the release of C3 from astrocytes, which simultaneously communicate with microglial C3aR and neuronal C3aR to dynamically regulate microglial phagocytosis and impair dendritic morphology as well as synaptic function, subsequently deteriorate cognitive function. The damaged neurons in turn trigger more astrocytes and active more microglia. Complement-dependent intercellular crosstalk is critical to promote the pathogenic cycle, and the feedforward loop can be blocked effectively by C3aR inhibition (118, 119).

Astrocytes are major sources of many chemokines, such as CCL2, CXCL1, CXCL10, and CXCL12 (120–122), and microglia express some corresponding chemokine receptors, such as CCL2, CXCL12 (123, 124), and so on. This implicates a strong association between microglia and astrocytes.

In summary, astrocytes, one of the important components of the NVU, communicate simultaneously with both neurons and blood vessels as versatile cells to maintain the function of neurons and the blood–brain barrier, whose subtle changes are captured and responded to by astrocytes, and even transferred to microglia. In early mild cognitive impairment, astrocytes may be the primary responsibility for this, but, in moderate or severe cognitive impairment such as AD, amounts of accompanied neurons death or apoptosis may also directly activate microglia, as microglia are more sensitive to pathogens/damage and trigger more reactive astrocytes via inflammatory signals, which can be amplified not only by the self-feedback loop of HMGB1 but also by the unique anatomy structure of astrocytes. Although both microglia and astrocytes own their functional characteristics, they can achieve the immune "optimization" through their mutual communication and cooperation in neuroinflammation.

The communications of microglia and astrocytes is illustrated in Figure 3.

FIGURE 3 | The communications of microglia and astrocytes. Pathogens/damage trigger M1-like microglia via TLR4. During the neuroinflammation induced by LPS or

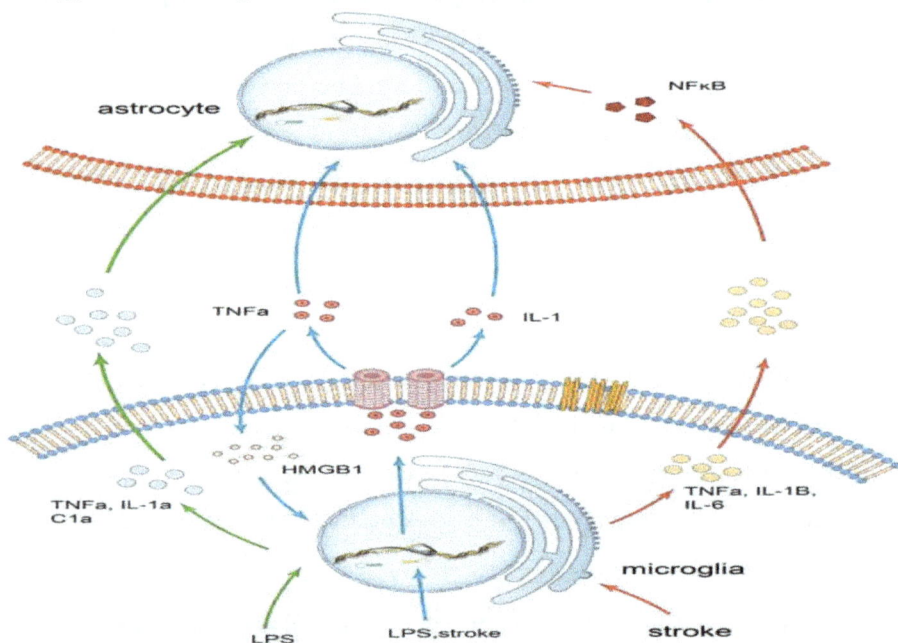

stroke, Microglia are more sensitive to pathogens/damage, firstly activated, and secrete the common "molecular signals," such as IL-1 and TNF-a, to trigger reactive astrocytes.

Different types of insults release different combinations of these molecules, which in turn trigger different responses. It has been demonstrated that inflammation factors induced by LPS, such as TNF-α, IL-1a, and C1a, can trigger reactive astrocytes. In stroke, however, the inflammatory factors secreted by activated microglia(M1), such as TNF-α, IL-1β, and IL-6, are significantly elevated.

Recombinant human HMGB1 (rhHMGB1) can trigger microglial activation via the TLR4 and increase production of TNF-α, which in turn stimulates microglia to release large amounts of HMGB1 to active more microglia. There seems to be self-feedback loop in the activation process of microglia.

Different Pathogens/Damage and Different Effects

The inflammatory effects of the central nervous system depend on several parameters, including the types and severity of pathogens/damage, glial cell types, a variety of combinations   of signal molecules (including chemokines, cytokines, etc.), and timeline of the response, etc. (112, 125, 126).

Zamanian et al. showed that reactive astrocytes induced by LPS or ischemic stroke upregulate over 1,000 genes, and genomic profiling has shown that both gene representation and fold induction correspond to individual injuries. Some of the upregulated genes are unique to the LPS subtype (A1) or the middle cerebral artery occlusion (MCAO) subtype (A2). For example, the three genes, including Ptx3, S1Pr3, and tweak, are markers for the MCAO subtype (A2), while H2-D1 and Serping1 are markers for the LPS subtype (A1) of reactive astrocytes. H2-D1 was induced 30-fold by LPS but only 3-fold by MCAO. Serping1 was induced 6.5-fold after MCAO and 34-fold after LPS (5). These data indicate that different pathogens/damage can induce different phenotypes of astrocytes. This may closely relate to the different interaction between the activated astrocytes and microglia, which contain different combinations of molecule signals. It has been demonstrated that inflammation factors induced by LPS, such as TNF-α, IL-1a, and C1al, can trigger reactive astrocytes (11). In stroke, the inflammatory factors secreted by activated microglia (M1), such as TNF-α, IL-1β and IL-6, are significantly elevated (77, 78, 127). Furthermore, a recent clinical inflammatory factor test is about the relationship of inflammatory markers and severity of ICH, and this test displayed that high TNF-a is closely associated with the size of edema around the hematoma and increase of early hematoma, leading to poor functional recovery and high mortality (128). These studies imply the different types and severities of insults release different combinations or levels of these molecule signals, which in turn trigger different responses.

Thus, different pathogens/damage correspond to different phenotypes of glia cells. Even the same pathogens/damage with the different levels of stimulation, the activated levels and phenotypic timeline of glia cell are also different. In the pathology of neuroinflammation induced by LPS, the pathogen is stronger, M1/A1 are primary, and it is critical to suppress the pro- inflammatory or shorten the phase. While sterile inflammation induced by stroke, such as cerebral infarction or hemorrhage, it may be beneficial to moderately attenuate the activation levels and shorten the timeline of M1/A1 or strengthen A2/M2, some studies and experiments have confirmed this (85, 129-131). In degenerative disease, such as AD, it may be beneficial to enhance the A2/M2 for brain repair and functional recovery. While in autoimmune diseases such as multiple sclerosis, autoimmune encephalitis, attenuating M1/A1 in time may be more beneficial (132–139).

SUMMARY AND OUTLOOK

Neuroinflammation is dynamic with the regulation of pro and anti-inflammatory signals. The activation and interaction of glial cells play a crucial role at different stages of pathology in CNS disorders. Microglia are more sensitive to pathogens or damage, firstly activated (M1) like "pioneers," monitoring and transmitting "danger" via the common molecule signals to trigger reactive astrocytes (A1). Astrocytes with dominant quantity may be "reserve forces" and amplify the neuroinflammation, owing to their syncytium of the structure, and function, and strategic position to mobilize peripheral immunity. Although inflammation signals between microglia and astrocytes may share the common inflammatory signals, such as IL- 1 and TNF-α, different pathogens and pathological conditions may correspond to different inflammatory signals (TNF-α, IL-1β, and IL-6 are significantly elevated in stroke, while TNF-α, IL-1a, and C1a induced by LPS can trigger markedly reactive astrocytes), and different strategies may be required. As the pathology further progresses, the communication between M2 and A2 significantly promote neuronal survival and repair. In addition, astrocytes, as one of the essential components of the neurovascular unit (NVU), communicate simultaneously with both neurons and blood vessels as versatile cells to maintain the function of neurons and the BBB; their subtle changes are identified and responded by astrocytes and even transferred to microglia. Activated microglia and reactive astrocyte may achieve the immune "optimization" through mutual communication and cooperation in neuroinflammation. Inflammation signals between microglia and astrocytes can be amplified not only by the self-feedback loop of microglial activation but also by the unique anatomy structure of astrocytes in the immune network (140-148). With advancements in technology, the interaction of microglia and astrocytes may be an effective and accurate therapeutic target in the future.

REFERENCES:

1. DiSabato DJ, Quan N, Godbout JP. Neuroinflammation: the devil is in the details.

J Neurochem. (2016) 139:136–53. doi: 10.1111/jnc.13607

2. Anrather J, Iadecola C. Inflammation and stroke: an overview.Neurotherapeutics. (2016) 13:661–70. doi: 10.1007/s13311-016-0483-x

3. Hu X, Leak RK, Shi Y, Suenaga J, Gao Y, Zheng P, et al. Microglial and macrophage polarization-new prospects for brain repair. Nat Rev Neurol. (2015) 11:56–64. doi: 10.1038/nrneurol.2014.207

4. Xiong XY, Liu L, Yang QW. Functions and mechanisms of microglia/macrophages in neuroinflammation and neurogenesis after stroke. Prog Neurobiol. (2016) 142:23–44. doi: 10.1016/j.pneurobio.2016. 05.001

5. Zamanian JL, Xu L, Foo LC, Nouri N, Zhou L, Giffard RG, et al. Genomic analysis of reactive astrogliosis. J Neurosci. (2012) 32:6391–410. doi: 10.1523/JNEUROSCI. 6221-11.2012

6. Jha MK, Lee WH, Suk K. Functional polarization of neuroglia: implications in neuroinflammation and neurological disorders. Biochem Pharmacol. (2016) 103:1–16. doi: 10.1016/j.bcp.2015. 11.003

7. Lan X, Han X, Li Q, Yang QW, Wang J. Modulators of microglial activation and polarization after intracerebral haemorrhage. Nat Rev Neurol. (2017) 13:420–33. doi: 10.1038/nrneurol.2017.69

8. Shi Y, Yamada K, Liddelow SA, Smith ST, Zhao L, Luo W, et al. ApoE4 markedly exacerbates tau-mediated neurodegeneration in a mouse model of tauopathy. Nature. (2017) 549:523–7. doi: 10.1038/nature24016

9. Liddelow SA, Barres BA. Reactive astrocytes: production, function, and therapeutic potential. Immunity. (2017) 46:957–67. doi: 10.1016/j.immuni.2017.06.006

10. Jha MK, Jo M, Kim JH, Suk K. Microglia-astrocyte crosstalk: an intimate molecular conversation. Neuroscientist. (2019) 25:227–40. doi: 10.1177/ 107385841 8783959

11. Liddelow SA, Guttenplan KA, Clarke LE, Bennett FC, Bohlen CJ, Schirmer L, et al. Neurotoxic reactive astrocytes are induced by activated microglia. Nature. (2017) 541:481–7. doi: 10.1038/nature21029

12. Kirkley KS, Popichak KA, Afzali MF, Legare ME, Tjalkens RB. Microglia amplify inflammatory activation of astrocytes in manganese neurotoxicity. J Neuroinflammation. (2017) 14:99. doi: 10.1186/s12974-017-0871-0

13. Litwin M, Radwanska A, Paprocka M, Kieda C, Dobosz T, Witkiewicz W, et al. The role of FGF2 in migration and tubulogenesis of endothelial progenitor cells in relation to pro-angiogenic growth factor production. Mol Cell Biochem. (2015) 410:131–42. doi: 10.1007/s11010-015-2545-5

14. Pascual O, Ben Achour S, Rostaing P, Triller A, Bessis A. Microglia activation triggers astrocyte-mediated modulation of excitatory neurotransmission. Proc Natl

Acad Sci USA. (2012) 109: E197–205. doi: 10.1073/pnas.1111098109

15. del Zoppo GJ. The neurovascular unit in the setting of stroke. J Intern Med.(2010) 267:156–71. doi: 10.1111/j.1365-2796. 2009. 02199.x

16. Muoio V, Persson PB, Sendeski MM. The neurovascular unit–concept review.Acta Physiologica. (2014) 210:790–8. doi: 10.1111/apha.12250

17. Sa-Pereira I, Brites D, Brito MA. Neurovascular unit: a focus on pericytes.

Mol Neurobiol. (2012) 45:327–47. doi: 10.1007/s12035-012-8244-2

18. Carmichael ST. Emergent properties of neural repair: elemental biology to therapeutic concepts. Ann Neurol. (2016) 79:895-906. doi: 10.1002/ana.24653

19. Obermeier B, Daneman R, Ransohoff RM. Development, maintenance and disruption of the blood-brain barrier. Nat Med.(2013) 19:1584–96. doi: 10.1038/nm.3407

20. Rajasekaran SA, Beyenbach KW, Rajasekaran AK. Interactions of tight junctions with membrane channels and transporters. Biochim Biophys Acta. (2008) 1778:757–69. doi: 10.1016/j.bbamem.2007.11.007

21. Liebner S, Dijkhuizen RM, Reiss Y, Plate KH, Agalliu D, Constantin G. Functional morphology of the blood-brain barrier in health and disease. Acta Neuropathol. (2018) 135:311–36. doi: 10.1007/s00401-018-1815-1

22. Argaw AT, Asp L, Zhang J, Navrazhina K, Pham T, Mariani JN, et al. Astrocyte-derived VEGF-A drives blood-brain barrier disruption in CNS inflammatory disease. J Clin Invest. (2012) 122:2454–68. doi: 10.1172/jci60842

23. Argaw AT, Gurfein BT, Zhang Y, Zameer A, John GR. VEGF-mediated disruption of endothelial CLN-5 promotes blood-brain barrier breakdown. Proc Natl Acad Sci USA. (2009) 106:1977–82. doi: 10.1073/pnas.08086 98106

24. Filosa JA, Morrison HW, Iddings JA, Du W, Kim KJ. Beyond neurovascular coupling, role of astrocytes in the regulation of vascular tone. Neuroscience. (2016) 323:96–109. doi: 10.1016/j.neuroscience.2015.03.064

25. Yang S, Chen Y, Deng X, Jiang W, Li B, Fu Z, et al. Hemoglobin-induced nitric oxide synthase overexpression and nitric oxide production contribute to blood-brain barrier disruption in the rat. J Mol Neurosci. (2013) 51:352– 63. doi: 10.1007/s12031-013-9990-y

26. Skoff RP. Gliogenesis in rat optic nerve: astrocytes are generated in a single wave before oligodendrocytes. Dev. biol. (1990) 139:149–68.doi:10.1016/0012-1606(90)90285-q

27. Sofroniew MV, Vinters HV. Astrocytes: biology and pathology. Acta Neuropathol. (2010) 119:7–35. doi: 10.1007/s00401-009-0619-8

28. Santello M, Cali C, Bezzi P. Gliotransmission and the tripartite synapse. Adv Exp Med Biol. (2012) 970:307–31. doi: 10.1007/978-3-7091-0932-8_14

29. Lopez-Bayghen E, Ortega A. Glial glutamate transporters: new actors in brain signaling. IUBMB Life. (2011) 63:816–23. doi: 10.1002/iub.536

30. Bushong EA, Martone ME, Jones YZ, Ellisman MH. Protoplasmic astrocytes in CA1 stratum radiatum occupy separate anatomical domains. J Neurosci. (2002) 22:183–92. doi: 10.1523/jneurosci.22-01-00183.2002

31. Halassa MM, Fellin T, Haydon PG. The tripartite synapse: roles for gliotransmission in health and disease. Trends Mol Med. (2007) 13:54- 63. doi: 10.1016/j.molmed. 2006.12.005

32. Allen NJ, Bennett ML, Foo LC, Wang GX, Chakraborty C, Stephen J, et al. Astrocyte glypicans 4 and 6 promote formation of excitatory synapses via GluA1 AMPA receptors. Nature. (2012) 486:410–4. doi: 10.1038/nature11059

33. Wang AT, Lee SS, Sigman M, Dapretto M. Developmental changes in the neural basis of interpreting communicative intent. Soc Cogn Affect Neurosci. (2006) 1:107–21. doi: 10.1093/scan/nsl018

34. Charveriat M, Naus CC, Leybaert L, Saez JC, Giaume C. Connexin- dependent neuroglial networking as a new therapeutic target. Front Cell Neurosci. (2017) 11:174. doi: 10.3389/fncel.2017.00174

35. Giaume C. Astroglial wiring is adding complexity to neuroglial networking.Front Neuroenerget. (2010) 2:123. doi: 10.3389/fnene.2010.00129

36. Tanigami H, Okamoto T, Yasue Y, Shimaoka M. Astroglial integrins in the development and regulation of neurovascular units. Pain Res Treat. (2012) 2012:964652. doi: 10.1155/2012/964652

37. Pekny M, Nilsson M. Astrocyte activation and reactive gliosis. Glia. (2005) 50:427–34. doi: 10.1002/glia.20207

38. Iliff JJ, Wang M, Liao Y, Plogg BA, Peng W, Gundersen GA, et al. A paravascular pathway facilitates CSF flow through the brain parenchyma and the clearance of interstitial solutes, including amyloid beta. Sci. Transl. Med. (2012) 4:147ra11. doi: 10.1126/scitranslmed.3003748

39. Plog BA, Nedergaard M. The glymphatic system in central nervous system health and disease: past, present, and future. Annu Rev Pathol. (2018) 13:379–94. doi: 10.1146/annurev-pathol-051217-111018

40. Verkhratsky A, Nedergaard M. The homeostatic astroglia emerges from evolutionary specialization of neural cells. Philos Trans Royal Soc London Ser B Biol Sci. (2016) 371:428. doi: 10.1098/rstb.2015.0428

41. Bechmann I, Galea I, Perry VH. What is the blood-brain barrier (not)? Trends Immunol. (2007) 28:5–11. doi: 10.1016/j.it.2006.11.007

42. Ransohoff RM, Brown MA. Innate immunity in the central nervous system. J Clin Invest. (2012) 122:1164–71. doi: 10.1172/jci58644

43. Farina C, Aloisi F, Meinl E. Astrocytes are active players in cerebral innate immunity. Trends Immunol. (2007) 28:138–45. doi: 10.1016/j.it.2007.01.005

44. Klein RS, Hunter CA. Protective and pathological immunity during central nervous system infections. Immunity. (2017) 46:891–909. doi: 10.1016/j.immuni. 2017.06.012

45. Lyck L, Santamaria ID, Pakkenberg B, Chemnitz J, Schroder HD, Finsen B, et al. An empirical analysis of the precision of estimating the numbers of neurons and glia in human neocortex using a fractionator-design with sub-sampling. J Neurosci Methods. (2009) 182:143–56. doi: 10.1016/j.jneumeth.2009.06.003

46. Pelvig DP, Pakkenberg H, Stark AK, Pakkenberg B. Neocortical glial cell numbers in human brains. Neurobiol Aging. (2008) 29:1754– 62. doi: 10.1016/j. neurobiol aging. 2007.04.013

47. Alliot F, Godin I, Pessac B. Microglia derive from progenitors, originating from the yolk sac, and which proliferate in the brain. Brain Res Dev Brain Res. (1999) 117:145–52. doi: 10.1016/s0165-380600113-3

48. da Fonseca AC, Matias D, Garcia C, Amaral R, Geraldo LH, Freitas C, et al. The impact of microglial activation on blood-brain barrier in brain diseases. Front Cell Neurosci. (2014) 8:362. doi: 10.3389/fncel.2014.00362

49. Pont-Lezica L, Bechade C, Belarif-Cantaut Y, Pascual O, Bessis A. Physiological roles of microglia during development. J Neurochem. (2011) 119:901–8. doi: 10.1111/j.1471-4159. 2011.07504.x

50. Nimmerjahn A, Kirchhoff F, Helmchen F. Resting microglial cells are highly dynamic surveillants of brain parenchyma in vivo. Science. (2005) 308:1314– 8. doi: 10.1126/science.1110647

51. Schafer DP, Stevens B. Phagocytic glial cells: sculpting synaptic circuits in the developing nervous system. Curr Opin Neurobiol. (2013) 23:1034–40. doi: 10.1016 /j. conb.2013.09.012

52. Block ML, Hong JS. Chronic microglial activation and progressive dopaminergic neurotoxicity. Biochem Soc Trans. (2007) 35:1127– 32. doi: 10.1042/bst0351127

53. Farfara D, Lifshitz V, Frenkel D. Neuroprotective and neurotoxic properties of glial cells in the pathogenesis of Alzheimer's disease. J Cell Mol Med. (2008) 12:762–80. doi: 10.1111/j.1582-4934.2008. 00314.x

54. Colombo E, Farina C. Astrocytes: key regulators of neuroinflammation. Trends Immunol. (2016) 37:608–20. doi: 10.1016/j.it.2016.06.006

55. Mracsko E, Veltkamp R. Neuroinflammation after intracerebral hemorrhage. Front Cell Neurosci. (2014) 8:388. doi: 10.3389/fncel.2014. 00388

56. Ohnishi M, Katsuki H, Fukutomi C, Takahashi M, Motomura M, Fukunaga M, et al. HMGB1 inhibitor glycyrrhizin attenuates intracerebral hemorrhage-induced injury in rats. Neuropharmacology. (2011) 61:975– 80. doi: 10.1016/j.neuropharm.

2011.06.026

57. Dudvarski Stankovic N, Teodorczyk M, Ploen R, Zipp F, Schmidt MHH. Microglia-blood vessel interactions: a double- edged sword in brain pathologies. Acta Neuropathol. (2016) 131:347–63. doi: 10.1007/s00401-015-1524-y

58. Block ML, Zecca L, Hong JS. Microglia-mediated neurotoxicity: uncovering the molecular mechanisms. Nat Rev Neurosci. (2007) 8:57–69. doi: 10.1038/nrn2038

59. Orihuela R, McPherson CA, Harry GJ. Microglial M1/M2 polarization and metabolic states. Br J Pharmacol. (2016) 173:649–65. doi: 10.1111/bph.13139

60. Boche D, Perry VH, Nicoll JA. Review: activation patterns of microglia and their identification in the human brain. Neuropathol Appl Neurobiol. (2013) 39:3–18. doi: 10.1111/nan.12011

61. Pan J, Jin JL, Ge HM, Yin KL, Chen X, Han LJ, et al. Malibatol A regulates microglia M1/M2 polarization in experimental stroke in a PPAR gamma-dependent manner. J Neuroinflammation. (2015) 12:51.doi:10.1186/s12974-015-0270-3

62. Ajmone-Cat MA, Mancini M, De Simone R, Cilli P, Minghetti L. Microglial polarization and plasticity: evidence from organotypic hippocampal slice cultures. Glia. (2013) 61:1698–711. doi: 10.1002/glia.22550

63. Lampron A, Elali A, Rivest S. Innate immunity in the CNS: redefining the relationship between the CNS and Its environment. Neuron. (2013) 78:214–32. doi: 10.1016/j.neuron.2013.04.005

64. David S, Kroner A. Repertoire of microglial and macrophage responses after spinal cord injury. Nat Rev Neurosci. (2011) 12:388–99. doi: 10.1038/nr n3053

65. Ramaglia V, Baas F. Innate immunity in the nervous system. In: Verhaagen J, Hol EM, Huitenga I, Wijnholds J, Bergen AB, Boer GJ, et al., editors. Neurotherapy: Progress in Restorative Neuroscience and Neurology. Amsterdam: Elsevier Science Bv (2009). p. 95–123.

66. Anderson MA, Burda JE, Ren Y, Ao Y, O'Shea TM, Kawaguchi R, et al. Astrocyte scar formation aids central nervous system axon regeneration. Nature. (2016) 532:195–200. doi: 10.1038/nature17623

67. Sofroniew MV. Astrogliosis.Cold Spring Harb. Perspect. Biol. (2014) 7: a020420. doi: 10.1101/cshperspect. a020420

68. Gundersen GA, Vindedal GF, Skare O, Nagelhus EA. Evidence that pericytes regulate aquaporin-4 polarization in mouse cortical astrocytes. Brain Struct Funct. (2014) 219:2181–6. doi: 10.1007/s00429-013-0629-0

69. Lunde LK, Camassa LM, Hoddevik EH, Khan FH, Ottersen OP, Boldt HB, et al. Postnatal development of the molecular complex underlying astrocyte polarization. Brain Struct Function. (2015) 220:2087– 101. doi: 10.1007/s00429-014-0775-z

70. Mathiisen TM, Lehre KP, Danbolt NC, Ottersen OP. The perivascular astroglial sheath provides a complete covering of the brain microvessels: an electron microscopic 3D reconstruction. Glia. (2010) 58:1094–103. doi: 10.1002/glia.20990

71. Paulson OB, Kanno I, Reivich M, Sokoloff L. History of international society for cerebral blood flow and metabolism. J Cerebral Blood Flow Metab. (2012) 32:1099–106. doi: 10.1038/jcbfm.2011.183

72. Magaki SD, Williams CK, Vinters HV. Glial function (and dysfunction) in the normal and ischemic brain. Neuropharmacology. (2018) 134:218– 25. doi: 10.1016/j.neuropharm.2017.11.009

73. Wang J, Dore S. Heme oxygenase-1 exacerbates early brain injury after intracerebral haemorrhage. Brain. (2007) 130:1643– 52. doi: 10.1093/brain/awm095

74. Xue M, Del Bigio MR. Intracerebral injection of autologous whole blood in rats: time course of inflammation and cell death. Neurosci Lett. (2000) 283:230– 2. doi: 10.1016/s0304-3940 00971-x

75. Wu H, Zhang Z, Hu X, Zhao R, Song Y, Ban X, et al. Dynamic changes of inflammatory markers in brain after hemorrhagic stroke in humans: a postmortem study. Brain Res. (2010) 1342:111–7. doi: 10.1016/j.brainres.2010.04.033

76. Zhang Z, Liu Y, Huang Q, Su Y, Zhang Y, Wang G, et al. NF-kappaB activation and cell death after intracerebral hemorrhage in patients. Neurol Sci. (2014) 35:1097–102. doi: 10.1007/s10072-014-1657-0

77. Liesz A, Middelhoff M, Zhou W, Karcher S, Illanes S, Veltkamp R. Comparison of humoral neuroinflammation and adhesion molecule expression in two models of experimental intracerebral hemorrhage. Exp Transl Stroke Med. (2011) 3:11. doi: 10.1186/2040-7378-3-11

78. Matsushita H, Hijioka M, Ishibashi H, Anan J, Kurauchi Y, Hisatsune A, et al. Suppression of CXCL2 upregulation underlies the therapeutic effect of the retinoid Am80 on intracerebral hemorrhage in mice. J Neurosci Res. (2014) 92:1024–34. doi: 10.1002/jnr.23379

79. Lin S, Yin Q, Zhong Q, Lv FL, Zhou Y, Li JQ, et al. Heme activates TLR4-mediated inflammatory injury via MyD88/TRIF signaling pathway in intracerebral hemorrhage. J Neuroinflammation. (2012) 9:46. doi: 10.1186/1742-2094-9-46

80. Wasserman JK, Zhu X, Schlichter LC. Evolution of the inflammatory response in the brain following intracerebral hemorrhage and effects of delayed minocycline treatment. Brain Res. (2007) 1180:140–54. doi: 10.1016/j.brainres.2007.08.058

81. Xie RX, Li DW, Liu XC, Yang MF, Fang J, Sun BL, et al. Carnosine attenuates brain oxidative stress and apoptosis after intracerebral hemorrhage in rats. Neurochem Res. (2017) 42:541–51. doi: 10.1007/s11064-016-2104-9

82. Clausen BH, Lambertsen KL, Babcock AA, Holm TH, Dagnaes-Hansen F, Finsen B. Interleukin-1beta and tumor necrosis factor-alpha are expressed by different subsets

of microglia and macrophages after ischemic stroke in mice. J Neuroinflammation. (2008) 5:46. doi: 10.1186/1742-2094-5-46

83. Clausen BH, Lambertsen KL, Dagnaes-Hansen F, Babcock AA, von Linstow CU, Meldgaard M, et al. Cell therapy centered on IL-1Ra is neuroprotective in experimental stroke. Acta Neuropathol. (2016) 131:775– 91. doi: 10.1007/s00401-016-1541-5

84. Michelucci A, Heurtaux T, Grandbarbe L, Morga E, Heuschling P. Characterization of the microglial phenotype under specific pro-inflammatory and anti-inflammatory conditions: effects of oligomeric and fibrillar amyloid-beta. J Neuroimmunol. (2009) 210:3–12. doi: 10.1016/j.jneuroim.2009.02.003

85. Lambertsen KL, Clausen BH, Babcock AA, Gregersen R, Fenger C, Nielsen HH, et al. Microglia protect neurons against ischemia by synthesis of tumor necrosis factor. J Neurosci. (2009) 29:1319–30. doi: 10.1523/jneurosci.5505-08.2009

86. Wang JM, Jiang C, Zhang K, Lan X, Chen XM, Zang WD, et al. Melatonin receptor activation provides cerebral protection after traumatic brain injury by mitigating oxidative stress and inflammation via the Nrf2 signaling pathway. Free Radic Biol Med. (2019) 131:345–55. doi: 10.1016/j.freeradbiomed.2018.12.014

87. Chen SH, Oyarzabal EA, Sung YF, Chu CH, Wang Q, Chen SL, et al. Microglial regulation of immunological and neuroprotective functions of astroglia. Glia. (2015) 63:118–31. doi: 10.1002/glia.22738

88. Lambertsen KL, Meldgaard M, Ladeby R, Finsen B. A quantitative study of microglial-macrophage synthesis of tumor necrosis factor during acute and late focal cerebral ischemia in mice. J Cereb Blood Flow Metab. (2005) 25:119–35. doi: 10.1038/sj.jcbfm.9600014

89. Mayne M, Fotheringham J, Yan HJ, Power C, Del Bigio MR, Peeling J, et al. Adenosine A2A receptor activation reduces proinflammatory events and decreases cell death following intracerebral hemorrhage. Ann Neurol. (2001) 49:727–35. doi: 10.1002/ana.1010

90. Luheshi NM, Rothwell NJ, Brough D. Dual functionality of interleukin-1 family cytokines: implications for anti-interleukin-1 therapy. Br J Pharmacol. (2009) 157:1318–29. doi: 10.1111/j.1476-5381.2009. 00331.x

91. Vezzani A, Conti M, De Luigi A, Ravizza T, Moneta D, Marchesi F, et al. Interleukin-1beta immunoreactivity and microglia are enhanced in the rat hippocampus by focal kainate application: functional evidence for enhancement of electrographic seizures. J Neurosci. (1999) 19:5054–65.

92. Wagner KR, Beiler S, Beiler C, Kirkman J, Casey K, Robinson T, et al. Delayed profound local brain hypothermia markedly reduces interleukin- 1beta gene expression and vasogenic edema development in a porcine model of intracerebral hemorrhage. Acta Neurochir Suppl. (2006) 96:177–82. doi: 10.1007/3-211-30714-1_39

93. Xi G, Hua Y, Keep RF, Younger JG, Hoff JT. Systemic complement depletion

diminishes perihematomal brain edema in rats. Stroke. (2001) 32:162– 7. doi: 10.1161/ 01.Str.32.1.162

94. Aronowski J, Hall CE. New horizons for primary intracerebral hemorrhage treatment: experience from preclinical studies. Neurol Res. (2005) 27:268– 79. doi: 10.1179/016164105x 25225

95. Ekdahl CT, Kokaia Z, Lindvall O. Brain inflammation and adult neurogenesis: the dual role of microglia. Neuroscience. (2009) 158:1021–9. doi: 10.1016/ j.neuroscience. 2008.06.052

96. Sansing LH, Harris TH, Welsh FA, Kasner SE, Hunter CA, Kariko K. Toll-like receptor 4 contributes to poor outcome after intracerebral hemorrhage. Ann Neurol. (2011) 70:646–56. doi: 10.1002/ana. 22528

97. Holm TH, Dræby D, Owens T. Microglia are required for astroglial toll-like receptor 4 response and for optimal TLR2 and TLR3 response. (2012) 60:630–8. doi: 10.1002/ glia.22296

98. Tarassishin L, Suh HS, Lee SC. LPS and IL-1 differentially activate mouse and human astrocytes: role of CD14. Glia. (2014) 62:999–1013. doi: 10.1002/glia.22657

99. Teh DBL, Prasad A, Jiang W, Ariffin MZ, Khanna S, BelorkarA, et al. Transcriptome analysis reveals neuroprotective aspects of human reactive astrocytes induced by Interleukin 1 beta. Sci Rep-Uk. (2017) 7. doi: 10.1038/s41598-017-13174-w

100. Yang C-M, Hsieh H-L, Yu P-H, Lin C-C, Liu S-W. IL-1 beta induces MMP-9-dependent brain astrocytic migration via transactivation of PDGF receptor/NADPH oxidase 2-derived reactive oxygen species signals. Mol Neurobiol. (2015) 52:303–17. doi: 10.1007/s12035-014-8838-y

101. Buffo A, Rolando C, Ceruti S. Astrocytes in the damaged brain: molecular and cellular insights into their reactive response and healing potential. Biochem Pharmacol. (2010) 79:77–89. doi: 10.1016/j.bcp.2009.09.014

102. Gao T-L, Yuan X-T, Yang D, Dai H-L, Wang W-J, Peng X, et al. Expression of HMGB1 and RAGE in rat and human brains after traumatic brain injury. J Trauma Acute Care Surgery. (2012) 72:643– 9. doi: 10.1097/TA.0b013e31823c54a6

103. Hayakawa K, Qiu J, Lo EH. Biphasic actions of HMGB1 signaling in inflammation and recovery after stroke. Ann N Y Acad Sci. (2010) 1207:50–7. doi: 10.1111/j.1749-6632.2010. 05728.x

104. Kim J-B, Sig Choi J, Yu Y-M, Nam K, Piao C-S, Kim S-W, et al. HMGB1, a novel cytokine-like mediator linking acute neuronal death and delayed neuroinflammation in the postischemic brain. J Neurosci. (2006) 26:6413-21. doi: 10.1523/jneurosci.3815-05.2006

105. Murakami K, Koide M, Dumont TM, Russell SR, Tranmer BI, Wellman GC. Subarachnoid hemorrhage induces gliosis and increased expression of the pro-

inflammatory cytokine high mobility group box 1 protein. Transl Stroke Res. (2011) 2:72–9. doi: 10.1007/s12975-010-0052-2

106. Lei C, Lin S, Zhang C,Tao W, Dong W, Hao Z,et al. High- mobility group box1 protein promotes neuroinflammation after intracerebral hemorrhage in rats. Neuroscience. (2013) 228:190–9. doi: 10.1016/j.neuroscience.2012.10.023

107. Wu H, Wu T, Han X, Wan J, Jiang C, Chen W, et al. Cerebroprotection by the neuronal PGE (2) receptor EP2 after intracerebral hemorrhage in middle-aged mice. J Cerebral Blood Flow Metab. (2017) 37:39– 51. doi: 10.1177/0271678x15625351

108. Zhao X, Wu T, Chang C-F, Wu H, Han X, Li Q, et al. Toxic role of prostaglandin E-2 receptor EP1 after intracerebral hemorrhage in mice. Brain Behav Immunity. (2015) 46:293–310. doi: 10.1016/j.bbi.2015.02.011

109. Wang R, Zhang Q, Yang S, Guo Q. TNF-alpha induces the release of high mobility group protein B1 through p38 mitogen-activated protein kinase pathway in microglia. Zhong nan da xue xue bao Yi xue ban. (2015) 40:967– 72. doi: 10.11817/j.issn.1672-7347.2015.09.004

110. Yang Q-W, Lu F-L, Zhou Y, Wang L, Zhong Q, Lin S, et al. HMBG1 mediates ischemia-reperfusion injury by TRIF-adaptor independent Toll- like receptor 4 signaling. J Cerebral Blood Flow Metab. (2011) 31:593– 605. doi: 10.1038 /jcbfm. 2010.129

111. Peng J, Zhou F, Wang Y, Xu Y, Zhang H, Zou F, et al. Differential response to lead toxicity in rat primary microglia and astrocytes. Toxicol Appl Pharmacol. (2019) 363:64–71. doi: 10.1016/j.taap.2018. 11.010

112. Davalos D, Grutzendler J, Yang G, Kim JV, Zuo Y, Jung S, et al. ATP mediates rapid microglial response to local brain injury in vivo. Nat Neurosci. (2005) 8:752–8. doi: 10.1038/nn1472

113. Shinozaki Y, Shibata K, Yoshida K, Shigetomi E, Gachet C, Ikenaka K, et al. Transformation of astrocytes to a neuroprotective phenotype by microglia via P2Y (1) receptor downregulation. Cell Rep. (2017) 19:1151-64. doi:10.1016/ j.celrep. 2017.04. 047

114. Norden DM, Fenn AM, Dugan A, Godbout JP. TGF beta produced by IL-10 redirected astrocytes attenuates microglial activation. Glia. (2014) 62:881–95. doi: 10.1002/glia.22647

115. Burda JE, Sofroniew MV. Reactive gliosis and the multicellular response to CNS damage and disease. Neuron. (2014) 81:229-48. doi: 10.1016/j.neuron.2013.12. 034

116. D'Orleans-Juste P, Ndunge OBA, Desbiens L, Tanowitz HB, Desruisseaux MS. Endothelins in inflammatory neurological diseases. Pharmacol Ther. (2019) 194:145– 60. doi: 10.1016/j.pharmthera.2018.10.001

117. Stephan AH, Barres BA, Stevens B. The complement system: an unexpected role in synaptic pruning during development and disease. In: Hyman SE, editor. Annual

Review of Neuroscience. (2012). p. 369-89.

118. Lian H, Litvinchuk A, Chiang ACA, Aithmitti N, Jankowsky JL, Zheng H. Astrocyte-microglia cross talk through complement activation modulates amyloid pathology in mouse models of Alzheimer's disease. J Neurosci. (2016) 36:577–89. doi: 10.1523/jneurosci.2117-15.2016

119. Lian H, Yang L, Cole A, Sun L, Chiang ACA, Fowler SW, et al. NF kappa B-activated astroglial release of complement C3 compromises neuronal morphology and function associated with Alzheimer's disease. Neuron. (2015) 85:101–15. doi: 10.1016/j.neuron.2014.11.018

120. Allaman I, Belanger M, Magistretti PJ. Astrocyte-neuron metabolic relationships: for better and for worse. Trends Neurosci. (2011) 34:76–87. doi:10.1016/j.tins.2010.12.001

121. Rosell A, Vilalta A, Garcia-Berrocoso T, Fernandez-Cadenas I, Domingues-Montanari S, Cuadrado E, et al. Brain perihematoma genomic profile following spontaneous human intracerebral hemorrhage. PLoS ONE. (2011) 6:16750. doi: 10.1371/journal.pone.0016750

122. McKimmie CS, Graham GJ. Astrocytes modulate the chemokine network in a pathogen-specific manner. Biochem Biophys Res Commun. (2010) 394:1006–11. doi: 10.1016/j.bbrc.2010.03.111

123. Luo X, Tai WL, Sun L, Pan Z, Xia Z, Chung SK, et al. Crosstalk between astrocytic CXCL12 and microglial CXCR4 contributes to the development of neuropathic pain. Mol Pain. (2016) 12. doi: 10.1177/1744806916636385

124. Xu JW, Dong HQ, Qian QQ, Zhang X, Wang YW, Jin WJ, et al. Astrocyte- derived CCL2 participates in surgery-induced cognitive dysfunction and neuroinflammation via evoking microglia activation. Behav Brain Res. (2017) 332:145–53. doi: 10.1016/j.bbr.2017.05.066

125. Liu GJ, Nagarajah R, Banati RB, Bennett MR. Glutamate induces directed chemotaxis of microglia. Eur J Neurosci. (2009) 29:1108-18. doi: 10.1111/j.1460-9568.2009. 06659.x

126. Carpentier PA, Palmer TD. Immune influence on adult neural stem cell regulation and function. Neuron. (2009) 64:79–92. doi: 10.1016/j.neuron.2009.08.038

127. Lambertsen KL, Biber K, Finsen B. Inflammatory cytokines in experimental and human stroke. J Cereb Blood Flow Metab. (2012) 32:1677–98. doi: 10.1038/ jcbfm.2012.88

128. Bernstein JE, Savla P, Dong F, Zampella B, Wiginton JGT, Miulli DE, et al. Inflammatory markers and severity of intracerebral hemorrhage. Cureus.(2018) 10:e3529. doi: 10.7759/cureus.3529

129. Fernandez-Lopez D, Faustino J, Klibanov AL, Derugin N, Blanchard E, Simon F, et al. Microglial cells prevent hemorrhage in neonatal focal arterial stroke. J Neurosci.

(2016) 36:2881–93. doi: 10.1523/jneurosci.0140- 15.2016

130. Wang G, Wang L, Sun Xg, Tang J. Haematoma scavenging in intracerebral haemorrhage: from mechanisms to the clinic. J Cell Mol Med. (2018) 22:768– 77. doi: 10.1111/jcmm.13441

131. Wang G, Guo Z, Tong L, Xue F, Krafft PR, Budbazar E, et al. TLR7 (Toll-Like Receptor 7) facilitates heme scavenging through the BTK (Bruton Tyrosine Kinase)-CRT (Calreticulin)-LRP1 (Low-Density Lipoprotein Receptor- Related Protein-1)-Hx (Hemopexin) pathway in murine intracerebral hemorrhage. Stroke. (2018) 49:3020–9. doi: 10.1161/strokeaha.118.022155

132. Chen Z, Zhong D, Li G. The role of microglia in viral encephalitis: a review. J Neuroinflammation. (2019). 16:76. doi: 10.1186/s12974-019- 1443-2

133. Maragakis NJ, Rothstein JD. Mechanisms of disease: astrocytes in neurodegenerative disease. Nat Clin Practice Neurol. (2006) 2:679– 89. doi: 10.1038/ncpneuro0355

134. Iadecola C. The neurovascular unit coming of age: a journey through neurovascular coupling in health and disease. Neuron. (2017) 96:17-42. doi: 10.1016/j.neuron.2017. 07.030

135. Pannell M, Meier MA, Szulzewsky F, Matyash V, Endres M, Kronenberg G, et al. The subpopulation of microglia expressing functional muscarinic acetylcholine receptors expands in stroke and Alzheimer's disease. Brain Struct Funct. (2016) 221:1157–72. doi: 10.1007/s00429-014-0962-y

136. Jha MK, Kim JH, Song GJ, Lee WH, Lee IK, Lee HW, et al. Functional dissection of astrocyte-secreted proteins: implications in brain health and diseases. Prog Neurobiol. (2018) 162:37-69. doi: 10.1016/j.pneurobio.2017.12.003

137. Frei K, Bodmer S, Schwerdel C, Fontana A. Astrocyte-derived interleukin 3 as a growth factor for microglia cells and peritoneal macrophages. J Immunol. (1986) 137:3521-7.

138. Nichols MR, St-Pierre MK, Wendeln AC, Makoni NJ, Gouwens LK, Garrad EC, et al. Inflammatory mechanisms in neurodegeneration. J Neurochem. (2019) 149:562–81. doi: 10.1111/jnc.14674

139. Wolters FJ, Ikram MA. Epidemiology of dementia: the burden on society, the challenges for research. Method Mol Biol. (2018) 1750:3– 14. doi: 10.1007/978-1-4939-7704-8_1

140. Michinaga S, Seno N, Fuka M, Yamamoto Y, Minami S, Kimura A, et al. Improvement of cold injury-induced mouse brain edema by endothelin ETB antagonists is accompanied by decreases in matrixmetalloproteinase 9 and vascular endothelial growth factor-A. Eur J Neurosci. (2015) 42:2356– 70. doi: 10.1111/ejn.13020

141. Wu Y, Dissing-Olesen L, MacVicar BA, Stevens B. Microglia: dynamic mediators of synapse development and plasticity. Trends Immunol. (2015) 36:605–13. doi:

10.1016/j.it.2015.08.008

142. Bell-Temin H, Culver-Cochran AE, Chaput D, Carlson CM, Kuehl M, Burkhardt BR, et al. Novel molecular insights into classical and alternative activation states of microglia as revealed by stable isotope labeling by amino acids in cell culture (SILAC)-based proteomics. Mol Cell Proteomics. (2015) 14:3173–84. doi: 10.1074/ mcp.M115. 053926

143. Becerra-Calixto A, Cardona-Gómez GP. The role of astrocytes in neuroprotection after brain stroke: potential in cell therapy. Front Mol Neurosci. (2017) 10:88. doi: 10.3389/fnmol.2017. 00088

144. Krasemann S, Madore C, Cialic R, Baufeld C, Calcagno N, El Fatimy R, et al. The TREM2-APOE pathway drives the transcriptional phenotype of dysfunctional microglia in neurodegenerative diseases. Immunity. (2017) 47:566–81.e9. doi: 10. 1016/j.immuni. 2017.08.008

145. Polanco JC, Li C, Bodea LG, Martinez-Marmol R, Meunier FA, Gotz J. Amyloid-beta and tau complexity–towards improved biomarkers and targeted therapies. Nat Rev Neurol. (2018) 14:22–39. doi: 10.1038/nrneurol.2017.162

146. Nakanishi M, Niidome T, Matsuda S, Akaike A, Kihara T, Sugimoto H. Microglia-derived interleukin-6 and leukaemia inhibitory factor promote astrocytic differentiation of neural stem/progenitor cells. Eur J Neurosci. (2007) 25:649–58. doi: 10.1111/j.1460-9568.2007. 05309.x

147. Christopherson KS, Ullian EM, Stokes CC, Mullowney CE, Hell JW, Agah A, et al. Thrombospondins are astrocyte-secreted proteins that promote CNS synaptogenesis. Cell. (2005) 120:421–33. doi: 10.1016/j.cell.2004.12.020

148. Harada K, Kamiya T, Tsuboi T. Gliotransmitter release from astrocytes: functional, developmental, and pathological implications in the brain. Front Neurosci. (2015) 9:499. doi: 10.3389/fnins.2015.00499

FUNDING

Financial support was from the National Natural Science Foundation of China (Project no. 81771294).

DECLARATION: This chapter was authored by Li-rong Liu, Jia-chen Liu, Jin-shuang Bao, Qin-qin Bai and Gai-qing Wang published as "Interaction of microglia and astrocytes in the neurovascular unit" in "Frontiers in Immunology", 2020;11:1024

CHAPTER 8:

Low-density lipoprotein receptor-related protein-1 Facilitates Heme Scavenging after Intracerebral Hemorrhage

ABSTRACT:

Heme-degradation after erythrocyte lysis plays an important role in the pathophysiology of intracerebral hemorrhage. Low-density lipoprotein receptor-related protein-1 is a receptor expressed predominately at the neurovascular interface, which facilitates the clearance of the hemopexin and heme complex. In the present study, we investigated the role of low-density lipoprotein receptor-related protein-1 in heme removal and neuroprotection in a mouse model of intracerebral hemorrhage. Endogenous low-density lipoprotein receptor-related protein-1 and hemopexin were increased in ipsilateral brain after intracerebral hemorrhage, accompanied by increased hemoglobin levels, brain water content, blood–brain barrier permeability and neurological deficits. Exogenous human recombinant low-density lipoprotein receptor-related protein-1 protein reduced hematoma volume, brain water content surrounding hematoma, blood–brain barrier permeability and improved neurological function three days after intracerebral hemorrhage. The expression of malondialdehyde, fluoro-Jade C positive cells and cleaved caspase 3 was increased three days after intracerebral hemorrhage in the ipsilateral brain tissues and decreased with recombinant low-density lipoprotein receptor-related protein-1. Intracerebral hemorrhage decreased and recombinant low-density lipoprotein receptor-related protein-1 increased the levels of superoxide dismutase 1. Low-density lipoprotein receptor-related protein-1 siRNA reduced the effect of human recombinant low-density lipoprotein receptor-related protein-1 on all outcomes measured.

Collectively, our findings suggest that low-density lipoprotein receptor-related protein-1 contributed to heme clearance and blood–brain barrier protection after intracerebral hemorrhage. The use of low-density lipoprotein receptor-related protein-1 as supplement provides a novel approach to ameliorating intracerebral hemorrhage brain injury via its pleiotropic neuroprotective effects.

KEY WORDS: Intracerebral hemorrhage; blood–brain barrier permeability; brain edema, heme scavenging; low-density lipoprotein receptor-related protein-1

Introduction

Intracerebral hemorrhage (ICH) is the most common type of hemorrhagic stroke and has the highest mortality rate of all stroke subtypes.1,2 The rapid accumulation of blood within the brain parenchyma leads to the disruption of the normal anatomy and results in an increase of local pressure.3 Following the initial ictus, the resulting hematoma triggers a series of secondary brain injury events. The extravasated blood and its components trigger the formation of brain swelling, tissue death, and impose a strong cytotoxic, pro-oxidative, and proinflammatory insult to the adjacent

tissue which can be observed within minutes after the initial ICH event.3,4 These conditions can result in damage to surrounding neuronal tissue and the blood–brain barrier (BBB), thus increasing edema formation and decreasing neurological functions.

Blood plasma components present in the brain tissue early after the ICH injury include blood-derived coagulation factors, complement components, immunoglobulins, and other bioactive molecules considered to be toxic substances that generate tissue damage.3,5,7 Hemoglobin (Hb) and its degradation products, heme and iron, are potent cytotoxic components that can induce cell death and disrupt the BBB.8 The prominent mechanism of Hb toxicity is via the generation of free radicals (mainly through a Fenton-type mechanism) and the resulting oxidative damage to proteins, nucleic acids, carbohydrates, and lipids.2,4,9,10 The removal of the hematoma and its blood components may be a key strategy to ameliorating the brain injury and improving recovery following ICH.

Low-density lipoprotein receptor-related protein-1 (LRP1) is a transmembrane receptor expressed on several cells types including macrophages, hepatocytes, neurons, vascular endothelial cells, pericytes, smooth muscle cells, and astrocytes.11,13 The receptor has been identified to have a multifunctional role as a cargo transporter, signaling receptor for lipid endocytosis, and protein scavenging.14,15 A key function defined for LRP1 has been its integral role with inducing systemic heme clearance. Free heme is highly toxic due to its oxidative and proinflammatory effects. LRP1 has been identified as a receptor for free heme, hemopexin (Hx), and the Hx–heme complex. Hx is a high-affinity heme scavenging protein found prominently in plasma and cerebrospinal fluid that binds with heme to form the Hx–heme complex. The formation of the Hx–heme complex facilitates the cellular metabolism of heme, also decreasing available free heme levels, thus preventing its cytotoxic effects.16 LRP1 have been recently identified as a primary receptor responsible for uptake of Hx–heme complexes in humans.17 Upon binding of heme–Hx to LRP1, the complex becomes internalized via endocytosis into cells.

Inside the cell, the heme–Hx complex is dissociated by lysosomal activity. Heme is catabolized by heme oxygenases into biliverdin, carbon monoxide, and iron.18,19

LRP1 is upregulated in neurons and astrocytes as a response to increased iron concentration20 and its expression correlated with iron status.21 There are indications that the activation of LRP1 scavenging system in humans has favorable effects after subarachnoid hemorrhage (SAH).22 Effects of the activation of LRP1 system after ICH have not been evaluated yet and the findings, as mentioned above, let us hypothesize that the activation of the LRP1 system will have beneficial, clinically translatable effects after ICH.

In this study, we suggest that elevating LRP1 activity will increase Hx–heme clearance, therefore reducing cytotoxic cell death and improving BBB integrity after ICH in a collagenase infusion model in mice.

Materials and methods

Animals Eight-week-old male CD1 mice (weight $30g \pm 5g$;Charles River, Wilmington, MA) were housed in a vivarium for a minimum of three days before surgery with a 12 h light/dark cycle and ad libitum access to food and water. All procedures in this study were approved by the Institutional Animal Care and Use Committee at Loma Linda University and comply with the National Institutes of Health's Guide for the Care and Use of Laboratory Animals, and the manuscript adheres to the ARRIVE (Animal Research: Reporting of In Vivo Experiments) guidelines for reporting animal experiments.

Experimental design

The experiments were performed in a mouse model of ICH. A total of 134 mice were used. Animals were randomly divided into different experimental groups. Animals, which died before final assessment, were replaced. There were no significant differences in the mortality rate between the different experimental groups.

Seventeen animals are designated for sham, 22 for ICH by collagenase (i.c.), 19 for ICH +vehicle (saline, intracerebroventricular (i.c.v).), 18 for

ICH +human LRP1 recombinant protein (50 ng, i.c.v.), 19 for ICH +control siRNA (control siRNA, i.c.v.), 19 for ICH +LRP1 (100 pmol LRP1 siRNA, i.c.v.), and 20 for ICH +LRP1 siRNA+ human LRP1 recombinant protein (100 pmol LRP1 siRNA, i.c.v.; 50 ng r-LRP1, i.c.v.) were used.

Experiment 1 was to characterize the time course of endogenous changes in LRP1 and Hx levels in ipsilateral/right hemisphere at 1, 3, 7, and 14 days after ICH. Twenty-seven mice were randomized into five groups: sham, ICH-1d, ICH-3d, ICH-7d and ICH-14d (n=5/group). Two mice in ICH group died during surgery, one on days 1 and 2 each.

Experiment 2 was to evaluate the role of LRP1 in the pathophysiology of ICH. First, we tested the effect of the exogenous LRP1 (recombinant human LRP1 protein; r-LRP1). Fifty-seven mice were used in the following groups: sham (n=17), ICH+ vehicle (n=19), ICH+ r-LRP1 (n=18). r-LRP1 recombinant protein (50 ng in 1 ml saline; MyBioSource) was administered by i.c.v injection 20 min before the induction of ICH. The vehicle group was treated with the same volume of saline. Second, we investigated whether inhibition of LRP1 (LRP1 siRNA) mediates the repression of LRP1-Hx signaling. Thirty mice in two additional groups were added: ICH+ control siRNA (n=19) and ICH+ LRP1 siRNA (n=19). The 100 pmol of LRP1 siRNA (mouse, Santa Cruz Biotechnology) was dissolved in 1ml of sterilized RNase free water and injected intracerebroventricularly 24 h before ICH.23 The same volume of control siRNA (negative controls, Santa Cruz Biotechnology) was administered as a control. Third, we tested the effects of LRP1 using siRNA mediated LRP1 gene silencer and r-LRP1 protein. An additional group of ICH+ LRP1 siRNA+ r-LRP1 (n=20) was added.

ICH surgery

Experimental ICH was induced by intrastriatal injection of collagenase

(0.075 units in 0.5 ml saline, VII-S; Sigma, St Louis, MO, USA) into the basal ganglia as we have previously described.24 Briefly, mice were anesthetized with an intraperitoneal injection of ketamine (100 mg/kg) and xylazine (10 mg/kg) and positioned prone in a stereotaxic head frame (Stoelting, Wood Dale, IL, USA). An electronic thermostat-controlled warming blanket was used to maintain the core temperature at 37℃. A cranial burr hole (1 mm) was drilled and a 26-gauge needle on a 10 ml Hamilton syringe was inserted stereotactically into the right basal ganglia (coordinates: 0.9mm posterior to the bregma, 1.5mm lateral to the midline, and 4mm below the dura mater). The collagenase was infused at a rate of 0.25 ml/min over 2 min with an infusion pump (Stoelting, Harvard Apparatus, USA). The needle was left in place for an additional 10 min after injection to prevent possible leakage of the collagenase solution. After removal of the needle, the burr hole was closed using bone wax, the incision was sutured, and the mice were allowed to recover. Sham-operated mice were subjected to needle insertion only. Vital signs were monitored throughout surgery and recovery. At every time point (6 h, 1, 3, 7,and 14 days) after surgery, neurological functions were assessed. Following neurofunctional testing, the animals were euthanized for measurements of brain water content, hematoma volume, BBB permeability (Evans blue assay), Western blot, and immunohistochemistry assay as described below.

Intracerebroventricular injection

According to the manufacturer's instructions, 100 pmol of control or LRP1 siRNA or 50 ng r-LRP123 was dissolved in 1 ml of sterile 0.9% saline and stereotactically injected into the right lateral ventricle at a rate of 0.25 ml/min (coordinates: 0mm bregma, 1mm lateral, and 3.5mm ventral) using a 26-gauge needle. The control and LRP1 siRNA were administered 24 h before the induction of ICH and r-LRP1 30 min before ICH.

Neurobehavior exams

Neurobehavior tests were assessed at 24 and 72 h after the ICH surgery by an independent researcher blinded to the procedure. Three tests were implemented to evaluate neurological deficits: (1) modified Garcia test, (2) wire hang, and (3) beam balance. The modified Garcia exam was composed of seven subtests which were each scored out of three points (total=21points). The test included were (i) spontaneous activity, (ii) response to vibrissae touch, (iii) body proprioception, (iv) symmetry in the movement of four limbs, (v) forepaw outstretching, (vi) lateral turning, and (vii) climbing. Higher scores indicate greater neurofunction (healthy mouse).

Wire hanging and beam balance tests were performed as previously described.23 Bridges between platforms were built with wire (length, 50 cm; diameter,1 mm) and beam (length, 90 cm; diameter, 1 cm). Mice were put on the center of the wire or beam and allowed to reach the platform. Mice were observed for both their time and behavior until they reached one platform and scored according to six grades. The test was repeated three times, and an average score was taken (minimum score=0; maximum score (healthy mouse) =5). All behavioral tests were conducted by the investigator, blinded to the experiment groups.

Brain water content

The brain water content and neurological deficits were evaluated as previously described using the wet/dry method.25 Briefly, mice were euthanized under deep anesthesia. Brains were removed immediately and divided into five parts: ipsilateral and contralateral basal ganglia, ipsilateral and contralateral cortex, and cerebellum. The cerebellum was used as an internal control for brain water content. Tissue samples were weighed on an electronic analytical balance (APX-60, Denver Instrument) to the nearest 0.1mg to obtain the wet weight. The tissue was then dried at 100℃ for 48 h to determine the dry weight.

Brain water content (%) was calculated as ((wet weight-dry weight)/wet weight) *100.

Evans blue extravasation

BBB permeability using Evans blue extravasation was evaluated as previously described.26 A 2% solution of Evans blue dye in normal saline (4 ml/kg of body weight) was injected into the jugular vein. After allowing it to circulate for 1 h, the mice were transcardially perfused with 100 ml of ice-cold phosphate-buffered saline (PBS). The brain tissue was removed and divided into right and left hemispheres, frozen in liquid nitrogen, and stored at -80℃ until analysis. The samples were homogenized in 1100 ml of PBS, sonicated, and centrifuged (30 min, 15,000 r/min, 4℃). The supernatant was collected and for each 500 ml sample an equal amount of 50% trichloroacetic acid was added.

The samples were incubated over night at 4℃ and then centrifuged (30 min, 15,000 r/min, 4℃). Evans blue stain was measured by spectrophotometer (Thermo ScientificTM GENESYS 10 S UV-Vis spectrophotometer, USA) at 610nm and quantified according to a standard curve. These data were calculated as mg of Evans blue dye/g of tissue and represented as a ratio compared to sham.

Hemoglobin assay

For hematoma evaluation, supernatant collection was completed using the same method as the Evans blue extravasation. Following the supernatant collection, Drabkin's reagent (0.4 ml, Sigma-Aldrich) was added to 0.1 ml supernatant aliquots and allowed to rest for 15 min at room temperature, protected from light.

Optical density was measured and recorded at 540nm with a spectrophotometer (Thermo ScientificTM GENESYS 10S UV-Vis spectrophotometer, USA). These procedures yielded a linear relationship between measured hemoglobin concentrations in perfused brain and the volume of added blood on a standard curve.

Western blot

Western Blot was performed for proteins as previously described.23,25 Briefly, the right cerebral hemispheres were homogenized, and protein concentration was acquired for each sample using a detergent compatible assay (Bio-Rad, Philadelphia, PA). Protein samples (50 mg) were loaded on a tris-glycine gel, electrophoresed, and transferred to a nitrocellulose membrane.

Membranes were incubated overnight at 4℃ with the primary antibodies: rabbit polyclonal anti-LRP1 (1:300,000 abcam), rabbit polyclonal anti-Hx (1:2000 abcam), rabbit polyclonal anti-malondialdehyde (MDA, 1:5000 abcam), rabbit polyclonal anti-superoxide dismutase 1 (SOD1, 1:2000 Santa Cruz Bio) and rabbit polyclonal anti-caspase 3 (1:1000 cell signaling).The same membrane was probed with an antibody against b-actin (Santa Cruz, 1:5000) as an internal control after being stripped. Incubation with secondary antibodies (Santa Cruz Biotech) was done for 1 h at room temperature. Immunoblots were then probed with an ECL Plus chemiluminescence reagent kit (Amersham Biosciences, Arlington Heights, IL) and visualized with an imaging system (Bio-Rad, Versa Doc, model 4000). Data were analyzed using Image J software.

Immunohistochemistry

Immunohistochemistry was performed as described previously.27 The brains were cut into 10 mm thick coronal sections in a cryostat (CM3050S;

Leica Microsystems). The sections were incubated overnight at 4℃ with the following primary antibodies: rabbit anti-LRP1 (1:100), goat anti-ionized calcium-binding adaptor molecule 1 (Iba1, 1:100, Abcam), goat anti-Glial fibrillary acidic protein (GFAP, 1:100, Santa Cruz), goat polyclonal anti-Von Willebrand Factor (vWF, 1:100, Abcam), and rabbit anti-Hx (1:100) followed by incubation with appropriate FITC-conjugated or Alexa Fluor-conjugated secondary antibodies (Jackson Immuno Research). Negative control staining was performed by omitting the primary antibody. Perihemorrhagic area of the brain coronal sections was visualized with a fluorescence microscope (Olympus BX51).

Fluoro-Jade C (FJC) staining (Biosensis) was used to identify irreversibly degenerating neurons.28 Following manufacturer's protocol, the sections were rinsed in basic alcohol for 5 min followed by a 2 min rinse in 70% alcohol. The sections were then briefly rinsed in distilled water and incubated in 0.06% potassium permanganate for 10 min, and then briefly rinsed in distilled water to remove excess potassium permanganate.

Samples were then incubated in 0.0001% FJC stain in 0.1% acetic acid for 10 min. Following FJC labeling, the sections were rinsed three times in distilled water for 5 min each, air dried for 10 min, cleared in xylene, and covered with DPX.

Statistics

Quantitative data are presented as mean±SD. Oneway ANOVA for multiple comparisons with Tukey's post-hoc test were used to determine the differences of brain water content, neurological deficits, and Western blot assay among all groups at each time point. A $p < 0.05$ was considered statistically significant.

Results

Mortality

All sham-operated mice survived. The total operative mortality of mice was about 9% (n=12). The mortality was not significantly different among the experimental groups (data not shown).

Endogenous LRP1 and Hx expression increased after ICH

Western blot showed a significant increase in LRP1 and Hx protein expression within ipsilateral brain tissues at 1, 3, 7 and 14 days after ICH compared to sham (p<0.05, Figure 1(a) and (b)). The expression levels reached amaximum at three to seven days following ICH.

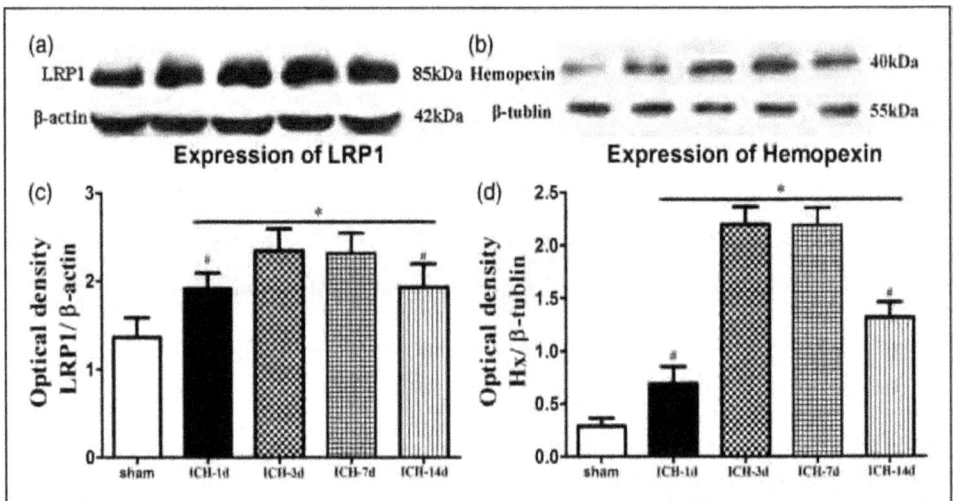

Figure 1. Time course in protein levels of LRP1 and hemopexin changes within ipsilateral brain tissues after ICH (a and b). Quantitative analysis with Western blot shows that LRP1 and hemopexin levels increased at 1, 3, 7 days and 14 days after ICH (c and d; n=5/group). One-way ANOVA followed by Tukey's test were used.*p<0.05 versus sham; #p<0.05 versus ICH-3d.

r-LRP1 improved neurobehavior following ICH

ICH+ vehicle animals scored significantly lower compared to sham mice in all neurobehavior tests performed at each time point (p<0.05, Figure 2(a) to (c)). In all neurobehavior tests, all groups were significant to sham at 6, 24, and 72 h after ICH (p<0.05). However, compared with ICH+ vehicle, r-LRP1 showed significant improvement in the modified Garcia test and the wire Hang 72 h after ICH (p<0.05, Figure 2(a) and (c)) but not in the beam balance test (p>0.05, Figure 2(b)) (n¼18/group). LRP1 siRNA countered the beneficial effect of the r-LRP1 on neurological outcome and did not reach significance against ICH+ vehicle at three days after ICH (p>0.05, Figure 2(a) and (c)). Following these results, we choose to examine the mechanism of LRP1 three days after ICH for future studies.

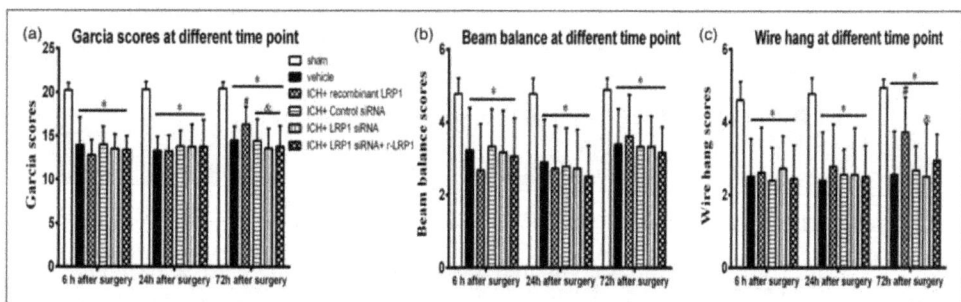

Figure 2. Effect of LRP1 on modified Garcia test, balance beam test and wire hang test 6, 24 and 72 h after ICH (a to c). (n=18/group). One-way ANOVA followed by Tukey tests were used. *p<0.05 versus sham; #p<0.05 versus vehicle; &p<0.05 versus human recombinant LRP1-treated ICH.

r-LRP1 decreases hematoma volume, BBB permeability, and brain water content three days following ICH

All groups showed a significant increase in hemoglobin levels, Evans blue extravasation, and brain water content compared with sham (p<0.05, Figure 3(a) to (d)). r-LRP1 significantly reduced hematoma volume, brain water content and BBB permeability compared with the ICH+ vehicle group (p<0.05, Figure 3(a) to (d)). LRP1 siRNA and control siRNA countered the beneficial effect of the r-LRP1on ICH (p>0.05). r-LRP1 was not able to reverse the effects of LRP1siRNA and did not reach significance against vehicle (p>0.05, Figure 3(a) to (d)).

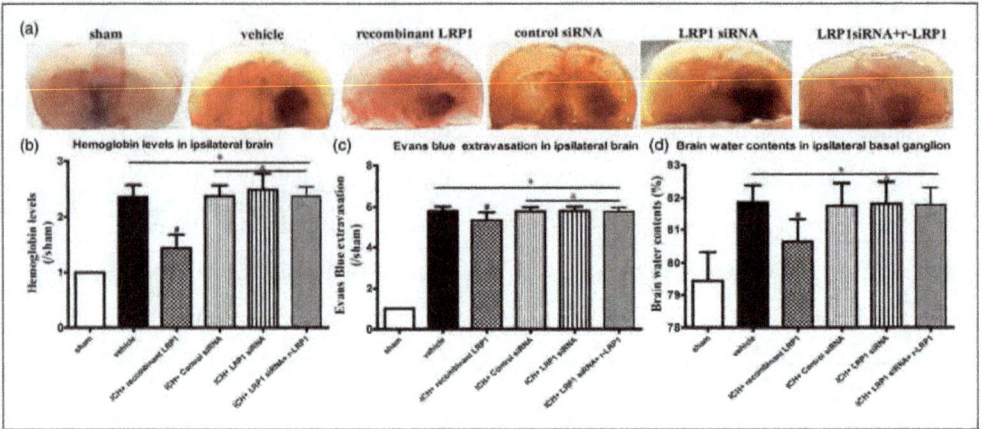

Figure 3. Effect of LRP1 on hematoma volume, blood–brain barrier permeability and brain water content 72 h after ICH (a to d). One-way ANOVA followed by Tukey tests were used. $*p<0.05$ versus sham; $\#p<0.05$ versus vehicle; $\&p<0.05$ versus human recombinant LRP1-treated ICH.

r-LRP1 increases Hx–heme scavenging three days after ICH

Western blot analysis was done on LRP1 and Hx on ipsilateral brain tissue. LRP1 was significantly elevated in ICH+ vehicle, ICH+ r-LRP1, and ICH+ control siRNA groups compared to sham ($p<0.05$, Figure 4(a)). Exogenous administration r-LRP1 showed significantly higher protein expression of LRP1 compared to vehicle ($p<0.05$). LRP1 siRNA given alone and with r-LRP1 displayed decreased expression compared to vehicle ($p<0.05$) and were not significantly changed compared to sham ($p>0.05$). Control siRNA did not show any difference when compared to vehicle ($p>0.05$). Hx was significantly elevated for all groups compared to the sham group ($p<0.05$, Figure 4(b)). ICH with the r-LRP1 treatment showed significant elevation of Hx expression when compared to vehicle ($p<0.05$).

However, LRP1 siRNA was able to reverse this effect when given with r-LRP1 on Hx expression and was no longer significant to vehicle ($p>0.05$). LRP1 siRNA and control siRNA without r-LRP1 did not show any changes compared to vehicle ($p>0.05$).

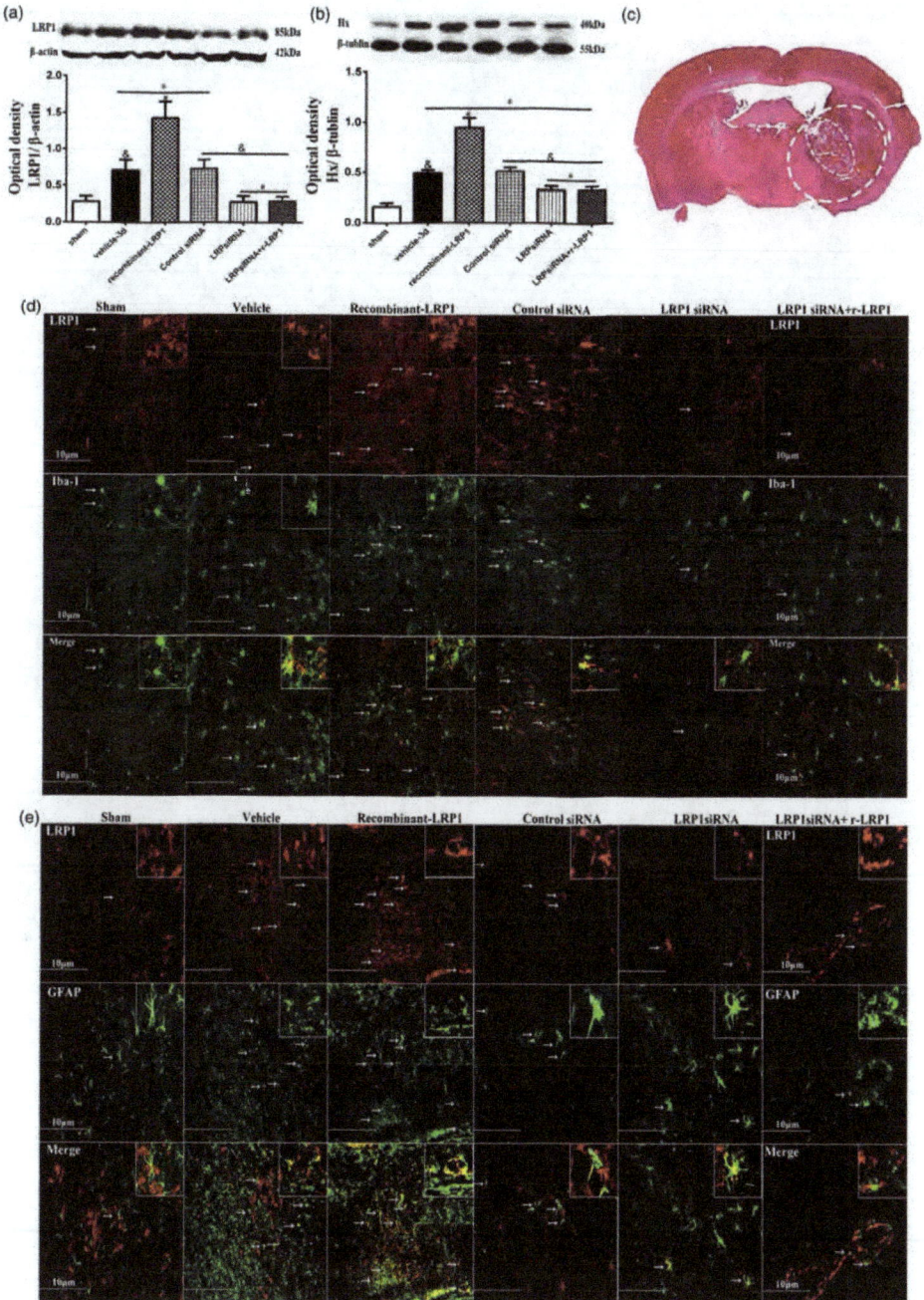

Figure 4. Effect of LRP1 on hemopexin associated with ICH 72 h after surgery. Representative images are shown of Western blot assay for LRP1 and hemopexin (Hx) level within ipsilateral brain tissues (a and b) (n=5/group). One-way ANOVA followed by Tukey tests were used. *p<0.05 versus sham; #p<0.05 versus vehicle; &p<0.05 versus human recombinant LRP1-treated ICH.

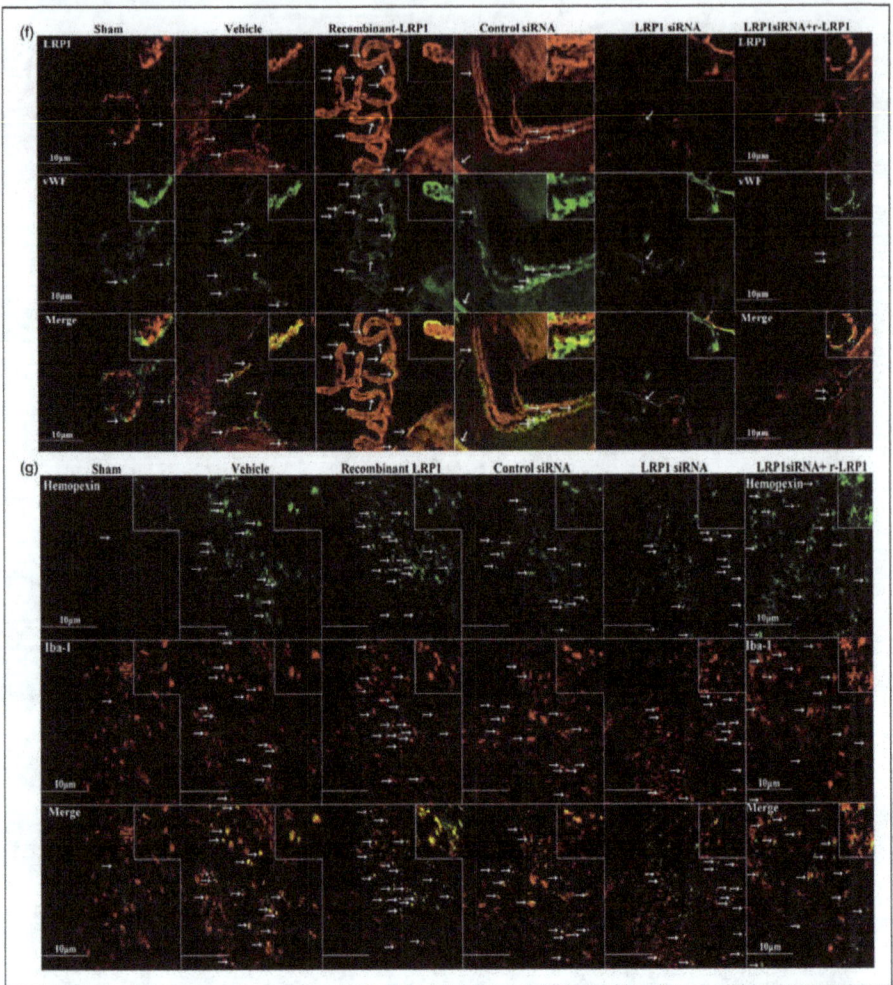

Figure 4. continued. Representative immunohistochemistry microphotographs of LRP1 and hemopexin with Iba-1 (d and g), LRP1 and GFAP (e), LRP1 and vWF (f) within perihematoma brain tissues (c) revealed that LRP1 and Hx expression were colocalized with microglia (scale bar: 10 mm).

Double immunofluorescence staining was completed in the perihematoma brain tissue (Figure 4(c), large dash line circle is perihematoma, small dash line circle is hematoma). Fluorescent staining found that LRP1 was colocalized with microglia (Iba-1), astrocytes (GFAP), and endothelial cells of the brain vessels (vWF; Figure 4(d) to (f)). Additionally, fluorescence of LRP1 revealed increased expression in vehicle, r- LRP1, and control siRNA groups while showing decreased expression in LRP1 siRNA and LRP1 siRNA with r-LRP1 groups, confirming similar Western blot results. Hx was also found to be colocalized with microglia and was increased in all groups compared to sham (Figure 4(g)).

r-LRP1 decreases oxidative stress and neuronal apoptosis after ICH

Compared with vehicle-treated ICH, Western blot analysis found that exogenous r-LRP1 treatments reduced protein expression of MDA, caspase 3, and cleaved caspase 3 and increased SOD1 expression ($p<0.05$, Figure 5(a) to (f)). r-LRP1 given with LRP1 siRNA results show that these protective effects tended to be reversed and were no longer significant to vehicle for all proteins ($p>0.05$). LRP1 and control siRNA groups without r-LRP1 did not display any changes compared to vehicle ($p>0.05$). All groups subjected to ICH displayed significantly different protein expression compared to sham animals ($p<0.05$).

FJC staining with neuron-specific nuclear antigen (NeuN) was used to determine apoptosis of neurons. It was found that fewer cells displayed FJC in the r-LRP1 treatment group compared to vehicle suggesting a decrease in cell death. Additionally, fewer FJC cells co-stained with NeuN were seen to express FJC in the r-LRP1 group suggesting less neuronal apoptosis. FJC with NeuN staining also reveals elevated neuron apoptosis in LRP1 and control siRNA groups. ICH animals given LRP1 siRNA and r-LRP1 together also display higher apoptosis of neurons compared to the sham group. However, this also shows that r-LRP1 was not able to reverse the effects of LRP1 siRNA to decrease apoptosis.

Double immunofluorescence staining of FJC with NeuN was done and found not only in degenerating nerve cell bodies but also in periventricular or perivascular cell bodies, microglias, and blood cells (Figure 5(g)). The images showed the similar trend of abovementioned results by Western blot.

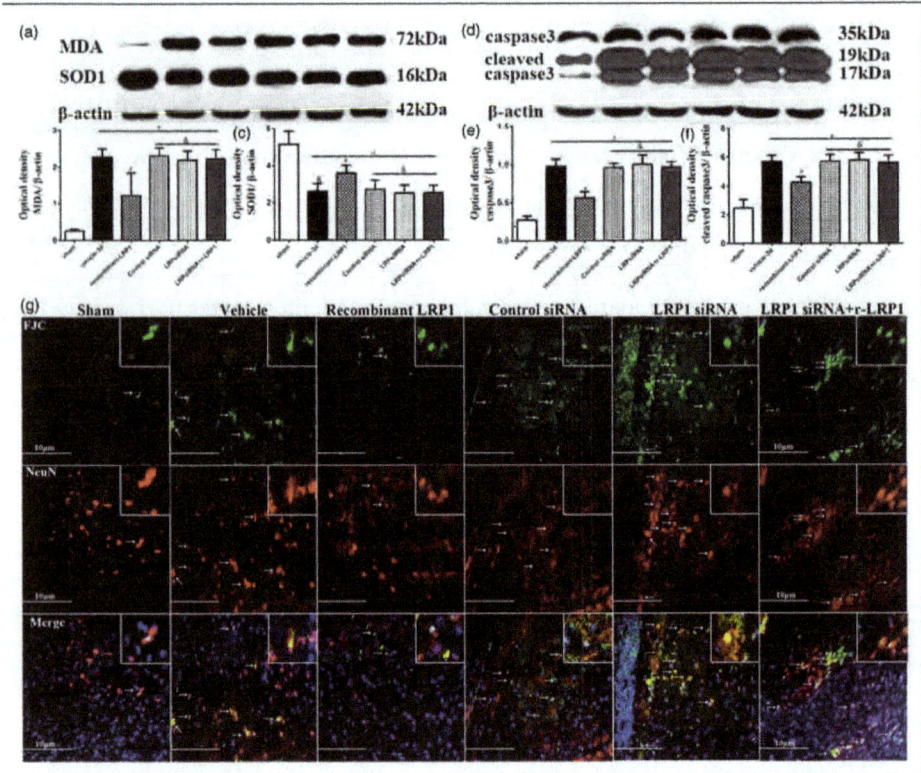

Figure 5. Effect of LRP1 on oxidative stress and neuronal apoptosis associated with ICH 72 h after surgery. Compared with the vehicle-treated ICH, rhLRP1 reduced levels of malondialdehyde (MDA; a and b), caspase 3 (d and e), cleaved caspase 3 (d and f) and elevated SOD1 (a and c) by ICH, the protective effects of which tended to be reversed by siRNA for LRP1 administration (n=5/group). One-way ANOVA followed by Tukey tests were used. *p<0.05 versus sham; #p<0.05 versus vehicle; &p<0.05 versus human recombinant LRP1-treated ICH. FJC staining with immunofluorescence to NeuN was found not only in degenerating nerve cell bodies but also in periventricular or perivascular cell bodies, microglias and blood cells (g). Arrows indicate cells with positive staining. Scale bar: 10 mm.

Discussion

In the present study, we have made the following observations:(1) endogenous LRP1 and Hx levels were significantly elevated in ipsilateral brain tissues at 1 day and up to 14 days after surgery in a mouse collagenase ICH model; they reached a peak at days three to seven after ICH. (2) Neurobehavior test scores lowered 6 h, 24 h, and three days after ICH compared with sham mice; hemoglobin levels, brain edema, and BBB permeability elevated three days after ICH; (3) exogenous human recombinant LRP1 protein significantly attenuated hematoma volume, ICH-induced brain edema, BBB permeability and neurological deficits at three days after ICH; (4) siRNA of LRP1 reversed the benefits of recombinant LRP1 on neurological outcomes at three days after ICH; (5) the improved outcomes by exogenous human recombinant LRP1 were associated with enhanced heme scavenging and less oxidative stress (MDA/SOD1) along with brain cells injury (FJC, caspase 3, and cleaved caspase 3 level) inipsilateral brain tissues three days after ICH; (6) siRNA for LRP1 partially offset the neuroprotection (heme phagocytosis, oxidative stress, and brain cells injury) provided by recombinant LRP1 3 days after ICH. These results demonstrate that LRP1 is involved in heme scavenging and BBB protection in adjacent hematoma brain tissues after ICH.

A central pathophysiologic event after ICH is the massive release of heme from red blood cells into the extracellular space. Free heme triggers oxidative stress and is highly proinflammatory.29 It has been demonstrated previously that the concentration of both nonheme iron and iron-handling proteins significantly increased three days after ICH.30,31 Therefore, the potential beneficial effects of the heme scavenging in the study were evaluated at day 3 after ICH induction. Following ICH, lysed erythrocytes and hemoglobin degradation products resulted in delayed edema and BBB disruption.32,33 The amplified processes of injury in ICH may be due to heme-catalyzed oxidative stress and lipid peroxidation then trigger apoptosis after ICH.34 FJC possesses a highest affinity for the endogenous neurodegeneration molecules,35 it is a reliable and effective marker of neuronal cell death.36 Neuronal death after ICH is mediated in part by apoptotic mechanisms.34 Caspase-dependent mechanisms play a crucial role in the lesion development caused by the blood effect on brain tissue.37 We found there were higher levels of MDA, caspase 3, cleaved caspase 3, and FJC-labeled neurons accompanied by increased hemoglobin levels, brain water contents, and Evans blue extravasation three days after ICH in the ipsilateral tissues of ICH animal, suggesting that the increased oxidative stress, apoptosis, and neurons death followed with high hematoma volume, cerebral edema, and BBB disruption occurred three days after ICH. Meanwhile, there were a decrease in neurobehavior test scores and SOD1 levels, it suggested an impairment in neurological function and antioxidation. After hemolysis and the subsequent release of heme from hemoglobin, several pathways are employed to transport and metabolize this heme and its iron moiety to protect the brain from potential oxidative stress.38 Oxidative stress is thought to be a key reason for delayed injury after ICH, which is likely due to free-Fe catalyzed free radical reactions. Such events include oxidative stress mediated by free Fe that originated from hemoglobin breakdown. Therefore, minimizing the damage caused by oxidative stress following hemoglobin breakdown and Fe release is a major therapeutic target.39 The only known Hx:heme receptor is the LRP1, also known as a2 macroglobulin receptor or CD 91, acts as a heme scavenger, a signaling receptor and transports multiple binding partners, including apoE, a-2-macroglobulin, tissue plasminogen activator, plasminogen activator inhibitor-1, factor VIII, lactoferrin, and Ab, which is the main efflux pump of Ab from the brain to the blood.40,43 In humans, LRP1 is a major Ab clearance receptor in cerebral vascular smooth muscle cell, and a disturbance of this pathway contributes to Ab accumulation.42 Deletion of LRP1 significantly alters the integrity of neuronal membranes, dendritic spines, and synapses in adult mice.44 Meanwhile, deletion of macrophage LRP1 creates an imbalance between efferocytosis and apoptosis susceptibility resulting in enhanced inflammation, lesion cell death, and plaque necrosis.45 LRP1 is ubiquitously expressed and has a low affinity for the Hx/heme complex. In the present study, there were significant increases in the Hx and LRP1 protein levels at 1 day and up to 14 days after ICH, the results showed that accumulation of heme in ICH triggered its removal-signaling pathway. Meanwhile, we found that LRP1 is expressed in cerebrovasculature, in particular in choroid plexus, perivascular microglias, and foot process of astroglias, which showed that LRP1 took part in transvascular scavenging system through BBB in brain. The results showed that LRP1 (specially expressed in choroid plexus) should play an important role in scavenging heme in this in vivo ICH model. Drug delivered through the CSF compartment could penetrate into the brain parenchyma and circulate into blood along CSF flow tracks.46 We hypothesize that due to the massive release of heme following ICH, LRP1 system is completely saturated and is unable to scavenge heme. Similar hypothesis regarding saturation of LRP1 system in human patients after SAH was discussed previously.22 Accumulation of the free heme accelerates tissue damage by promoting peroxidative reactions and activation of inflammatory cascades.47 Increasing the capacity of the system via administration of the recombinant LRP1 seemed to be a promising and clinical relevant approach. So we use recombinant LRP1 to enhance LRP1 expression at the BBB.

Intracerebroventricular human recombinant LRP1 administration reduced hematoma volumes, brain edema, BBB permeability as well as oxidative stress, apoptosis, neuron death, and better neurological scores three days after ICH, thus demonstrating a beneficial overall outcome after ICH. Inhibition of LRP1 expression with RAP (a specific LRP1 receptor antagonist) and LRP1 siRNA (LRP1 knockdown) could significantly block LRP1 function and significantly blocked both basal and intravenous immunoglobulin (IVIG)-induced Ab efflux from inner to outer chambers.48 In vivo LRP1 knock-out mice demonstrated that Ab clearance in brain is impaired49 and a significant neurodegeneration in the hippocampus and cortex in the absence of amyloid pathology.44 Consistent with this, our study used intracerebroventricular LRP1siRNA administration and found suppressed LRP1 expression in brain and further reversed the protective effect of exogenous human recombinant LRP1, confirming the protective role of LRP1 in ICH pathological progression.

Taken together, the release of cell-free heme is a major pathological factor after ICH, which leads to the oxidative stress, increased inflammation, apoptosis and consequently to the disruption of BBB, development of brain edema and impairment of neurological functions.

Pharmacological manipulations increasing heme–Hx clearance represent a novel, clinical relevant strategy that is able to attenuate the ICH-induced pathophysiology. Our results demonstrated that recombinant LRP1 administration resulted in the raise of LPR1 positive cell number, which is a sign of the activation of heme–Hx clearance system. The activation of the heme–Hx system resulted in SOD1 upregulation and subsequently in the decrease of oxidative stress as well as attenuation of post-ICH apoptosis. This beneficial effects of LRP1 administration improved BBB integrity, resulted in the attenuation of brain edema formation and in the improvement of neurological functions.

In conclusion, signaling through LRP1 appears to be a common platform controlling heme scavenging after ICH. Our study underscores the role of LRP1 achieved by local administration of human recombinant LRP1 in the setting of ICH. Selective LRP1 blockade partially reversed the neuroprotective effects associated with LRP1 supplement. LRP1 may offer pleiotropic protective effects through promoting heme resolution and diminishing brain edema after ICH and may thus prove beneficial to post-ICH outcomes.

Funding

This study was supported by NIH P01 NS082184-01 to JHZ.

Declaration of conflicting interests

The author(s) declared no potential conflicts of interest with respect to the research, authorship, and/or publication of this article.

Authors' contributions

GW conducted the experiments, analyzed data and drafted the manuscript. AM worked on the research design, experiments and manuscript preparation. AS, YO, PY and EB participated in the conduction of the experiments. DN helped in neurobehavioral tests and manuscript preparation. JHZ and JT worked on research design, data analysis and interpretation, and manuscript preparation.

REFERENCES:

1. Schlunk F and Greenberg SM. The pathophysiology of intracerebral hemorrhage formation and expansion. Transl Stroke Res 2015; 6: 257–263.

2. Chen S, Yang Q, Chen G, et al. An update on inflammation in the acute phase of intracerebral hemorrhage. Transl Stroke Res 2015; 6: 4–8.

3. Aronowski J and Zhao X. Molecular pathophysiology of cerebral hemorrhage: Secondary brain injury. Stroke 2011; 42: 1781–1786.

4. Baechli H, Behzad M, Schreckenberger M, et al. Blood constituents trigger brain swelling, tissue death, and reduction of glucose metabolism early after acute subdural hematoma in rats. J Cereb Blood Flow Metab 2010; 30: 576–585.

5. Wagner KR, Sharp FR, Ardizzone TD, et al. Heme and iron metabolism: Role in cerebral hemorrhage. J Cereb Blood Flow Metab 2003; 23: 629–652.

6. Xi G, Keep RF and Hoff JT. Mechanisms of brain injury after intracerebral haemorrhage. Lancet 2006; 5: 53–63.

7. Wang J and Dore S. Inflammation after intracerebral hemorrhage. J Cereb Blood Flow Metab 2007; 27:894–908.

8. Wang G. The pathogenesis of edema and secondary insults after ICH. In: Chaudhary V (ed) Intracerebral hemorrhage. Rijeka, Croatia: IN TECH, 2014, pp. 25–40.

9. Xiong XY, Wang J, Qian ZM, et al. Iron and intracerebral hemorrhage: from mechanism to translation. Transl Stroke Res 2014; 5: 429–441.

10. Zhao X and Aronowski J. Nrf2 to pre-condition the brain against injury caused by products of hemolysis after ICH. Transl Stroke Res 2013; 4: 71–75.

11. Zlokovic BV. Neurodegeneration and the neurovascular unit. Nat Med 2010; 16: 1370–1371.

12. Sagare AP, Deane R and Zlokovic BV. Low-density lipoprotein receptor-related protein 1: a physiological abeta homeostatic mechanism with multiple therapeutic opportunities. Pharmacol Ther 2012; 136: 94–105.

13. Ramanathan A, Nelson AR, Sagare AP, et al. Impaired vascular-mediated clearance of brain amyloid beta in Alzheimer's disease: the role, regulation and restoration of lrp1. Front Aging Neurosci 2015; 7: 136.

14. Lillis AP, Van Duyn LB, Murphy-Ullrich JE, et al. Ldl receptor-related protein 1: unique tissue-specific functions revealed by selective gene knockout studies. Physiol Rev 2008; 88: 887–918.

15. Ramanathan A, Nelson AR, Sagare AP, et al. Impaired vascular-mediated clearance of brain amyloid beta in Alzheimer's disease: the role, regulation and restoration of lrp1. Front Aging Neurosci 2015; 7: 136.

16. Nielsen MJ, Moller HJ and Moestrup SK. Hemoglobin and heme scavenger receptors. Front Aging Neurosci 2010; 12: 261–273.

17. Hvidberg V, Maniecki MB, Jacobsen C, et al. Identification of the receptor scavenging hemopexin heme complexes. Blood 2005; 106: 2572–2579.

18. Kumar S and Bandyopadhyay U. Free heme toxicity and its detoxification systems in human. Toxicol Lett 2005; 157: 175–188.

19. Piccard H, Van den Steen PE and Opdenakker G. Hemopexin domains as multifunctional liganding modules in matrix metalloproteinases and other proteins.

J Leukoc Biol 2007; 81: 870–892

20. Xu H, Perreau VM, Dent KA, et al. Iron regulates apolipoprotein expression and secretion in neurons and astrocytes. J Alzheimers Dis 2016; 51: 471–487.

21. Cao C, Pressman EK, Cooper EM, et al. Placental heme receptor lrp1 correlates with the heme exporter flvcr1 and neonatal iron status. Reproduction 2014; 148: 295–302.

22. Garland P, Durnford AJ, Okemefuna AI, et al. Heme hemopexin scavenging is active in the brain and associates with outcome after subarachnoid hemorrhage.Stroke 2016; 47: 872–876.

23. Wu B, Ma Q, Suzuki H, et al. Recombinant osteopontin attenuates brain injury after

intracerebral hemorrhage in mice. Neurocrit Care 2011; 14: 109–117.

24. Manaenko A, Lekic T, Ma Q, et al. Hydrogen inhalation ameliorated mast cell-mediated brain injury after intracerebral hemorrhage in mice. Crit Care Med 2013; 41: 1266–1275.

25. Manaenko A, Fathali N, Chen H, et al. Heat shock protein 70 upregulation by geldanamycin reduces brain injury in a mouse model of intracerebral hemorrhage. Neurochem Int 2010; 57: 844–850.

26. Manaenko A, Chen H, Kammer J, et al. Comparison evans blue injection routes: intravenous versus intraperitoneal, for measurement of blood-brain barrier in a mice hemorrhage model. J Neurosci Methods 2011; 195:206–210.

27. Huang L, Sherchan P, Wang Y, et al. Phosphoinositide 3-kinase gamma contributes to neuroinflammation in a rat model of surgical brain injury. J Neurosci 2015; 35:10390–10401.

28. Guo H, Liu J, Van Shura K, et al. N-acetyl-aspartylglutamate and inhibition of glutamate carboxypeptidases protects against soman-induced neuropathology. NeuroToxicology 2015; 48: 180–191.

29. Hu X, Tao C, Gan Q, et al. Oxidative stress in intracerebral hemorrhage: sources, mechanisms, and therapeutic targets. Oxid Med Cell Longev 2016; 2016: 3215391.

30. Wu J, Hua Y, Keep RF, et al. Iron and iron-handling proteins in the brain after intracerebral hemorrhage. Stroke 2003; 34: 2964–2969.

31. Nakamura T, Keep RF, Hua Y, et al. Deferoxamine induced attenuation of brain edema and neurological deficits in a rat model of intracerebral hemorrhage. J Neurosurg 2004; 100: 672–678.

32. Qing WG, Dong YQ, Ping TQ, et al. Brain edema after intracerebral hemorrhage in rats: the role of iron overload and aquaporin 4. J Neurosurg 2009; 110: 462–468.

33. Huang FP, Xi G, Keep RF, et al. Brain edema after experimental intracerebral hemorrhage: Role of hemoglobin degradation products. J Neurosurg 2002; 96: 287–293.

34. Matsushita K, Meng W, Wang X, et al. Evidence for apoptosis after intercerebral hemorrhage in rat striatum. J Cereb Blood Flow Metab 2000; 20: 396–404.

35. Xuan W, Vatansever F, Huang L, et al. Transcranial low level laser therapy improves neurological performance in traumatic brain injury in mice: effect of treatment repetition regimen. PLoS One 2013; 8: e53454.

36. Chidlow G, Wood JP, Sarvestani G, et al. Evaluation of fluoro-jade C as a marker of degenerating neurons in the rat retina and optic nerve. Exp Eye Res 2009; 88:426–437.

37. Alessandri B, Nishioka T, Heimann A, et al. Caspasedependent cell death involved in brain damage after acute subdural hematoma in rats. Brain Res 2006; 1111:196–202.

38. Wagner KR, Sharp FR, Ardizzone TD, et al. Heme and iron metabolism[colon] role in cerebral hemorrhage. J Cereb Blood Flow Metab 2003; 23: 629–652.

39. Hackett MJ, DeSouza M, Caine S, et al. A new method to image heme-fe, total Fe, and aggregated protein levels after intracerebral hemorrhage. ACS Chem Neurosci 2015; 6: 761–770.

40. Lin L and Hu K. Lrp-1: functions, signaling and implications in kidney and other diseases. Int J Mol Sci 2014; 15: 22887–22901.

41. Sagare A, Deane R, Bell RD, et al. Clearance of amyloid beta by circulating lipoprotein receptors. Nat Med 2007; 13: 1029–1031.

42. Kanekiyo T, Liu CC, Shinohara M, et al. Lrp1 in brain vascular smooth muscle cells mediates local clearance of alzheimer's amyloid-beta. J Neurosci 2012; 32: 16458–16465.

43. Storck SE, Meister S, Nahrath J, et al. Endothelial lrp1 transports amyloid-beta1-42 across the blood-brain barrier. J Clin Invest 2016; 126: 123–136.

44. Liu Q, Trotter J, Zhang J, et al. Neuronal lrp1 knockout in adult mice leads to impaired brain lipid metabolism and progressive, age-dependent synapse loss and neurodegeneration. J Neurosci 2010; 30: 17068–17078.

45. Yancey PG, Blakemore J, Ding L, et al. Macrophage lrp-1 controls plaque cellularity by regulating efferocytosis and akt activation. Arterioscler Thromb Vasc Biol 2010; 30: 787–795.

46. Kuo A and Smith MT. Theoretical and practical applications of the intracerebroventricular route for CSF sampling and drug administration in CNS drug discovery research: a mini review. J Neurosci Methods 2014; 233:166–171.

47. Belcher JD, Beckman JD, Balla G, et al. Heme degradation and vascular injury. Antioxid Redox Signal 2010; 12: 233–248.

48. Gu H, Zhong Z, Jiang W, et al. The role of choroid plexus in IVIG-induced beta-amyloid clearance. Neuroscience 2014; 270: 168–176.

49. Kanekiyo T, Cirrito JR, Liu CC, et al. Neuronal clearance of amyloid-beta by endocytic receptor lrp1. J Neurosci 2013; 33: 19276–19283.

DECLARATION: This chapter was authored by Gaiqing Wang, Anatol Manaenko, Anwen Shao, Yibo Ou, Peng Yang, Enkhjargal Budbazar, Nowrangi Derek, John H. Zhang and Jiping Tang published as "low-density lipoprotein receptor-related protein-1 Facilitates Heme Scavenging after Intracerebral Hemorrhage in Mice" in "Journal of cerebral blood flow and metabolism",2017; 37(4): 1299-1310

CHAPTER 9:

TLR7 facilitates heme scavenging through the BTK-CRT-LRP1-Hx pathway in murine intracerebral hemorrhage

ABSTRACT:

Background and Purpose—Heme and iron are considered to be key factors responsible for secondary insults after intracerebral hemorrhage (ICH). Our previous study showed that LRP1 (low-density lipoprotein receptor–related protein-1)–Hx (hemopexin) facilitates removal of heme. The TLR7 (Toll-like receptor 7)–BTK (Bruton tyrosine kinase)–CRT (calreticulin) pathway regulates the expression of LRP1-Hx. This study is designed to clarify whether TLR7 activation facilitates heme scavenging and to establish the potential role of the BTK-CRT-LRP1-Hx signaling pathway in the pathophysiology of ICH.

Methods—ICH was induced by stereotactic, intrastriatal injection of type VII collagenase. Mice received TLR7 agonist (imiquimod) via intraperitoneal injection after ICH induction. TLR7 inhibitor (ODN2088), BTK inhibitor (LFM-A13), and CRT agonist (thapsigargin) were given in different groups to further evaluate the underlying pathway. Mice were randomly divided into sham, ICH+vehicle (normal saline), ICH+ Imiquimod (2.5, 5, and 10 μg/g), ICH+ODN2088, ICH+LFM-A13, ICH+ thapsigargin, and ICH+ODN2088+thapsigargin. Imiquimod was administered twice daily starting at 6 hours after ICH; ODN2088 was administered by intracerebroventricular injection at 30 minutes, and LFM-A13 or thapsigargin was administered by intraperitoneal injection at 3 hours after ICH induction. Neurological scores, cognitive abilities, as well as brain edema, blood-brain barrier permeability, hemoglobin level, brain expression of TLR7/BTK/CRT/LRP1/Hx were analyzed.

Results—Low dosage imiquimod significantly attenuated hematoma volume, brain edema, BBB permeability, and neurological deficits after ICH. Imiquimod also increased protein expressions of TLR7, BTK, CRT, LRP1, and Hx; ODN2088 reduced TLR7, BTK, CRT, LRP1, and Hx expressions.

Conclusions—TLR7 plays an important role in heme scavenging after ICH by modulating the BTK-CRT-LRP1-Hx pathway. TLR7 may offer protective effects by promoting heme resolution and reduction of brain edema after ICH.

Visual Overview—An online visual overview is available for this article. (Stroke. 2018;49:3020-3029. DOI: 10.1161/STROKEAHA.118.022155.)

Visual Abstract

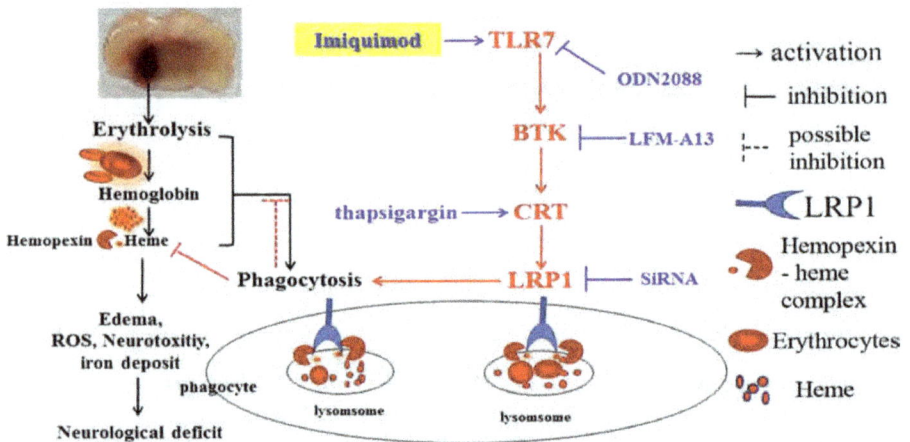

CRT is also considered to be an early eat-me signal that enhances the phagocytosis by activating the internalization receptor LRP1 on the phagocyte. BTK directly phosphorylates CRT and localize with LRP1 at the cell surface. TLR7 activates BTK and clears heme-Hemopexin by LRP1. Our study highlights the role of TLR7, evaluated by administration of TLR7 agonist, Imiquimod and TLR7 inhibitor, ODN2088 in murine ICH. Imiquimod facilitates heme scavenging and exert neuroprotective effects after ICH via activation of the BTK-CRT- LRP1-Hx pathway then diminishing brain edema after ICH. Selective TLR7 inhibition partially reversed the effects associated with imiquimod.

KEY WORDS: Bruton tyrosine kinase; calreticulin; heme scavenging; imiquimod; intracerebral hemorrhage; toll-like receptor

Hemoglobin degradation products, such as heme and iron, are potent cytotoxic molecules that induce oxidative stress, cell death, disruption of the blood-brain barrier (BBB) and are therefore considered key factors responsible for secondary insults after intracerebral hemorrhage (ICH).1 The human body's primary defense mechanism against heme cytotoxicity is provided by Hx (hemopexin), a serum, and neuronal glycoprotein that binds the heme molecule with high affinity, thereby mitigating its prooxidant effects.2 The heme-Hx complex is then endocytosed by cells expressing the LRP1 (low-density lipoprotein receptor–related protein-1).1,3 Indeed, LRP1 was found to be the main receptor binding heme-Hx, thereby enabling its systemic clearance.4 The heme-Hx-LRP1 complex (LRP1 is also known as CD91) facilitates heme scavenging through microglia/macrophages.5 Recently, we have demonstrated that activation of the LRP1 system results in neuroprotection after experimental ICH.1 To further pursue this concept of neuroprotection, we aimed to explore potential pharmacological targets activating LRP1 as a novel therapeutic strategy for ICH.

CRT (calreticulin) is a calcium-binding protein primarily located within the endoplasmic reticulum of phagocytes. Surface-exposed CRT enhances phagocytosis by activating the internalization of LRP1.6 BTK (Bruton tyrosine kinase) phosphorylates and thereby activates CRT. Accordingly, in the absence of BTK, CRT fails to activate LRP1 internalization at the cell surface, which indicates its importance in regulating phagocytosis via the CRT/LRP1 axis.7 It has been shown that TLR7 (Toll-like receptor7) stimulation activates BTK, which leads to phosphorylation of CRT and to clearance of heme-Hx by the cell-surface receptor LRP1.7 Therefore, we hypothesize that TLR7 agonism will activate the BTK-CRT-LRP1 pathway resulting in heme-Hx scavenging, thereby facilitating neuroprotection after experimental ICH.

Methods

The original data of this current study can be obtained from the corresponding author on request. All animals were randomized to the control and experimental groups and neurobehavioral testing, as well as quantitative data collection, was conducted in a blinded fashion (animals and sample tubes were marked by numbers, without any identifiers of group allocation).

Animals

All procedures in this study were approved by the Institutional Animal Care and Use Committee at Loma Linda University and comply with the National Institutes of Health's Guide for the Care and Use of Laboratory Animals. Eight-week-old male CD1 mice (weight 30±5g;Charles River, Wilmington, MA) were housed in a 12-hour light/dark cycle at controlled temperature and humidity with unlimited access to food and water.

ICH Model

The procedure for inducing ICH by stereotactic injection of bacterial collagenase (0.075 U dissolved in 0.5 μL saline, VII-S; Sigma, St Louis, MO) into the basal ganglia were performed as described in our previous publication.1 Sham-operated mice were subjected to needle insertion only. Vital signs were monitored throughout surgery and recovery period. Neurofunctional testing was performed at preselected time points after ICH induction (6 hours, as well as 1, 3, 7, 14, and 28 days). After neurofunctional testing, animals were euthanized, and brain tissues were collected for measurements of brain water content, hematoma volume,

BBB permeability (Evans Blue assay), Western blot, and immunohistochemistry assay as described below.

Experimental Design

Experiments were performed implementing a mouse model of ICH,as shown in Tables I and II in the online-only Data Supplement.

Animals were divided into different experimental groups. A total of 231 mice were used. Animals which died before final assessment were replaced. There were no significant differences in the mortality rates between the different experimental groups.

Experiment 1

For our initial outcome evaluation, 177 mice were divided into 5 groups (Table I in the online-only Data Supplement): sham, ICH+vehicle (sterile normal saline), ICH+imiquimod (2.5, 5, and 10 μg/g). The treatment consisted of TLR7 agonist, imiquimod, which was administered twice daily by intraperitoneal injections starting at 6 hours after ICH for 14 days. Neurofunctional testing (modified Garcia test, beam balance, and wire hang tests) and brain edema were evaluated at 24 and 72 hours after ICH; BBB permeability and hemoglobin levels were measured at 24 hours, as well as at 3, 7, and 14 days after ICH. Iron contents were measured at 28 days after

ICH. Long-term neurofunctional tests (Morris water maze) were conducted between 23 and 28 days after ICH induction. The vehicle group received the same volume of normal saline.

Experiment 2

For further evaluation of the pharmacological mechanism, 54 mice were used (Table II in the online-only Data Supplement). We tested the effect of the TLR7 agonist (imiquimod) and its inhibitor (ODN2088). Thirty-three mice were used for the following groups: sham (n=8), ICH+vehicle (n=8), ICH+imiquimod (2.5 μg/g, every 12 hours, intraperitoneally, n=8), ICH+ODN2088 (n=9),ODN2088 (2 μg in 1 μL normal saline, Invivogen, San Diego, CA) was administered by intracerebroventricular injection 30 minutes after the induction of ICH. We then aimed to investigate whether the neuroprotective effects of TLR7 are mediated through BTK-CRT-LRP1-Hx signaling. Twenty-one mice in 3 additional groups were included: ICH+BTK inhibitor (LFM-A13; n=6); ICH+CRT agonist (thapsigargin; n=6 ICH+ODN2088+thapsigargin (n=9). LFM-A13(25 mg/kg in 1 μL saline, every 12 hours; Sigma, St. Louis, MO) or thapsigargin (2 mg/kg in 1 μL saline; once a day; Sigma) was administered by intraperitoneal injection 3 hours after ICH. The expressions of TLR7/BTK/CRT/LRP1/Hx were evaluated by Western blot analysis. TLR7 expression was also visualized with immunohistochemistry staining.

Intracerebroventricular Injection

As previously described,1 2 μg ODN2088 was dissolved in 1 μL of sterile normal saline and stereotactically injected into the right lateral ventricle at a rate of 0.25 μL/min (coordinates from Bregma: 0 mm anterior, 1 mm right lateral, and 3.5 mm ventral) using a 26-gauge needle. ODN2088 and its control (1 μL normal saline) was administered 24 hours before induction of ICH.

Neurobehavioral Tests

As previously described,1 before euthanasia for tissue collection, all animals were subjected to neurofunctional assessments using the modified Garcia, wire hang, and beam balance tests. The modified Garcia test involves a 21-point sensorimotor assessment that includes 7 individual tests. Each test has a score ranging from 0 to 3, with a maximum score of 21. The individual tests evaluate spontaneous activity, response to side stroking, vibrissae touch, limb symmetry, climbing, lateral turning, and forelimb walking. The wire hang and beam balance tests involve either a wire or a beam connecting 2 platforms at either side. Mice were placed on the center of the wire or beam and allowed to reach the platform. The time to reach a platform, as well as the rodent's behavior, was scored. Scores ranged from 0 to 5, with 5 being the best possible test performance.

Morris water maze test was performed to evaluate the effects of the treatment on spatial learning and memory after ICH. This test was conducted in a round pool (100 cm diameter, 60 cm deep) filled with 22°C water rendered opaque with nontoxic white paint.

A 10 cm escape platform was submerged 1 cm below the water surface, and the pool was divided into 4 quadrants. Five platform zones (1 in each quadrant and 1 in the center of the pool) were specified in each trial. Mice were tested on days 23 to 28 after ICH. In a conditioning trial, each mouse was released into the pool for 90 seconds, guided to the hidden platform, and allowed to remain there for 15s.

On each of the 4 consecutive testing days, mice were released from one of 4 cardinal drop points. For each trial, mice were placed into the water, facing the edge of the pool, and were allowed to search for the platform for a maximum of 90 s. Mice were placed on the platform for 15 s if they did not find the platform before returning to their heated cages. An overhead camera recorded swim paths.

The SMART software (San Diego Instruments, San Diego, CA) analyzed escape latency, swim distances, and linger time in target zones for all trials.

Measurement of Brain Water Content

The brain water content was measured as previously reported using the wet weight/dry weight method.1 Brain specimen was weighed on an electronic analytical balance (APX-60, Denver Instrument,Bohemia, NY) to the nearest 0.1 mg to obtain the wet weight. The tissue was then dried at 100°C for 48 hours to determine the dry weight. Brain water content (%) was calculated as ([wet weight−dry weight]/wet weight)100.

Evans Blue Extravasation

BBB permeability using Evans Blue extravasation was evaluated as previously described.1 A 2% solution of Evans Blue Dye in normal saline (4 mL/kg of body weight) was injected into the jugular vein.

After allowing the dye to circulate for 1 hour, the mice were transcardially perfused with 100 mL of ice-cold PBS. The brain was removed and divided into right and left hemispheres, frozen in liquid nitrogen, and stored at −80°C until analysis. The samples were homogenized in 1100 µL of PBS, sonicated, and centrifuged (30 minutes, 15 000 rcf, 4°C). The supernatant was collected, and for each 500 µL sample, an equal amount of 50% trichloroacetic acid was added. Evans Blue was measured by spectrophotometer (GENESYS 10S UV-Vis spectrophotometer; Thermo Fisher Scientific) at 610 nm and quantified according to a standard curve. The data was calculated as µg of Evans Blue dye/g of tissue and represented as a ratio compared with sham.

Values were calculated from spectrophotometer×2/brain weight, then compared with sham values.

Hemoglobin Assay

For hematoma evaluation, supernatant was collected using the same method as for the Evans Blue assay.1 Drabkin reagent (0.4 mL; Sigma-Aldrich) was added to 0.1 mL supernatant aliquots and allowed to rest for 15 minutes at room temperature, protected from light. Optical density was measured and recorded at 540 nm with a spectrophotometer (GENESYS

10S UV-Vis spectrophotometer; Thermo Fisher Scientific). These procedures yielded a linear relationship between measured hemoglobin concentrations in perfused brain tissues and the volume of added blood on a standard curve.

Western Blot

Western Blot was performed to measure protein expressions as previously described.1 Protein samples (50 μg) were loaded on a Tris-glycine gel, electrophoresed, and transferred to a nitrocellulose membrane. Membranes were incubated overnight at 4°C with the primary antibodies: rabbit polyclonal anti-TLR7 (1:5000; Abcam, Cambridge, MA), rabbit monoclonal anti-BTK (1:4000; Cell Signaling, Danvers, MA), rabbit polyclonal anti-CRT (1:5000; Abcam), rabbit polyclonal anti-LRP1 (1:300000, Abcam), and rabbit polyclonal anti-Hx (1:2000; Abcam). The same membrane was probed with an antibody against β-actin (1:5000; Santa Cruz Biotechnology, Santa Cruz, CA) or tubulin (1:5000; Santa Cruz Biotechnology) as an internal control after being stripped. Incubation with secondary antibodies (Santa Cruz Biotechnology) was done for 1 hour at room temperature. Immunoblots were then probed with an enhanced chemiluminescence (ECL Plus reagent kit; Amersham Biosciences, Arlington Heights, IL) and visualized with an imaging system (Versa Doc, Model 4000; Bio-Rad Laboratories, Hercules,CA). Data were analyzed using Image J software.

Immunohistochemistry

Immunohistochemistry was performed as previously described.8 Whole brains were cut into 10-μm thick coronal sections in a cryostat (CM3050S; Leica Microsystems, Wetzlar, Germany). The sections were incubated overnight at 4°C with the following primary antibodies: rabbit anti-TLR7 (1:100; Abcam), goat anti-Iba1 (ionized calcium-binding adaptor molecule

1, 1:100; Abcam), goat anti-GFAP (glial fibrillary acidic protein, 1:100; Santa Cruz), mouse anti RECA-1 (rat endothelial cell antibody 1, 1:100; Abcam), and rabbit anti-NeuN (neuronal nuclei, 1:100; Abcam) followed by incubation with appropriate fluorescein isothiocyanate–conjugated or Alexa Fluor-conjugated secondary antibodies (Jackson ImmunoResearch Laboratories, West Grove, PA). Negative control staining was performed by omitting the primary antibody. Perihemorrhagic areas of the brain coronal sections were visualized with a fluorescence microscope (BX51; Olympus Corporation, Tokyo, Japan).

Iron Staining and Iron Content

Iron staining and iron content were evaluated as previously described.9 Brain sections were stained with Perls Prussian blue to identify ferric ion (Fe^{3+}) deposits. Briefly, brain sections were rinsed in distilled water and immersed in Perls solution (1% potassium ferrocyanide and 1% HCl [v/v]) for 20 minutes. All slides were rinsed with distilled water, then counterstained with nuclear fast red dye for 5 minutes.

According to the protocol of the commercially available Iron Assay Kit (ab83366; Abcam), brain tissues were homogenized on ice and prepared per instructions (1 mg of brain tissue diluted in 1mL of double-distilled water). The brain tissue homogenates were centrifuged for 20 minutes at 2000g. Supernatant was removed and stored in aliquots at −20°C. The included Iron Standard solution was diluted as per protocol (2–10 nmol/well) and the Iron Reducer (5 μL) was added to 0.1 mL supernatant aliquots or the standard solution and incubated for 30 minutes at room temperature, protected from light. Iron Probe (100 μL) was then added to each well containing the Iron Standard solution or the samples. Optical density was measured and recorded at 570 nm with an automated ELISA reader (iMarkTM Microplate Absorbance Reader, Bio-Rad Laboratories).

These procedures yielded a linear relationship between measured iron concentrations in brain samples and the Iron Standard curve. Total iron contents of the samples were acquired from the standard curve.

Statistical Analysis

Quantitative data are presented as mean±SD. One-way ANOVA for multiple comparisons with Tukey post hoc test was used to determine the differences of brain water contents and Western blot assay among all groups at each time point. Two-way ANOVA with Bonferroni post-test was used to assay the differences of neurological deficits. $P<0.05$ was considered statistically significant.

Results

Mortality

All sham-operated mice survived. The total operative mortality of mice subjected to ICH was 8.2 % (n=19). The mortality was not significantly different among the experimental groups (data not shown).

TLR7 Agonist, Imiquimod, Decreased Hematoma Volume and Ameliorated BBB Disruption and Brain Edema

All ICH groups showed a significant increase in brain water content, hemoglobin levels, and Evans blue extravasation when compared with sham at 24 hours after surgery ($P<0.05$, Figure 1A,1C, and 1D). Imiquimod 5 and 10 μg/g treatment resulted in lower hemoglobin levels at 24 hours after collagenase injection when compared to the vehicle group; however, there were no significant differences between imiquimod 2.5 μg/g treatment and the vehicle group. Imiquimod 2.5 and 5 μg/g treatment reduced hemoglobin levels (hematoma volumes) at 72 hours after collagenase injection compared with the vehicle group (Figure 1D), but only 2.5 μg/g imiquimod reduced brain water content and BBB permeability at 24 and 72 hours after ICH when compared with the ICH+vehicle group (P<0.05, Figure 1A–1C).

Low-Dose Imiquimod Improved Short-Term Neurological Deficits After ICH

ICH+vehicle animals scored significantly lower compared to sham mice in all neurofunctional tests performed at each time point (p<0.05). Compared with ICH+vehicle, TLR7 agonist, Imiquimod treatment resulted in significant improvement of neurofunctional deficits evaluated with the modified Garcia test at 24 and 72 hours after ICH (p<0.05), but only low dose imiquimod showed improvement in the wire hang and beam balance tests at 72 hours after ICH induction (p<0.05).

Following these results, we chose 2.5 µg/g imiquimod to examine the long-term neurofunctional tests and the pharmacologic mechanisms of TLR7 at 72 hours after ICH for further studies.

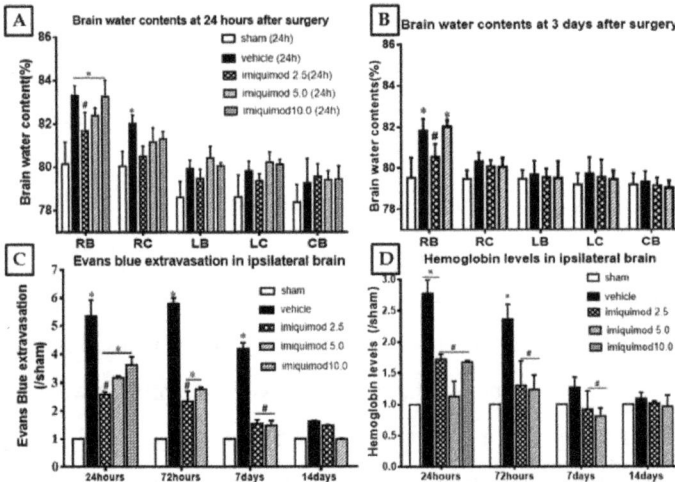

Figure 1. Effect of TLR7 (Toll-like receptor 7) agonist (imiquimod) on brain water content (A and B, n=6–7 per group), blood-brain barrier permeability (C,n=6–7 per group), hematoma volume (D, n=6–7 per group) at different time points after intracerebral hemorrhage (ICH). One-way ANOVA followed by Tukey tests were used. *P<0.05 vs sham, #P<0.05 vs ICH+vehicle.

Imiquimod improved long-term neurofunctional deficits following ICH

Results of the Morris Water Maze showed that low dose imiquimod improved the spacial memory after ICH ($p<0.05$, Fig. 2 A-D). A was visualization of swimming track and heat map; B was a mean latency to escape onto the platform; C was a mean swimming distances before escaping onto the platform; D was a mean searching times for the platform in the target quadrant in the probe trial on the 6th day. Specifically, Imiquimod-treated ICH mice showed shorter routes travelled compared with vehicle animals. During the first day of testing (with the platform being visible above the water surface), sham, imiquimod-treated and vehicle mice exhibited a similar latency to reach the platform. In subsequent testing (with the platform being hidden below the water surface), imiquimod-treated ICH mice showed a shorter latency to escape onto the platform on the 3rd and 4th day of the Water Maze experiments. Compared with vehicle animals, imiquimod-treated mice demonstrated a shorter swimming length before escaping onto the hidden platform on the 2nd and 4th day of testing. In the probe trial on the 6th day of testing, imiquimod-treated mice traveled significantly more within the target quadrant (where the rescue platform used to be) than vehicle animals.

Imiquimod reduced iron levels after ICH

Iron staining and iron contents were measured on day 28 after ICH induction, upon completion of Morris Water Maze testing. Imiquimod-treated ICH mice exhibited decreased iron contents in the ipsilateral brain hemispheres as compared to vehicle group ($p<0.05$, Fig.3).

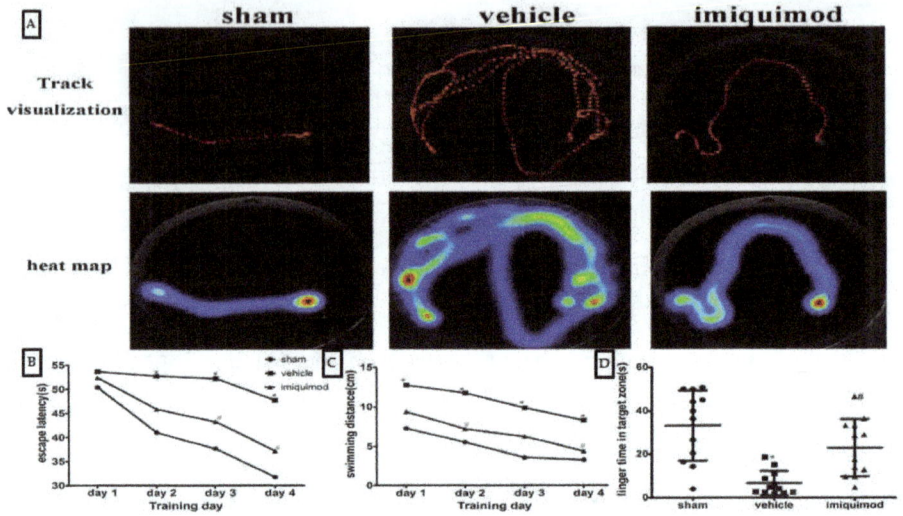

Figure 2. Morris Water Maze was tested in sham and imiquimod-treated (2.5 μg/g, twice a day) or vehicle solution injections from 23 to 28 d after intracerebral hemorrhage (ICH; n=7/group). *P<0.05 vs sham, #P<0.05 vs ICH+vehicle, (n=7/group), 2-way ANOVA, mean±SD, analysis by repeated measures ANOVA.

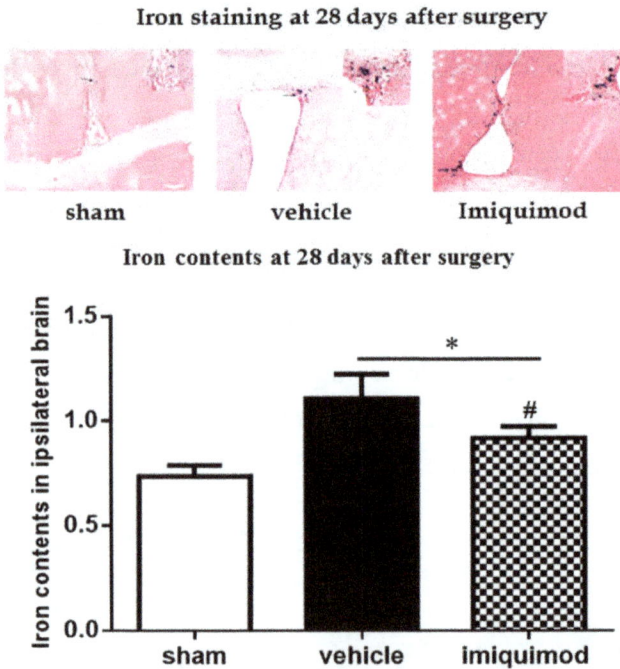

Figure 3. Iron staining and iron content assays at 28 d after intracerebral hemorrhage (ICH) induction. *P<0.05 vs sham, #P<0.05 vs ICH+vehicle, n=7 per group, 1-way ANOVA, Tukey multiple comparison test, mean±SD.

TLR7 treatment was mediated through BTK-CRT-LRP1-Hx signaling activation

Western blot analysis was implemented to measure the protein expression of TLR7, BTK, CRT, LRP1 and Hx within the ipsilateral brain hemisphere. TLR7, BTK, CRT, LRP1 and Hx were significantly elevated in ICH+ vehicle and ICH+ imiquimod groups when compared to sham ($p<0.05$, Fig.4-5). The BTK inhibitor (LFM-A13) did not show any difference in expression of TLR7 when compared to the vehicle group ($p>0.05$, Fig.4). TLR7 agonist (imiquimod) treatment resulted in significantly higher protein expression of TLR7, BTK, CRT, LRP1 and Hx when compared to its vehicle ($p<0.05$, Fig.4-5). TLR7 inhibitor (ODN2088) given alone displayed decreased expression of TLR7, BTK, CRT, LRP1 and Hx compared to its vehicle ($p<0.05$) and were similar to sham group ($p>0.05$, Fig.4-5). LFM-A13 administration resulted in a significant reduction of BTK, CRT, LRP1 and Hx expression when compared to vehicle ($p<0.05$, Fig.4-5) and were similar to sham group ($p>0.05$, Fig.4-5). The CRT agonist (Thapsigargin), when given alone, resulted in a significant elevation of CRT, LRP1 and Hx expression; however, ODN2088 combined with Thapsigargin still reduced TLR7, BTK, LRP1 and Hx expressions but demonstrated no change in CRT expression as compared to vehicle.

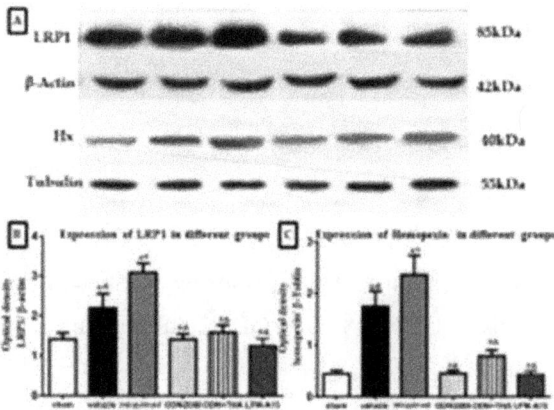

Figure 4. Effect of TLR7 (Toll-like receptor 7) agonist (imiquimod), TLR7 inhibitor (ODN2088) alone and with CRT (calreticulin) agonist (thapsigargin [THA]), BTK (Bruton tyrosine kinase) inhibitor (LFM-A13) on TLR7, BTK, and CRT at 72 h after ICH induction.

Figure 4. continued. Representative images are shown of Western blot assays for TLR7, BTK, and CRT levels within ipsilateral brain tissue (A–D, n=6–7 per group). One-way ANOVA followed by Tukey tests were used. *P<0.05 vs sham, #P<0.05 vs ICH+vehicle, and P<0.05 vs ICH+imiquimod.

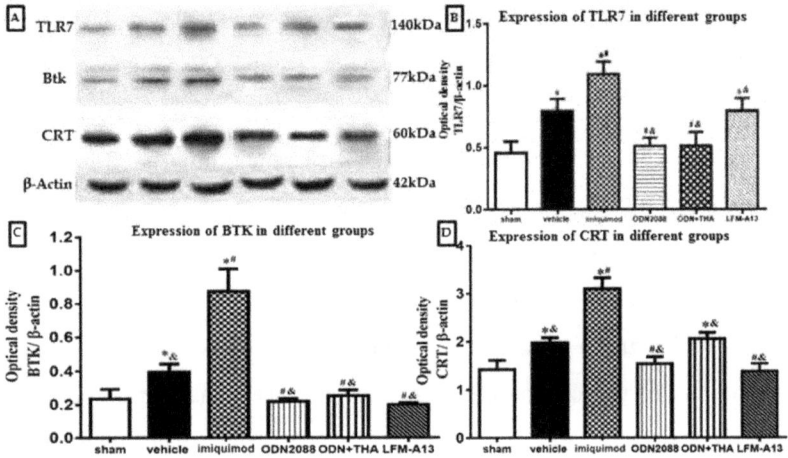

Figure 5. Effect of TLR7 (Toll-like receptor 7) agonist (imiquimod), TLR7 inhibitor (ODN2088) alone and with CRT (calreticulin) agonist (thapsigargin [THA]), BTK (Bruton tyrosine kinase) inhibitor (LFM-A13) on LRP1 (low-density lipoprotein receptor–related protein-1) and Hx(hemopexin) at 72 h after ICH induction. Representative images are shown of Western blot assays for LRP1 and Hx levels within ipsilateral brain tissue (A–C, n=6–7 per group). One-way ANOVA followed by Tukey tests were used. *P<0.05 vs sham, #P<0.05 vs ICH+vehicle, and P<0.05 vs ICH+ imiquimod.

Double immunofluorescence staining was completed in the perihematomal brain tissue (Fig. 6). Fluorescent staining demonstrated that TLR7 was expressed in microglia (Iba-1, Fig. 6A), astrocytes (GFAP, Fig. 6B), endothelial cells of brain vessels (RECA; Fig. 6C) and neurons (NeuN, Fig. 6D).

Additionally, fluorescence of TLR7 revealed increased expression in vehicle and Imiquimod-treated groups while showing decreased expression in animals that received ODN2088 and ODN2088 combined with Thapsigargin, thereby supporting the Western blot results.

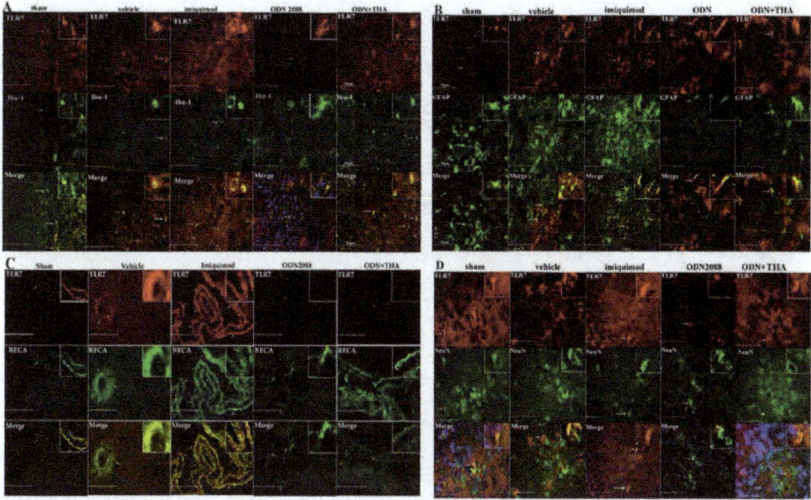

Figure 6. Representative immunohistochemistry microphotographs of TLR7 (Toll-like receptor 7) with Iba1 (ionized calcium-binding adaptor molecule 1; A),TLR7 and GFAP (glial fibrillary acidic protein; B), TLR7 and RECA (rat endothelial cell antibody; C) TLR7 and Neun (neuronal nuclei; D) within the perihematomal brain tissues in different groups (n=2 per group), which demonstrated that TLR7 was expressed in microglia, astroglia, endothelial cells and neurons (scale bar, 10 μm). THA indicates thapsigargin.

Discussion

In the present study, we have made the following observations: (1) The TLR7 agonist, Imiquimod significantly attenuated hematoma volume, ICH-induced brain edema, BBB permeability, and neurofunctional deficits at 24 hours and 3 days after ICH. (2) Imiquimod also improved spaceal memory and reduced iron levels in mice 28 days after ICH. (3) Endogenous TLR7, BTK, CRT, LRP1 and Hx levels were significantly elevated in the ipsilateral brain hemispheres at 3 days after ICH induction. (4) Imiquimod treatment resulted in increased protein expressions of TLR7, BTK, CRT, LRP1 and Hx, whereas the TLR7 inhibitor, ODN2088 resulted in decreased expressions of TLR7, BTK, CRT, LRP1 and Hx. (5) The BTK inhibitor, LFM-A13 reduced BTK, CRT, LRP1 and Hx expressions when compared to its vehicle but were similar to those of sham animals. (6) CRT agonist, Thapsigargin resulted in increased expressions of CRT, LRP1 and Hx. However, when combined with the TLR7 inhibitor, Thapsigargin did not elevate but decreased BTK, LRP1 and Hx expression compared to the vehicle group. These results suggest that TLR7 is involved in heme scavenging and BBB protection in adjacent hematoma brain tissues after ICH. The TLR7 agonist, Imiquimod facilitates heme-Hx scavenging and exert neuroprotective effects after ICH likely by modulating the BTK-CRT-LRP1-Hx pathway.

Our group has recently reported that LRP1 contributes to heme clearance and subsequent BBB protection after ICH by reinforcing the effect of Hx after ICH, signaling pathway through LRP1 appears to be a common platform modulating heme scavenging after ICH 1. Hx is a plasma glycoprotein able to bind heme with a high affinity 5, 10 which clears heme in a non-toxic form and transports it to the liver for catabolism and evacuation11. Therefore activating LRP1 could be a therapeutic strategy to scavenge toxic hematoma products after ICH.

Erythrophagocytosis can be mediated by the interaction between calreticulin (CRT) on the target cell and LRP1 (CD91/α2-macroglobulin receptor) on the macrophage12. CRT and LRP1 functions at the cell membrane and regulate uptake of apoptotic cells or debris. BTK is critical in regulating CRT-driven apoptotic cell uptake, as it directly phosphorylates CRT and without BTK, CRT fails to localize with LRP1 at the cell surface and at the phagocytic cup7. BTK plays a key role in macrophage stimulation by various Toll-like receptors (TLRs)13. TLRs are a class of pattern recognition receptors that play a bridging role in innate immunity and adaptive immunity 14. The stimulation of TLRs, leads to the initiation of intracellular signal transduction pathways regulating macrophagic activation and effector functions 15. TLR7, a member of TLR family, is an intracellular receptor expressed on the membrane of endosomes 14. TLR7 stimulation results in activation of BTK, which plays an important role in facilitating the tyrosine phosphorylation of CRT. Rectification of CRT via BTK is important for control of the trafficking of CRT within myeloid cells. Trafficking of CRT to the cell surface facilitates colocalization with the cell-surface receptor LRP1 7. Therefore, stimulation of TLR7 should activate phagocytosis through the BTK-CRT-LRP1 pathway. Consistent with this hypothesis, our study utilized TLR7 inhibitor, ODN2088 administration and with it found suppressed TLR7-BTK-CRT-LRP1-Hx expression in the brain. It further reversed the role of TLR7 agonist on the BTK-CRT-LRP1-Hx pathway, BTK inhibitor also suppressed CRT-LRP1-Hx expression, confirming the role of TLR7 in ICH through BTK-CRT-LRP1-Hx pathway.

Microglia and astrocytes are the major immune cells of the brain and express a full repertoire of TLR7 16, 17. TLR7 is expressed in brain capillary endothelial cells 18 as well as in peripheral neurons 19. Our results verified that TLR7 is mainly expressed on the dendrites of astroglia, endothelial cells and microglia, especially in the choroid plexus, the location of TLR7 sh owed that it should take an important role in trafficking heme in ICH model. TLR7-dependent astrocyte activation could be mediated by cytokines and chemokines that are produced following TLR7 stimulation in macrophages or microglia 17. Alternatively, TLR7-dependent activation of phagocytes may be direct, following endocytosis of the foreign microbes, necrotic cells, and debris. The main target cells of TLR7 agonists are dendritic cells, producing IFN-γ then acting on other immune cells 20. TLR7 agonist, Imiquimod is an immunomodulatory, synthetic small-molecule compound in the imidazoquinoline family that displays both antiviral and antitumor effec21-25. Imiquimod has been shown to activate a variety of genes associated with macrophage activation 26, 27. So imiquimod could induce leukocyte infiltration and inflammation then aggravated brain swelling 24. This could explain why the low but not the high dose of imiquimod is effective in our study, implementing experimental ICH in mice. The phagocytosis of Imiquimod in ICH could be explained by its induced substantial astrocyte responses in vivo 28. Our immunohistochemical staining demonstrated that Imiquimod enhanced the expression of TLR7 on astrocytes following ICH. Furthermore, our study used intraperitoneal Imiquimod administration and found activated TLR7 expression in the brain which further reduced heme levels then attenuated brain edema and BBB permeability around hematoma, confirming the protective role of TLR7 in ICH pathological progression.

In conclusion, our study highlights the role of TLR7, evaluated by administration of TLR7 agonist and TLR7 inhibitor in experimental murine ICH. Imiquimod facilitates heme scavenging and exert neuroprotective effects after ICH via activation of the BTK-CRT- LRP1-Hx pathway. Selective TLR7 inhibition partially reversed the effects associated with TLR7 agonist. Thus, TLR7 may offer protective effects through promoting heme scavenging and thereby diminishing brain edema after ICH, which may prove beneficial in post-ICH outcomes.

Sources of Funding:

This study was supported in part by a grant from National Natural Science Foundation of China (81771294)

Disclosures:

None

REFERENCE:

1. Wang G, Manaenko A, Shao A, Ou Y, Yang P, Budbazar E, et al. Low-density

lipoprotein receptor-related protein-1 facilitates heme scavenging after intracerebral hemorrhage in mice. J Cereb Blood Flow Metab. 2017;37:1299-1310

2. Chen L, Zhang X, Chen-Roetling J, Regan RF. Increased striatal injury and behavioral deficits after intracerebral hemorrhage in hemopexin knockout mice. J Neurosurg. 2011;114:1159-1167

3. Hvidberg V, Maniecki MB, Jacobsen C, Hojrup P, Moller HJ, Moestrup SK. Identification of the receptor scavenging hemopexin-heme complexes. Blood. 2005;106:2572-2579

4. Cao C, Pressman EK, Cooper EM, Guillet R, Westerman M, O'Brien KO. Placental heme receptor lrp1 correlates with the heme exporter flvcr1 and neonatal iron status. Reproduction. 2014;148:295-302

5. Aronowski J, Zhao X. Molecular pathophysiology of cerebral hemorrhage: Secondary brain injury. Stroke. 2011;42:1781-1786

6. Gardai SJ, McPhillips KA, Frasch SC, Janssen WJ, Starefeldt A, Murphy-Ullrich JE, et al. Cell-surface calreticulin initiates clearance of viable or apoptotic cells through trans-activation of lrp on the phagocyte. Cell. 2005;123:321-334

7. Byrne JC, Ni Gabhann J, Stacey KB, Coffey BM, McCarthy E, Thomas W, et al. Bruton's tyrosine kinase is required for apoptotic cell uptake via regulating the phosphorylation and localization of calreticulin. J Immunol. 2013;190:5207-5215

8. Huang L, Sherchan P, Wang Y, Reis C, Applegate RL, 2nd, Tang J, et al. Phosphoinositide 3-kinase gamma contributes to neuroinflammation in a rat model of surgical brain injury. J Neurosci. 2015;35:10390-10401

9. Wang G, Hu W, Tang Q, Wang L, Sun XG, Chen Y, et al. Effect comparison of both iron chelators on outcomes, iron deposit, and iron transporters after intracerebral hemorrhage in rats. Mol Neurobiol. 2016;53:3576-3585

10. Tolosano E, Altruda F. Hemopexin: Structure, function, and regulation. DNA Cell Biol. 2002;21:297-306

11. Schaer DJ, Vinchi F, Ingoglia G, Tolosano E, Buehler PW. Haptoglobin, hemopexin, and related defense pathways-basic science, clinical perspectives, and drug development. Front Physiol. 2014;5:415

12. Nilsson A, Vesterlund L, Oldenborg PA. Macrophage expression of lrp1, a receptor for apoptotic cells and unopsonized erythrocytes, can be regulated by glucocorticoids. Biochem Biophys Res Commun. 2012;417:1304-1309

13. Vijayan V, Baumgart-Vogt E, Naidu S, Qian G, Immenschuh S. Bruton's tyrosine kinase is required for tlr-dependent heme oxygenase-1 gene activation via nrf2 in macrophages. J Immunol. 2011;187:817-827

14. Chi H, Li C, Zhao FS, Zhang L, Ng TB, Jin G, et al. Anti-tumor activity of toll-like receptor 7 agonists. Front Pharmacol. 2017;8:304

15. Koprulu AD, Ellmeier W. The role of tec family kinases in mononuclear phagocytes. Crit Rev Immunol. 2009;29:317-333

16. Hanke ML, Kielian T. Toll-like receptors in health and disease in the brain: Mechanisms and therapeutic potential. Clin Sci (Lond). 2011;121:367-387

17. Peterson KE, Du M. Innate immunity in the pathogenesis of polytropic retrovirus infection in the central nervous system. Immunol Res. 2009;43:149-159

18. Lewis SD, Butchi NB, Khaleduzzaman M, Morgan TW, Du M, Pourciau S, et al. Toll-like receptor 7 is not necessary for retroviral neuropathogenesis but does contribute to virus-induced neuroinflammation. J Neurovirol. 2008;14:492-502

19. Karper JC, Ewing MM, Habets KL, de Vries MR, Peters EA, van Oeveren-Rietdijk AM, et al. Blocking toll-like receptors 7 and 9 reduces postinterventional remodeling via reduced macrophage activation, foam cell formation, and migration. Arterioscler Thromb Vasc Biol. 2012;32:24

20. Kobold S, Wiedemann G, Rothenfusser S, Endres S. Modes of action of tlr7 agonists in cancer therapy. Immunotherapy. 2014;6:1085-1095

21. Hemmi H, Kaisho T, Takeuchi O, Sato S, Sanjo H, Hoshino K, et al. Small anti-viral compounds activate immune cells via the tlr7 myd88-dependent signaling pathway. Nat Immunol. 2002;3:196-200

22. Palamara F, Meindl S, Holcmann M, Luhrs P, Stingl G, Sibilia M. Identification and characterization of pdc-like cells in normal mouse skin and melanomas treated with imiquimod. J Immunol. 2004;173:3051-3061

23. Imiquimod for superficial and in situ skin malignancy. Drug Ther Bull. 2009;47:113-116

24. Prins RM, Craft N, Bruhn KW, Khan-Farooqi H, Koya RC, Stripecke R, et al. The tlr-7 agonist, imiquimod, enhances dendritic cell survival and promotes tumor antigen-specific t cell priming: Relation to central nervous system antitumor immunity. J Immunol. 2006;176:157-164

25. Xiong Z, Ohlfest JR. Topical imiquimod has therapeutic and immunomodulatory effects against intracranial tumors. J Immunother. 2011;34:264-269

26. Buates S, Matlashewski G. Identification of genes induced by a macrophage activator, s-28463, using gene expression array analysis. Antimicrob Agents Chemother. 2001;45:1137-1142

27. Arevalo I, Ward B, Miller R, Meng TC, Najar E, Alvarez E, et al. Successful treatment of drug-resistant cutaneous leishmaniasis in humans by use of imiquimod, an immunomodulator. Clin Infect Dis. 2001;33:1847-1851

28. Butchi NB, Pourciau S, Du M, Morgan TW, Peterson KE. Analysis of the neuroinflammatory response to tlr7 stimulation in the brain: Comparison of multiple tlr7 and/or tlr8 agonists. J Immunol. 2008;180:7604-7612

DECLARATION: This chapter was authored by Gaiqing Wang, Zhenni Guo, Lusha Tong, Fang Xue, Paul R. Krafft, Enkhjargal Budbazar, John H. Zhang and Jiping Tang published as "TLR7 facilitates heme scavenging through the BTK-CRT-LRP1-Hx pathway in murine intracerebral hemorrhage" in "Stroke", 2018; 49(12):3020–3029

CHAPTER 10:

PPAR-γ promotes hematoma clearance through Haptoglobin-Hemoglobin-CD163 in a Rat Model of Intracerebral Hemorrhage

ABSTRACT:

Background and Purpose. PPAR-γ is a transcriptional factor which is associated with promoting hematoma clearance and reducing neurological dysfunction after intracerebral hemorrhage (ICH). Haptoglobin- (Hp-) hemoglobin- (Hb-) CD163 acts as a main pathway to Hb scavenging after ICH. The effect of PPAR-γ on the Hp-Hb-CD163 signaling pathway has not been reported. We hypothesized that PPAR-γ might protect against ICH-induced neuronal injury via activating the Hp-Hb-CD163 pathway in a rat ICH model.

Methods. 107 Sprague-Dawley rats were used in this research. They were randomly allocated to 4 groups as follows: sham group, vehicle group, monascin-treated group, and Glivec-treated group. Animals were euthanized at 3 days after the model was established successfully. We observed the effects of PPAR-γ on the brain water content, hemoglobin levels, and the expressions of CD163 and Hp in Western blot and real-time PCR; meanwhile, we measured hematoma volumes and edema areas by MRI scanning.

Results. The results showed that PPAR-γ agonist significantly reduced hematoma volume, brain edema, and hemoglobin after ICH. It also enhanced CD163 and Hp expression while PPAR-γ antagonist had the opposite effects.

Conclusions. PPAR-γ promotes hematoma clearance and plays a protective role through the Hp-Hb-CD163 pathway in a rat collagenase infusion ICH model.

KEY WORDS: Hematoma clearance; PPAR-γ; Hemoglobin; Haptoglobin; CD163; Monascin; Intracerebral hemorrhage

1. Introduction

In Western societies, intracerebral hemorrhage (ICH) takes up for 8–15% of all strokes and 20–30% in the Asian area, and there is no definite effective therapy so far [1, 2]. Understanding the complex pathophysiology of cerebral injury after ICH is crucial to developing new approaches to reduce the harmful impacts on ICH.

The occurrence of ICH begins with a vast release of blood within the brain parenchyma [3, 4]. Erythrocytes, as the major cellular components of the hematoma, dissolves and releases hemoglobin (Hb) which subsequently broke down into heme and iron after ICH within a few days [5]. These cytotoxins mainly cause secondary brain injury following ICH [6]. Haptoglobin-Hb-CD163 as well as hemopexin-heme-LRP1 (low-density lipoprotein receptor-related protein-1) is believed to be the most important endogenous scavenging pathway which participates in hematoma/blood component resolution following ICH [6]. The cell-free Hb can trigger oxidative damages caspase activation, blood-brain barrier disruption, and neuronal death and result in irreversible brain damages [7]. CD163, which is the only hemoglobin clearance receptor expressed in the mononuclear phagocyte system, is formed during the hemolysis of erythrocytes and mediates the endocytosis of the Hb, leading to the degradation of the ligand protein and cytoplasmic heme oxygenase [8]. Haptoglobin (Hp), which is a primary Hb-binding protein, attenuates the destructive effects of Hb in the plasma [6, 9, 10]. Superabundant Hb in the plasma can upregulate the expression of Hp and the Hb-Hp receptor CD163 in neurons [11]. Hp is bound to free Hb and once Hp-Hb complex is endocytosed by CD163 may cause an anti-inflammatory response. The Hp-Hb- CD163 acts as the main pathway inHbscavenging and exerts a pivotal protective role [9, 12].

PPAR-γ is a transcription factor which can regulate the expression of catalase and superoxide dismutase which are two important antioxidant genes [13, 14]. It is also associated with promoting hematoma clearance and reducing neurological dysfunction [15]. As a PPAR-γ agonist, monascin is the main component of red yeast rice with a Chinese traditional technique and has been shown to have a protective effect by promoting hematoma clearance and reducing cerebral edema in rats after ICH [13], but the specific mechanism of monascin in ICH has not been clarified so far.

We hypothesize that PPAR-γ will promote hematoma clearance via CD163 and Hp upregulation, therefore reducing brain edema and improving BBB integrity after ICH. So we designed the study to test the effect of PPAR-γ on the Hp-Hb-CD163 pathway through PPAR-γ agonist monascin and its antagonist Glivec which mediates PPAR-γ by declining the phosphorylation level [16] in a collagenase-induced ICH rat model.

2. Materials and Methods

2.1. Animal Preparation. This study used 107 male adult Sprague-Dawley rats, weighing about 250~300 g (from Shanxi Medical University Animal Laboratory). The protocol for using these animals was in accordance with the Animal Utilization and Management Committee which was made by Shanxi Medical University. All rats were available to get fodder and water freely in the research.

2.2. Animal Treatments and Experimental and Control Groups.

All rats were randomized to the following groups: sham operation group ($n = 25$), vehicle group ($n = 27$), monascin-treated group (10 mg/kg twice a day, $n = 26$), and Glivec-treated group (100 mg/kg/day, $n = 29$). Dead animals were replaced before final assessment. All gavages were administered by gastric perfusion 6 h after ICH until the endpoint.

2.3. Intracerebral Hemorrhage Model of Rats.

The intracerebral hemorrhage model was made by injecting collagenase IV to the corpus striatum under a head stereotaxic apparatus [13]. Briefly, experimental rats were anesthetized by hydrated chloric aldehyde (300–350 mg/kg) in an intraperitoneal injection method. After being anesthetized, rats were positioned in the stereotactic instrument (Jiangwan type 1 C Instrument, Shanghai, China). A 1mm needle was inserted through a cranial burr hole into the striatum to the following frame of references: 0.50mm anterior, 5.8mm ventral, and 2.3mm lateral to the bregma. Then, we used a 5 μL flatheaded microsyringe (Hamilton 600, Switzerland) to infuse 0.5U type IV collagenase (Sigma-Aldrich, USA) which was dissolved in 2.5 μL saline solution. After infusion, the needle needs to be maintained in there for extra 3 minutes and subsequently be pulled out slowly. In the sham group, 2.5 μL saline solution was infused using the same method. After the surgery, the hole in the skull was sealed and the scalp was well sutured. Animals were bred in a specific facility which was pathogen free. Besides, they can get food and water uncontrolled.

2.4. Brain Water Content.

The water content of rat brain tissue was performed as earlier described [13]. We used 4% chloral hydrate for intraperitoneal injection to deeply anesthetize the rat, and then the rat was decapitated to measure the cerebral water content. The brain tissue was removed from the skull rapidly and then divided into 4mm sections in the portion around the puncture point. All brain tissue samples we got from the ipsilateral basal ganglia were instantly weighed by an electric microbalance to know the wet weight (Ww). Then tissues were placed in a 100°C drying oven for 48 hours to desiccation. After that, we can obtain dry weight (Dw). The brain water content was calculated by the following formula: $(Ww-Dw)/Ww \times 100\%$.

2.5. Hemoglobin Assay.

Quantitation of brain hemoglobin after ICH was measured by hemoglobin assay under the guidance of the manufacturer's instructions. Briefly, successful modeling rats were sacrificed and the brain tissues were quickly removed and put into four glass dishes, respectively. A total of 1000 μL prerefrigerated PBS buffer was added into each glass dish. Brain tissue was smashed by sonication, collected in a centrifuged tube, and centrifuged at 4°C, 12000 rpm for 30 minutes. 25 μL of the supernatant of each group was put into a 96-well plate, and Drabkin's reagent was added to the supernatant in a ratio of 1: 4. After incubation for 5 minutes at room temperature, OD value was measured by a spectrophotometer in 400 nm. The OD value of each sample was calibrated by a blank group.

2.6. Expression of PPAR-γ, CD163, and Hp in Different Groups by Western Blot.

The brain tissue was smashed, and RIPA Lysis Buffer with PMSF was added for extracted total protein in each sample for Western blot analysis. Protein concentration was determined by a bicinchoninic acid (BCA) assay. 50 μg of each sample lysis was loaded on a 10% sodium dodecyl sulfate gel and electrophoresed in 90 volts for 2 hours. Belt was transferred to the polyvinylidene fluoride membrane after an electrophoresis process. Membranes were blocked with 5% BSA blocking buffer at 37°C for 2 hours and incubated with first antibodies: polyclonal anti-PPAR-γ of rabbit (1: 1000, Bioss), anti-CD163 of rabbit (1 : 500, Bioss), and polyclonal anti-Hp of rabbit (1 : 500, Bioss) at 4°C in a thermostat shaker overnight. Meanwhile, other membranes were probed with β-actin (1: 3000, Bioworld) as an internal control.

After being washed by the TBST buffer, all membranes were incubated with the second antibodies at 37°C for 2 hours.

Immunoreactive membranes were processed with an ECL Plus chemiluminescence assay kit. After that, it can be visualized through an imaging system (Bio-Rad, ChemiDoc). Finally, band intensities were normalizing with their internal controls, respectively, and digitizing using Image J software.

2.7. Measurements of Volume of Hematoma and Cerebral Edema by MRI. All rats were given brain MRI scan on a 1.5 T clinical scanner (GE Signa HDx, GE healthcare Milwaukee) with a knee coil 3 days post-ICH at the Second Hospital affiliated to Shanxi Medical University. During the MRI imaging scanning, rats were maintained well anesthetized after the use of 5% chloral hydrate with the prone position.

A series of MR sequences were acquired in our study, the protocol included T2-weighted imaging (T2WI) and T2 Flair to assess the edema, and scanning parameters [13] are listed as follows: repetition time (TR)/echo time (TE) = 2400/129 ms, field of view (FOV) = 18 × 18mm, slice thickness = 2.0mm, matrix size = 512 × 448, and interval = 0.2mm. In T2 fluid-attenuated inversion recovery (T2 Flair), TR/TE = 8502/128.6 ms, FOV= 12 × 12mm, slice thickness = 2.0mm, matrix size = 512 × 448, and interval = 0.2 mm. T2*-weighted imaging (T2*WI) and susceptibility weighted imaging (SWI) were used to determine the hematoma size; scan parameters are as follows: in T2*WI, TR/TE = 400/15 ms, FOV= 18 × 18mm, slice thickness =2.0 mm, matrix size = 448 × 384, interval = 0.2mm, and flip angle = 15°. In SWI: TR/TE = 49.9/4.5 ms, FOV=18 × 18mm, slice thickness = 1.5 mm, flip angle = 15°, and matrix size = 448 × 448. MRI postprocessing was performed on an off-line workstation by two experienced neurologists who were blinded to the group set and scan date. The absolute

volume of intracerebral hemorrhage area which contains the outer amount of edema and hematoma was adopted during the measurement process. The total value of the absolute volume was calculated by integrating injured areas of brain hemorrhage slices. All the assessments were repeated three times, respectively. The results were shown as the mean and standard deviation.

2.8. Assay of Haptoglobin and CD163 in Different Groups by Real-Time PCR.

The total RNA of different groups was extracted from the brain tissue surrounding hematoma by using TRIzol Reagent (Takara Inc., Japan) complied with the manufacturer's instructions. After completing the extraction process, total RNA was determined by Nano-drop 2000 (Thermo Fisher, USA) with the UV absorbance at 260nm to ensure purity. Complementary DNA was reverse transcribed by using a one-step PrimeScript™ RT Master Mix kit (Takara Inc., Japan), and a total of 20 μL reaction mixture system which contained 1 μg total RNA was carried out at 37°C for 15 minutes; finally, the complementary DNA was kept at a minus 80°C environment. Real-time PCR analysis was processed in a BIO-RAD iCycler Thermal Cycler for RT-PCR (Bio-rad, USA) with the complementary DNA and SYBR® Premix Ex Taq™ Kit (Takara Inc., Japan). Oligonucleotide PCR-based primers are as follows: haptoglobin: 5′-gaaaggcgctgtaagtcctg-3′ (forward primer) and 5′-tcctcttccagggtgaattg-3′(reverse primer) and CD163: 5′-gacagacccaacggcttaca-3′ (forward primer) and 5′-ggtcacaaaacttcaaccgga-3′(reverse primer). The experiment uses a 25 μL volume total reaction mixture reaction system which contains 2 μL of the diluted complementary DNA product, 12.5 μL of the SYBR Premix Ex Taq Mix (Takara Inc., Japan), 1 μL of forward/reverse primers, respectively, and 8.5 μL of RNase-free water. The condition of real-time PCR reaction was implemented as follows: predenaturation step was processed at 95°C for 1 minute. The extended process sets the denaturation at 95°C for 30 seconds and annealing and elongation at 55°C for 45 seconds, and the extended process was repeated for 40 cycles. Reverse transcription PCR was performed three times for each sample. To standardize the expression of haptoglobin and CD163 mRNA, the levels of the reference gene β-actin were determined for each sample parallelly. Expression of final results was ratios of the target gene copy numbers to β-actin transcripts. The expression of the targeted gene was computed by the 2−ΔΔCt method.

2.9. Statistical Analysis.

Quantitative data were sorted out as the mean ± SD. One-way ANOVA was taken for multiple comparisons. The SNK-q test was adopted for the comparison of the differences between groups of brain water content, hemoglobin levels, and real-time PCR assay, while the differences of MRI parameter and Western blot results were determined by Tukey's post hoc test. $p < 0.05$ was denoted the difference processing statistical significance among all groups.

3. Results

3.1. Mortality.

The overall mortality in operative rats was approximately 10.2% (n = 11). All the sham group rats survived, and there was no significant difference in the mortality of each group (data not shown).

3.2. PPAR-γ Agonist Monascin Decreased Brain Water Content.

All the operative groups showed a significant increase in brain water content when compared to the sham group ($*p < 0.05$ versus sham; Figure 1). PPAR-γ agonist monascin significantly lowed the water content of brain tissue around hematoma while PPAR-γ antagonist Glivec acted the opposite way, in comparison with the vehicle group (#$p < 0.05$; Figure 1).

3.3. PPAR-γ Agonist Monascin Reduced Hemoglobin Level.

The hemoglobin level of all the operative groups was obviously higher than that of the sham group ($*p < 0.05$; Figure 2). Compared to the vehicle group, monascin significantly decreased the level of hemoglobin (#$p < 0.05$ versus vehicle), while Glivec increased it (#$p < 0.05$ versus vehicle).

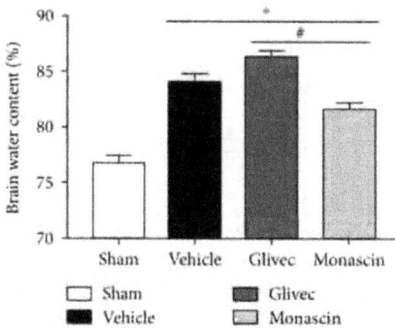

Figure 1: Effect of PPAR-γ on brain water content associated with ICH 3 days after surgery ($*p < 0.05$ versus sham; #$p < 0.05$ versus vehicle).

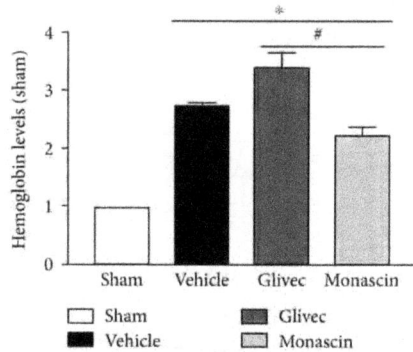

Figure 2: Effect of PPAR-γ on hemoglobin levels associated with ICH 3 days after surgery ($*p < 0.05$ versus sham; #$p < 0.05$ versus vehicle).

3.4. Effect of Monascin and Glivec on CD163 and Hp Expression following ICH.

The results of Western blot and PCR showed a significant increase in PPAR-γ, Hp, and CD163 expression within ipsilateral brain tissues after ICH when compared to sham (*p < 0.05, Figure 3). Compared to vehicle, monascin increased PPAR-γ, Hp, and CD163 expression with Western blot (#p < 0.05, Figures 3(a)–3(d)) and real-time PCR (#p < 0.05, Figures 3(e) and 3(f)). Meanwhile, the administration of Glivec downregulated the expression of PPAR-γ, Hp, and CD163 (#p < 0.05, Figure 3).

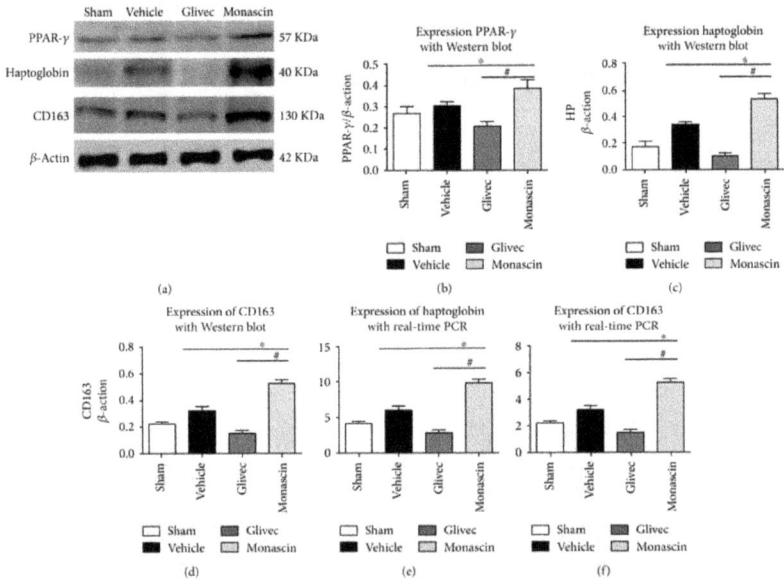

Figure 3: Effect of Glivec and monascin on PPAR-γ, haptoglobin, and CD163 associated with ICH 3 days after surgery. Representative images are shown of Western blot assay (a–d) and real-time PCR (e and f) for PPAR-γ, haptoglobin, and CD163 levels within ipsilateral brain tissues. One-way ANOVA followed by Tukey's tests was used. (*p < 0.05 versus sham; #p < 0.05 versus vehicle).

3.5. Monascin Decreased the Volume of Hematoma (T2*WI/SWI) and Brain Edema (T2WI/T2 Flair) in the Rat Model after ICH.

The volumes of hematoma and edema of all groups were measured at 3 days after modeling successfully (showed in Figure 4). The volume of hematoma

and edema was reduced in the monascin group compared to the vehicle group. While Glivec extended the volume of hematoma and edema 3 days after ICH. The link assay between brain edema and hematoma lesion showed a positive correlation between them (r = 0.989, p = 0.011).

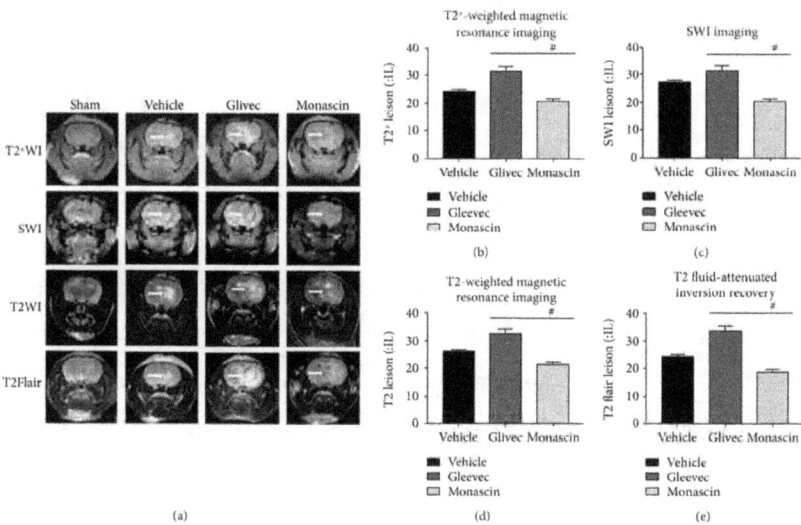

Figure 4: Effect of PPAR-γ on hematoma volume (a–c) and brain edema (a, d, and e) associated with ICH 3 days after surgery. Representative images are shown of T2*WI (a and b), SWI (a and c) for hematoma volume, T2WI (a and d), and T2 Flair (a and e) for brain edema within ipsilateral brain tissues. One-way ANOVA followed by Tukey's tests were used (#p < 0 05 versus vehicle).

4. Discussion

In our study, we demonstrated that PPAR-γ is neuroprotective through decreasing hematoma size and hemoglobin levels then reduced brain edema. PPAR- γ agonist monascin enhanced haptoglobin and CD163 expression whereas PPAR-γ antagonist Glivec had the opposite effects on a rat ICH model.

Intracerebral hemorrhage is a devastating disease, and there has been no specific therapy to reduce the mortality [17]. It started from the blood's massive release into the brain parenchyma [3, 11, 18]. The red blood cell (RBC) lyses within several days and releases Hb at the same time [6]. The hematoma is the culprit of brain insults after ICH, so how to effectively remove blood products is crucial in ICH-induced brain injury [19].

Hp is a glycoprotein which is abundant in the plasma [20]. It is mainly secreted by hepatocytes, and a mononuclear phagocyte system can also produce it [21]. The levels of Hp in the plasma increases to answer stress response and anti-inflammation, which bond to free Hb after cerebral hemorrhage [14, 19]. The formation of Hp-Hb complex protects Hb from oxidative modifications. Otherwise, oxidative modification can prevent the clearance processing and lead the releasing of free Hb into the circulation of the blood [22]. Besides, the Hp-Hb-CD163 complex has a high-affinity site for CD163 to recognize and promote hemoglobin clearance [8, 9, 14]. CD163 acts as a hemoglobin scavenger receptor. It is only expressed in the monocyte-macrophage system [9] and is a 130kDa transmembrane glycoprotein which can be combined with a variety of ligands. It also belongs to scavenger receptor superfamily class B [18]. CD163 is the cellular receptor target of Hp after ICH [10]. After recognization by the Hp-Hb complex, the Hp-Hb-CD163 complex system is formed during the hemolysis of erythrocytes and mediates the endocytosis of the hemoglobin, leading to the degradation of the lysosomal ligand protein [8]. The Hp-Hb-CD163 acts as the main pathway in Hb scavenging and exerts a pivotal protective role [9].

PPAR-γ is a transcription factor belonging to the nuclear hormone receptor superfamily. During the past years, the transcription factors of PPAR-γ [19,

23] were validated as important players in regulating phagocyte-mediated cleanup processes and able to promote endogenous hematoma absorption, decrease neuronal damage, and improve functional recovery in a rodent model of ICH [24]. It not only increased microglia-mediated phagocytosis of RBC in rat primary microglia in culture but also reduced the generation of peroxide during the phagocytic process [25]. The specific mechanism of PPAR-γ in ICH has not been completely clarified so far.

In the present study, we found that PPAR-γ agonist monascin is neuroprotective by decreasing the brain water content and the level of hemoglobin. Besides, it also enhanced CD163 and Hp expression in Western blot and real-time PCR results whereas Glivec reduced Hp and CD163 expression.

Magnetic resonance imaging (MRI) is a medical imaging technique and has been extensively used in the study of intracerebral hemorrhage [14]. It has high sensitivity for presenting the temporal and spatial shifts of hematoma and edema after ICH. At 3 days after surgery, we assessed the volume of hematoma and cerebral edema via T2*WI/SWI and T2WI/T2 FLAIR sequences [7]. The results showed PPAR-γ agonist monascin evidently reduced hematoma volume and cerebral edema after ICH, while the Glivec expanded the hematoma and edema areas.

Our results demonstrated that PPAR-γ agonist monascin decreased hematoma volume and brain edema in a collagenase-induced ICH rat model via histology, molecular biology, and MRI imaging methods. Meanwhile, monascin upregulated the expression of CD163 and Hp which belong to the endogenous hemoglobin scavenging system in ICH.

PPAR-γ activation reinforced microglia-induced erythrocyte phagocytosis. Our previous study demonstrated that PPAR-γ agonist improved outcome through reducing hematoma volume and edema formation following ICH

[13]. While macrophages play a central role in hematoma clearance, hemoglobin mostly remains encapsulated within erythrocytes until they are phagocytosed and degraded by microglia and infiltrating macrophages [1]. CD163, a hemoglobin scavenger receptor, is mainly expressed on macrophages/microglia, and it plays a major role in scavenging free hemoglobin released during erythrolysis after ICH. CD163 transports hemoglobin into microglia/macrophages and functions as a membrane-bound scavenger receptor for clearing extracellular haptoglobin-hemoglobin (Hp-Hb) complexes [11]. Excessive Hb upregulated the expression of Hp and the Hb/Hp receptor CD163 in vivo and in vitro. Free Hb binds to Hp and once Hp-Hb complex is endocytosed by CD163, which mediated the delivery of Hb to the macrophage, may fuel an anti-inflammatory response because heme metabolites have potent anti-inflammatory effects [6]. So PPAR-γ activation possibly reinforced microglia induced Hp-Hb complex phagocytosis through enhancing CD163 expression.

In conclusion, PPAR-γ promotes hematoma clearance and plays a protective role possibly through the Hp-Hb-CD163 pathway in a rat collagenase-induced ICH model. Monascin, as a PPAR-γ agonist, will be a potential medical treatment for ICH in the future.

Data Availability

The data used to support the findings of this study are available from the corresponding author upon request.

Conflicts of Interest

The authors declare that there is no conflict of interest regarding the publication of this paper.

Authors' Contributions

Gaiqing Wang and Tong Li contributed equally to this work.

Acknowledgments

This study was supported by a project from the National Natural Science Foundation of China (Project no. 81771294).

REFERENCES:

[1] R. Liu, S. Cao, Y. Hua, R. F. Keep, Y. Huang, and G. Xi, "CD163 expression in neurons after experimental intracerebral hemorrhage," Stroke, vol. 48, no. 5, pp. 1369–1375, 2017.

[2] J. Chen-Roetling and R. F. Regan, "Haptoglobin increases the vulnerability of CD163-expressing neurons to hemoglobin,"Journal of Neurochemistry, vol. 139, no. 4, pp. 586–595, 2016.

[3] X. Zhao, S. Song, G. Sun et al., "Neuroprotective role of haptoglobin after intracerebral hemorrhage," The Journal of Neuroscience, vol. 29, no. 50, pp. 15819–15827, 2009.

[4] S. Cao, M. Zheng, Y. Hua, G. Chen, R. F. Keep, and G. Xi, "Hematoma changes during clot resolution after experimental intracerebral hemorrhage," Stroke, vol. 47, no. 6, pp. 1626–1631, 2016.

[5] H. Zhao, X. Zhang, Z. Dai et al., "P2X7 receptor suppression preserves blood-brain barrier through inhibiting RhoA activation after experimental intracerebral hemorrhage in rats,"Scientific Reports, vol. 6, no. 1, article 23286, 2016.

[6] G. Wang, L. Wang, X. G. Sun, and J. Tang, "Haematoma scavenging in intracerebral haemorrhage: from mechanisms to the clinic," Journal of Cellular and Molecular Medicine, vol. 22, no. 2, pp. 768–777, 2017.

[7] X. Zhao, G. Sun, J. Zhang et al., "Transcription factor Nrf2 protects the brain from damage produced by intracerebral hemorrhage," Stroke, vol. 38, no. 12, pp. 3280–3286, 2007.

[8] J. H. Thomsen, A. Etzerodt, P. Svendsen, and S. K. Moestrup, "The haptoglobin-CD163-heme oxygenase-1 pathway for hemoglobin scavenging," Oxidative Medicine and Cellular Longevity, vol. 2013, Article ID 523652, 11 pages, 2013.

[9] J. Galea, G. Cruickshank, J. L. Teeling et al., "The intrathecal CD163-haptoglobin-hemoglobin scavenging system in subarachnoid hemorrhage," Journal of Neurochemistry, vol. 121, no. 5, pp. 785–792, 2012.

[10] J. L. Leclerc, A. S. Lampert, C. Loyola Amador et al., "The absence of the CD163 receptor has distinct temporal influences on intracerebral hemorrhage outcomes," Journal of Cerebral Blood Flow & Metabolism, vol. 38, no. 2, pp. 262–273, 2017.

[11] D. J. Schaer, A. I. Alayash, and P. W. Buehler, "Gating the radical hemoglobin to macrophages: the anti-inflammatory role of CD163, a scavenger receptor," Antioxidants & Redox Signaling, vol. 9, no. 7, pp. 991–999, 2007.

[12] C. J. Roche, D. Dantsker, A. I. Alayash, and J. M. Friedman, "Enhanced nitrite reductase activity associated with the haptoglobin complexed hemoglobin dimer: functional and antioxidative implications," Nitric Oxide, vol. 27, no. 1, pp. 32–39, 2012.

[13] J. Wang, G. Wang, J. Yi et al., "The effect of monascin on hematoma clearance and edema after intracerebral hemorrhage in rats," Brain Research Bulletin, vol. 134, pp. 24–29,2017.

[14] X. Wang, T. Mori, T. Sumii, and E. H. Lo, "Hemoglobin induced cytotoxicity in rat cerebral cortical neurons: caspase activation and oxidative stress," Stroke, vol. 33, no. 7,

pp. 1882–1888, 2002.

[15] J. Zhao, N. Kobori, J. Aronowski, and P. K. Dash, "Sulforaphane reduces infarct volume following focal cerebral ischemia in rodents," Neuroscience Letters, vol. 393, no. 2-3, pp. 108–112,2006.

[16] S. S. Choi, E. S. Kim, J. E. Jung et al., "PPARγ antagonist Gleevec improves insulin sensitivity and promotes the browning of white adipose tissue," Diabetes, vol. 65, no. 4, pp. 829–839, 2016.

[17] H. B. Brouwers and J. N. Goldstein, "Therapeutic strategies in acute intracerebral hemorrhage," Neurotherapeutics, vol. 9,no. 1, pp. 87–98, 2012.

[18] M. Roy-O'Reilly, L. Zhu, L. Atadja et al., "Soluble CD163 in intracerebral hemorrhage: biomarker for perihematomal edema," Annals of Clinical Translational Neurology, vol. 4, no. 11, pp. 793–800, 2017.

[19] J. Aronowski and X. Zhao, "Molecular pathophysiology of cerebral hemorrhage: secondary brain injury," Stroke, vol. 42, no. 6, pp. 1781–6, 2011.

[20] D. H. Ko, H. E. Chang, T. S. Kim et al., "A review of haptoglobin typing methods for disease association study and preventing anaphylactic transfusion reaction," BioMed Research International, vol. 2013, Article ID 390630, 6 pages, 2013.

[21] C. Burkard, S. G. Lillico, E. Reid et al., "Precision engineering for PRRSV resistance in pigs: macrophages from genome edited pigs lacking CD163 SRCR5 domain are fully resistant to both PRRSV genotypes while maintaining biological function," PLoS Pathogens, vol. 13, no. 2, article e1006206, 2017.

[22] C. A. Gleissner, I. Shaked, C. Erbel, D. Bockler, H. A. Katus, and K. Ley, "CXCL4 downregulates the atheroprotective hemoglobin receptor CD163 in human macrophages," Circulation Research, vol. 106, no. 1, pp. 203–211, 2010.

[23] X. Zhao, J. Grotta, N. Gonzales, and J. Aronowski, "Hematoma resolution as a therapeutic target: the role of microglia/macrophages," Stroke, vol. 40, no. 3, Supplement 1, pp. S92–S94, 2009.

[24] X. R. Zhao, N. Gonzales, and J. Aronowski, "Pleiotropic role of PPARγ in intracerebral hemorrhage: an intricate system involving Nrf2, RXR, and NF-κB," CNS Neuroscience & Therapeutics, vol. 21, no. 4, pp. 357–366, 2015.

[25] F. A. Monsalve, R. D. Pyarasani, F. Delgado-Lopez, and R. Moore-Carrasco, "Peroxisome proliferator-activated receptor targets for the treatment of metabolic diseases," Mediators of Inflammation, vol. 2013, Article ID 549627, 18 pages, 2013.

DECLARATION: This chapter was authored by Gaiqing Wang, Tong Li, Shu-na Duan, Liang Dong, Xin-gang Sun and Fang Xue published as "PPAR-γ promotes hematoma clearance through Haptoglobin-Hemoglobin-CD163 in a Rat Model of Intracerebral Hemorrhage" in "Behavioural Neurology", 2018; 2018: 764610

CHAPTER 11:

The effect of monascin on hematoma clearance and edema after intracerebral hemorrhage in rats

ABSTRACT:

Background and purpose: Intracerebral hemorrhage (ICH) is a particularly devastating form of stroke with high mortality and morbidity. Hematomas are the primary cause of neurologic deficits associated with ICH. The products of hematoma are recognized as neurotoxins and the main contributors to edema formation and tissue damage after ICH. Finding a means to efficiently promote absorption of hematoma is a novel clinical challenge for ICH. Peroxisome proliferator-activated receptor gamma (PPARγ) and nuclear factor erythroid 2-related factor 2 (Nrf2), had been shown that, can take potential roles in the endogenous hematoma clearance. However, monascin, a novel natural Nrf2 activator with PPARγ agonist, has not been reported to play a role in ICH. This study was designed to evaluate the effect of monascin on neurological deficits, hematoma clearance and edema extinction in a model of ICH in rats.

Methods: 164 adult male Sprague-Dawley (SD) rats were randomly divided into sham; vehicle; monascin groups with low dosages (1 mg/kg/day), middle dosages (5 mg/kg/day) and high dosages (10 mg/kg/day) respectively. Animals were euthanized at 1, 3 and 7 days following neurological evaluation after surgery. We examined the effect of monascin on the brain water contents, blood brain barrier (BBB) permeability and hemoglobin levels, meanwhile reassessed the volume of hematoma and edema around the hematoma by Magnetic Resonance Imaging (MRI) in each group.

Results: The high dosage of monascin significantly improved neurological deficits, reduced the volume of hematoma in 1–7 days after ICH, decreased BBB permeability and edema formation in 1–3 days following ICH.

Conclusion: Our study demonstrated that the high dosage of monascin played a neuroprotective role in ICH through reducing BBB permeability, edema and hematoma volume.

KEY WORDS: Intracerebral hemorrhage; Monascin; Hematoma clearance Neuroprotection; Magnetic resonance imaging

1. Introduction

ICH accounts for 8–15% of all strokes in Western societies and 20–30% among Asian populations, and most patients either die or are left with significant neurological deficit (Keep et al., 2012; Sangha and Gonzales, 2011). Clinical treatment of ICH presently consists of decompressive surgery in selected cases and supportive measures to reduce bleeding and control hypertension (Brouwers and Goldstein, 2012; Fischer et al., 2016). Given the enormity of the clinical problem, it is imperative that new therapeutic approaches should be developed to improve outcome following ICH.

During past years, the transcription factors of PPARγ (Aronowski and Zhao, 2011; Zhao et al., 2009) and Nrf2 (Zhao et al., 2015a,b) were received as important players in regulating phagocyte-mediated cleanup processes. PPARγ and Nrf2 play an important role in phagocytosis and hematoma clearance after ICH (Zhao et al., 2015a,b).

Monascin- a major component of red yeast rice, acts as a PPARγ agonist, were confirmed to regulate the expression of Nrf2 (Hsu et al., 2013,2014; Lee et al., 2011). Effects of monascin after ICH have not been evaluated yet and the findings, as mentioned above, let us hypothesize that monascin will have beneficial, clinically translatable effects after ICH.

In this study, we suggest that monascin will promote hematoma clearance via PPARγ and Nrf2 up-regulation, therefore reducing brain edema and improving BBB integrity after ICH in a collagenase infusion model in rats.

2. Material and methods

2.1. Animals

Twelve-week-old male SD rats (weight 275g ± 25 g, Animal Experimental Center of Shanxi Medical University) were used in this study. All experimental procedures were conducted in accordance with the Care and Use of Laboratory and approved by the Committee of Shanxi Medical University. Rats were given free access to food and water throughout the study.

2.2. Animal treatments and experimental groups

A total of 164 rats were used. Animals were randomly divided into the following groups: sham (n= 30); Vehicle (n = 34); ICH+ low dosage monascin (1 mg/kg/day, n = 34); ICH+ middle dosage monascin (5 mg/kg/day, n = 33); ICH+ high dosage monascin (10 mg/kg/day, n = 33). Each group was equally divided into three subgroups (point at 1, 3, 7 days after ICH). Animals, which died before final assessment, were replaced. All gavages were administered intragastrically 6 h after ICH and twice a day until the euthanasia point.

2.3. Intracerebral hemorrhage model in rats

Experimental ICH was induced by stereotactic-guided injection of collagenase type IV (0.5 units in 2 μl saline) into the basal ganglia areaas we previously described (Wang et al., 2016). The rats were fastened on a stereotaxic apparatus under chloral hydrate anesthesia (0.8 mg/kg intraperitoneally), exposed the skull and reveal bregma. A 1-mm cranial bur hole was drilled in the skull (coordinates: 1.0 mm posterior to the bregma, 3.0 mm lateral to the midline), and microinjector was inserted with collagenase infused into the right basal ganglia (5.8 mm deep from the dura mater). The needle was left in place for an additional 10 min after injection after injection to prevent "back-leakage" and then slowly withdrawn over 5 min. The Sham-operated rats were syringed with equivalent dosages physiological saline.

After the surgery, the skull hole was sealed with bone wax and the incision was closed with sutures. Animals were allowed to recover after successful ICH induction that was confirmed by Rosenberg's neurological score (Rosenberg et al., 1990).

2.4. Analysis of neurological deficit score

All behavioral tests were conducted in a quiet and low light room by an independent researcher blinded to the procedure by the Garcia test (Garcia et al., 1995; Wang et al., 2017). Neurological symptoms were calculated by combining the score as follows (score: 2–18): (1) spontaneous activity,

(2) symmetry in the movement of four limbs, (3) forepaw outstretching, (4) mesh wall climbing, (5) body proprioception, (6) response to vibrissae touch. Higher scores indicate greater neurofunction (healthy rat).

2.5. Brain water content

Animals were euthanized under deep anesthesia and decapitated for brain water content determination as previously described (Wang et al.,2017). The brains were quickly removed and cut into 4 mm sections around the puncture point. All specimens obtained from ipsilateral basal ganglion were immediately weighed on an analytical microbalance to obtain the wet weight. The tissue was then dried at 100 °C for 48 h to determine the dry weight. Brain water content was calculated as percentage of (Wet weight-Dry weight)/Wet weight × 100.

2.6. The blood brain barrier (BBB) permeability measurement

The vascular permeability of BBB was evaluated with Evans blue (EB) extravasation method (Manaenko et al., 2011). Three hours before each experiment, 2% EB (4 ml/Kg) was injected into the abdominal cavity. After the circulation period, the rats were perfused with 100 ml of ice-cold phosphate-buffered saline (PBS). The brain tissue was quickly removed. The samples were homogenized in 1100 μl of PBS, sonicated and centrifuged (30 min, 15,000 rcf, 4 °C). The supernatant was collected in aliquots. For each 500 μl sample an equal amount of 50% trichloroacetic acid was added, incubated over night by 4 °C and then centrifuged. Optical density was measured and recorded at 540 nm with a spectrophotometer. The dye content was expressed as ug/g of tissue weight and calibrated with a standard curve obtained from known amounts of the EB dye. The data was represented as a ratio compared to sham.

2.7. Hemoglobin assay

The supernatant collection was completed as the BBB permeability measurement. Following the supernatant collection, 100 μl supernatant aliquots was added to 400 μl Drabkin's reagent. The hemoglobin assay was measured by spectrophotometer at 540 nm.

2.8. Western blot

Western Blot was performed for proteins as previously described (Wang et al., 2017). Briefly, the right cerebral hemispheres were homogenized, and protein concentration acquired for each sample using a detergent compatible assay (Bio-Rad, Philadelphia, PA). Protein samples (50 μg) were loaded on a tris–glycine gel, electrophoresed, and transferred to a nitrocellulose membrane. Membranes were incubated overnight at 4 °C with the primary antibodies: rabbit polyclonal anti-PPARγ (1:750, abcam), anti-Nrf2 (1:1000, abcam). The same membrane was probed with an antibody against β-actin (1:3000, bioworld) as an internal control after being stripped. Incubation with secondary antibodies (bioworld) was done for 2 h at room temperature. Immunoblots were then probed with an ECL Plus chemiluminescence reagent kit (Amersham Biosciences, Arlington Heights, IL) and visualized with an imaging system (Bio-Rad, Versa Doc, model 4000). Data was analyzed using Alpha View software.

2.9. Assessments of hematoma volume and brain edema

The cranial MRI examinations were obtained on a 1.5T clinical scanner (GE SignaHDx, GE healthcare Milwaukee). A knee coil was used for radio frequency transmission and reception. Studies were performed at 1, 3, 7 days post-ICH. During the MRI experiments, anesthesia was maintained using 5% chloral hydrate, and placed in a prone position. After set-up, a series of MR images, including T2-weighted imaging (T2WI), T2 fluid attenuated inversion recovery (T2Flair), T2*-weighted imaging (T2*WI), and susceptibility-weighted imaging (SWI), were acquired.

The scan sequence and details were listed as follows: (1) T2WI:repetition time (TR)/echo time (TE) =2400/129.2 ms, matrix was = 512× 448, field of view (FOV) = 18× 18 mm, slice thickness =2.0 mm, interval =0.2 mm. (2) T2 Flair: TR/TE= 8502/128.6 ms, matrix was = 512× 448, FOV 12× 12 mm, slice thickness =2.0 mm, interval = 0.2 mm. (3) T2*WI: TR/TE = 400/15 ms, matrix was =448 × 384, FOV = 18× 18 mm, slice thickness =2.0 mm, interval = 0.2 mm, flip angle= 15°. (4) SWI: TR/TE= 49.9/4.5 ms, matrix was = 448× 448, FOV = 18× 18 mm, slice thickness = 1.5 mm, flip angle = 15°. Hematoma size was determined from T2*WI and SWI, T2WI and T2 Flair were used for edema quantification. The measurements were performed by an examiner blinded to the exam date using a computer-assisted image analysis program-Image J (Jack, 1994). The volumes were calculated by summation of lesion areas of all brain slices showing brain damage and integrated by slice thickness. The absolute volume of brainedema =the outer volume of brain edema −hematoma volume. All measurements were repeated three times and the mean value was used.

2.10. Statistical analysis

Quantitative data are presented as mean ± SD. One-way ANOVA for multiple comparisons with Tukey's post-hoc test were used to determine the differences of hemoglobin levels, brain water content, BBB permeability, neurological deficits, MRI parameters and western blot assay among all groups at each time point. $p < 0.05$ was considered statistically significant.

3. Results

3.1. Mortality

All sham-operated rats survived. The total operative mortality of rats was about 8.5% (n =14). The mortality was not significantly different among the experimental groups (data not shown).

3.2. Effect of monasin on PPARγ and Nrf2 expression following ICH

Western blot showed a significant increase in PPARγ and Nrf2 protein expression within ipsilateral brain tissues at 1 and 3 days after ICH with/without monascin compared to sham (p < 0.05, Fig. 1). Administration monascin (middle and high dosage) showed significantly higher protein expression of PPARγ and Nrf2 compared to vehicle (p < 0.05, Fig. 1).

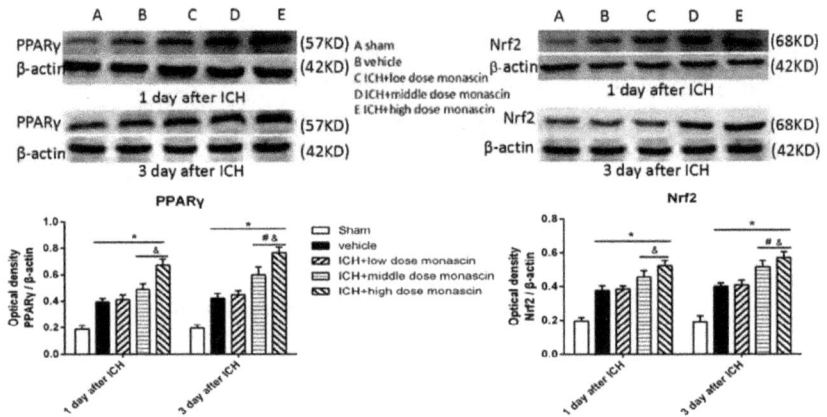

Fig. 1. Effect of Monascin (different dosages) on PPARγ and Nrf2 associated with ICH 24 h and 72 h after surgery. Representative images are shown of western blot assay for PPARγ and Nrf2 level within ipsilateral brain tissues. *p < 0.05 versus sham; #p < 0.05 versus former timepoint; & p < 0.05 versus vehicle.

3.3. High dosages monascin improved neurological functions and reduced hemoglobin levels at 1–7 days following ICH

All animals after ICH demonstrated significant neurological deficits and higher hemoglobin levels compared to sham (p < 0.05; Fig. 2). However, compared with ICH+ vehicle, the high dosages monascin showed significant improvement in the Garcia test and decrease in hemoglobin levels at each time point (p < 0.05 vs. Vehicle; Fig. 1). The middle dosages monascin animals slightly attenuated ICH-induced neurological deficits and hemoglobin levels at 3 and 7days post-ICH (p < 0.05 vs. Vehicle; Fig. 2).

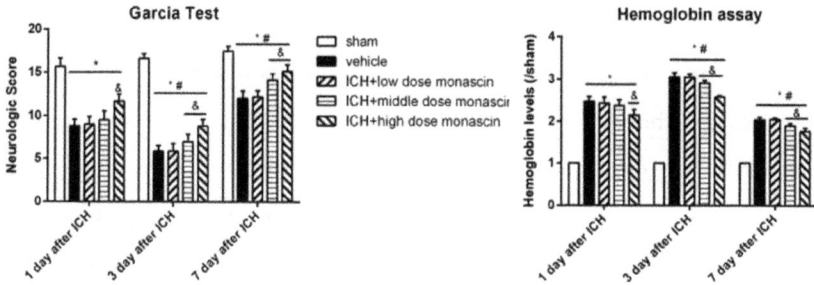

Fig. 2. Effect of monascin (different dosages) on Garcia test and hemoglobin levels 24 h, 72 h and 7 days after ICH. *p < 0.05 versus sham; #p < 0.05 versus former timepoint; & p < 0.05 versus vehicle.

3.4. High dosages monascin decreased brain water content and BBB permeability at 1–3 days following ICH

All groups showed a marked increase in perihematomal water content and Evans blue extravasation compared with sham (p < 0.05; Fig.3). High dosages monascin significantly reduced brain water content and BBB permeability in the ipsilateral basal ganglia compared with the ICH +Vehicle group at 1, 3 days after surgery (p < 0.05; Fig.3). Additionally, 7 days post-ICH, the Evans blue extravasation attenuated in all ICH animals (with or without treatment).

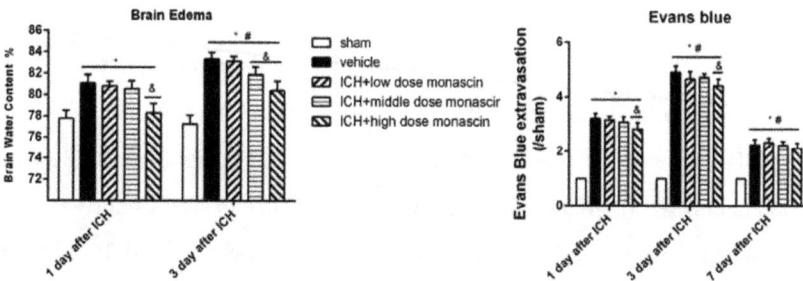

Fig. 3. Effect of monascin (different dosages) on brain water content and blood brain barrier permeability 24 h, 72 h and 7 days after ICH. *p < 0.05 versus sham; #p < 0.05 versus former timepoint; & p < 0.05 versus vehicle.

3.5. High dosages monascin narrowed the volume of hematoma (T2*WI/ SWI)

Hematoma volumes measured at 1, 3 and 7 days using T2*WI and SWI images are shown in Fig. 4. The images of monascin treatment groups showed the uniform trend of control groups. Compared with vehicle, hematoma volume in ICH +10 mg/kg monascin rats were significantly smaller than in the vehicle at 1, 3, 7 days (p < 0.05; Fig. 4). Meanwhile, the volume of hematoma were also reduced at 3–7 days after ICH + 5 mg/kg monascin (p < 0.05; Fig. 4).

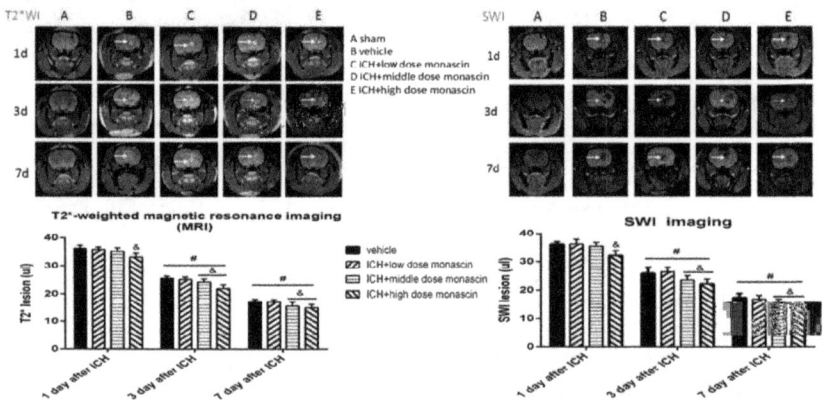

Fig. 4. Effect of monascin (different dosages) on hematoma volume by T2*WI and SWI 4 h, 72 h and 7 days after ICH. *p < 0.05 versus sham; #p < 0.05 versus former timepoint; & p < 0.05 versus vehicle.

3.6. High dosages monascin reduced the volume of edema (T2WI/T2 Flair)

Compared with sham group, the perihematomal edema volume measured by MRI increased in the first 24 h after ICH, reached its peak on 3 days, then declined. Given the high dosages of monascin can significantly reduce the volume of brain edema on 1–3 days versus vehicles (p < 0.05; Fig. 5).

In addition, there was a slight decrease at 3 days after ICH +5 mg/kg monascin (p < 0.05; Fig. 5).

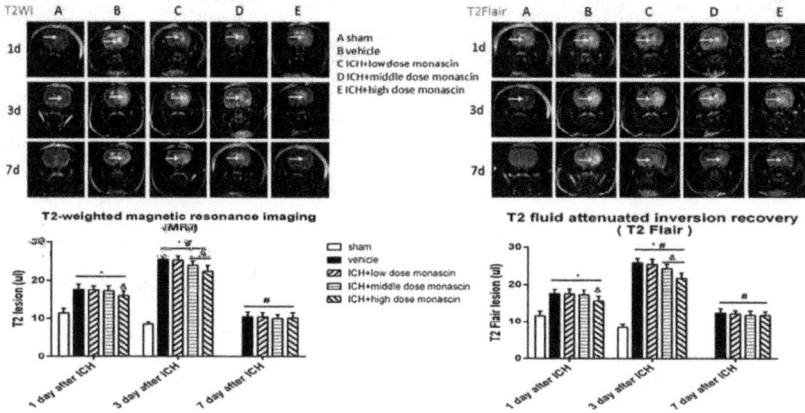

Fig. 5. Effect of monascin (different dosages) on edema volume by T2WI and T2 flair 24 h, 72 h and 7 days after ICH. *p < 0.05 versus sham; #p < 0.05 versus former timepoint; & p < 0.05 versus vehicle.

4. Discussion

In the present study, we found that endogenous PPARγ and Nrf2 levels were significantly elevated in ipsilateral brain tissues at 1 days and 3 days after surgery in a rat collagenase ICH model. And the high dosages monascin (10 mg/kg) appeared to be protective and improved neurological deficits were associated with enhanced PPARγ /Nrf2 expression along with hematoma scavenging, and less BBB disruption along with edema in ipsilateral brain tissues after ICH.

ICH remains a major public-health problem worldwide and is associated with a poor prognosis that is characterized by a high mortality rate and severe neurological dysfunction, for which specific therapies and treatments remain elusive (Brouwers and Goldstein, 2012; Fischer et al., 2016; Keep et al., 2012; Sangha and Gonzales,2011). Within hours to days after ICH, a secondary cause of injury is due to the presence of intraparenchymal blood. Extravasated erythrocytes in the hematoma undergo lysis, releasing hemoglobin, heme, and iron, thereby leading to further tissue damage, blood-brain barrier disruption, and edema (Aronowski and Zhao, 2011; Fang et al., 2013). To offset this process, phagocytic cells, including the brain's microglia and hematogenous macrophages, were beginning to take effect. CD36 in macrophages enhances the ability of microglia to phagocytose red blood cells, helps to improve hematoma resolution, and reduces ICH induced deficit in the model of ICH (Cho et al., 2005; Li et al., 2015). In particular, PPARγ and Nrf2 can upregulate CD36 expression in microglia/macrophages, leading to increased phagocytosis of blood products and more rapid hematoma resolution after intracerebral hemorrhage (Aronowski and Zhao, 2011; Zhao et al., 2007, 2009, 2015b).

Monascin- a major component of red yeast rice, acts as a PPARγ agonist (Lee et al., 2011), were confirmed to regulate the expression of Nrf2 (Hsu et al., 2013, 2014), leading to increased phagocytosis of blood products (Zhao et al., 2015a). Monascin, the natural edible pigment, which is made by unique fermentation technology in China. Monascus-fermented product has long been thought to possess both medicinal and edible purposes. Traditionally, monascin has been widely used as natural food colorant in East Asia for a long time particularly for Chinese food and cosmetics. Recently, monascin have been proven to significantly reduce the concentrations in serum of total cholesterol, triglycerides, and low-density lipoprotein cholesterol because it contains monacolinK (Endo and Monacolin, 1980; Lee et al., 2011, 2006). In addition, monascin is reported to have anti-cancer (Su et al., 2005), anti-infammation (Hsu et al., 2012), antimutagenic (Izawa et al., 1997) and prevent atherosclerosis (Lee et al., 2010). However, there is no report on the effects of monascin in ICH.

The injury after ICH is mainly divided into primary and secondary brain injury. The primary injury refers to the occupying effect of hematoma and the mechanical constriction (Forbes et al., 2003). The secondary is due to hematoma lysis, Inflammatory reaction, blood-brain barrier damage, brain edema, apoptosis after 24h (Keep et al., 2012; Zhou et al., 2014). Under physiological conditions, the blood brain barrier strictly controls the water soluble substances such as the electrolyte into the brain tissue. After ICH, the permeability increased and the barrier function was damaged. This may be related to a variety of factors, such as cerebral ischemia, inflammation, the contraction of capillary endothelial cells and so on (Xue and Del Bigio, 2000). After the treatment of high dosages monascin, the BBB permeability and brain edema were significantly decreased on 1–3 days after ICH compared with vehicle groups.

MRI as a noninvasive, in vivo, dynamic, multi parameter quantitative tool, has been widely used in the study of ICH (Knight et al., 2008). The foundation of MRI was related to the strong paramagnetic substances of hemoglobin (Schellinger et al., 2003). After successful modeling, T2WI, T2 Flair, T2*WI, SWI clearly showed the range of the brain lesions and the surrounding abnormal signal bands. We observed the changes of MRI images after ICH, Using T2*WI/SWI to calculate the volume of hematoma and T2WI/T2 FLAIR to measure the volume of brain edema. High dosages monascin can significantly reduce the volume of hematoma and perihematomal edema after ICH.

Taken together, hematoma is a major pathological factor after ICH, which gives rise to the damage of BBB, growth of brain edema and impairment of neurological functions. Pharmacological manipulations increasing hematoma clearance, represents a novel, clinical relevant strategy that is able to mitigate the ICH-induced pathophysiology. Our results demonstrated that monascin administration resulted in the protein increase of PPARγ and Nrf2, which are markers of the activation of hematoma clearance system. This beneficial effects of monascin administration improved BBB integrity, resulted in the attenuation of brain edema formation and in the improvement of neurological functions.

In conclusion, monascin (10 mg/kg) may offer protective effects through promoting hematoma resolution and diminishing brain edema after ICH and may thus prove beneficial to post-ICH outcomes.

Conflict of interest

None.

REFERENCES:

Aronowski, J., Zhao, X., 2011. Molecular pathophysiology of cerebral hemorrhage: secondary brain injury. Stroke 42 (6), 1781–1786.

Brouwers, H.B., Goldstein, J.N., 2012. Therapeutic strategies in acute intracerebral hemorrhage. Neurotherapeutics 9 (1), 87–98.

Cho, S., P.E, Febbraio, M., Anrather, J., Park, L., Racchumi, G., Silverstein, R.L., Iadecola, C., 2005. The class B scavenger receptor CD36 mediates free radical production and tissue injury in cerebral ischemia. J. Neurosci. 25 (10), 2504–2512.

Endo, K., Monacolin, A., 1980. a new hypocholesterolemic agent that specifically inhibits 3-hydroxy-3-methylglutaryl coenzyme A reductase. J. Antibiot. (Tokyo) 33 (3), 334–336.

Fang, H., W.P, Zhou, Y., Wang, Y.C., Yang, Q.W., 2013. Toll-like receptor 4 signaling in intracerebral hemorrhage-induced inflammation and injury. J. Neuroinflammation 10, 27.

Fischer, M., S.A, Lackner, P., Helbok, R., Beer, R., Pfausler, B., Schmutzhard, E., Broessner, G., 2017. Targeted temperature management in spontaneous intracerebral hemorrhage: a systematic review. Curr. Drug Targets 18(12):1430-1440.

Forbes, K.P., P.J, Heiserman, J.E., 2003. Diffusion-weighted imaging provides support for secondary neuronal damage from intraparenchymal hematoma. Neuroradiology 45 (6), 363–367.

Garcia, J.H., W.S, Liu, K.F., Hu, X.J., 1995. Neurological deficit and extent of neuronal necrosis attributable to middle cerebral artery occlusion in rats. Statistical validation. Stroke 26 (4), 627–634.

Hsu, W.H., Lee, B.H., Liao, T.H., Hsu, Y.W., Pan, T.M., 2012. Monascus-fermented metabolite monascin suppresses inflammation via PPAR-gamma regulation and JNK inactivation in THP-1 monocytes. Food Chem. Toxicol. 50 (5), 1178–1186.

Hsu, W.H., L.B, Li, C.H., Hsu, Y.W., Pan, T.M., 2013. Monascin and AITC attenuate methylglyoxal-induced PPAR gamma phosphorylation and degradation through inhibition of the oxidative stress/PKC pathway depending on Nrf2 activation. J. Agric. Food Chem. 61 (25), 5996–6006.

Hsu, W.H., L.B, Pan, T.M., 2014. Monascin attenuates oxidative stress-mediated lung inflammation via peroxisome proliferator-activated receptor-gamma (PPAR-gamma) and nuclear factor-erythroid 2 related factor 2 (Nrf-2) modulation. J. Agric. Food Chem. 62 (23), 5337–5344.

Izawa, S., H.N, Watanabe, T., Kotokawa, N., Yamamoto, A., Hayatsu, H., Arimotokobayashi, S., 1997. Inhibitory effects of food-coloring agents derived from Monascus on the mutagenicity of heterocyclic amines. J. Agric. Food Chem. 45,3980–3984.

Jack Jr., C.R., 1994. MRI-based hippocampal volume measurements in epilepsy. Epilepsia 35, 21–29.

Keep, R.F., H.Y, Xi, G., 2012. Intracerebral haemorrhage: mechanisms of injury. Lancet Neurol. 11 (8), 720–731.

Knight, R.A., H.Y, Nagaraja, T.N., Whitton, P., Ding, J., Chopp, M., Seyfried, D.M., 2008. Temporal MRI assessment of intracerebral hemorrhage in rats. Stroke 39 (9),2596–2602.

Lee, C.L., T.T, Wang, J.J., Pan, T.M., 2006. In vivo hypolipidemic effects and safety of low dosage Monascus powder in a hamster model of hyperlipidemia. Appl. Microbiol. Biotechnol. 70 (5), 533–540.

Lee, C.L., K.Y, Wu, C.L., Hsu, Y.W., Pan, T.M., 2010. Monascin and ankaflavin act as novel hypolipidemic and high-density lipoprotein cholesterol-raising agents in red mold dioscorea. J. Agric. Food Chem. 58 (16), 9013–9019.

Lee, B.H., H.W, Liao, T.H., Pan, T.M., 2011. The Monascus metabolite monascin against TNF-alpha-induced insulin resistance via suppressing PPAR-gamma phosphorylation in C2C12 myotubes. Food Chem. Toxicol. 49 (10), 2609–2617.

Li, X., M.E, Postupna, N., Montine, K.S., Keene, C.D., Montine, T.J., 2015. Prostaglandin E2 receptor subtype 2 regulation of scavenger receptor CD36 modulates microglial Abeta42 phagocytosis. Am. J. Pathol. 185 (1), 230–239.

Manaenko, A., C.H, Kammer, J., Zhang, J.H., Tang, J., 2011. Comparison Evans Blue injection routes: intravenous versus intraperitoneal, for measurement of blood-brain barrier in a mice hemorrhage model. J. Neurosci. Methods 195 (2), 206–210.

Rosenberg, G.A., M.-B, S., Wesley, M., Kornfeld, M., 1990. Collagenase-induced intracerebral hemorrhage in rats. Stroke 21 (5), 801–807.

Sangha, N., Gonzales, N.R., 2011. Treatment targets in intracerebral hemorrhage. Neurotherapeutics 8 (3), 374–387.

Schellinger, P.D., F.J, Hoffmann, K., Becker, K., Orakcioglu, B., Kollmar, R., Jüttler, E., Schramm, P., Schwab, S., Sartor, K., Hacke, W., 2003. Stroke MRI in intracerebral hemorrhage: is there a perihemorrhagic penumbra? Stroke 34 (7), 1674–1679.

Su, N.W., L.Y, Lee, M.H., Ho, C.Y., 2005. Ankaflavin from Monascus-fermented red rice exhibits selective cytotoxic effect and induces cell death on Hep G2 cells. J. Agric.Food Chem. 53 (6), 1949–1954.

Wang, G., Hu, W., Tang, Q., Wang, L., Sun, X.G., Chen, Y., et al., 2016. Effect comparison of both iron chelators on outcomes, iron deposit, and iron transporters after intracerebral hemorrhage in rats. Mol. Neurobiol. 53 (6), 3576–3585.

Wang, G., Manaenko, A., Shao, A., Ou, Y., Yang, P., Budbazar, E., et al., 2017. Low density lipoprotein receptor-related protein-1 facilitates heme scavenging after intracerebral hemorrhage in mice. J. Cereb. Blood Flow Metab. 37, 1299–1310.

Xue, M., Del Bigio, M.R., 2000. Intracortical hemorrhage injury in rats: relationship between blood fractions and brain cell death. Stroke 31 (7), 1721–1727.

Zhao, X., Sun, G., Zhang, J., Strong, R., Song, W., Gonzales, N., et al., 2007. Hematoma resolution as a target for intracerebral hemorrhage treatment: role for peroxisome proliferator-activated receptor gamma in microglia/macrophages. Ann. Neurol. 61,352–362.

Zhao, X.G.J., G.J, Gonzales, N., Aronowski, J., 2009. Hematoma resolution as a therapeutic target: the role of microglia/macrophages. Stroke 40 (3), 92–94.

Zhao, X., Sun, G., Ting, S.M., Song, S., Zhang, J., Edwards, N.J., et al., 2015a. Cleaning up after ICH: the role of Nrf2 in modulating microglia function and hematoma clearance. J. Neurochem. 133, 144–152.

Zhao, X.R., Gonzales, N., Aronowski, J., 2015b. Pleiotropic role of PPAR gamma in intracerebral hemorrhage: an intricate system involving Nrf2, RXR, and NF-kappaB. CNS Neurosci. Ther. 21, 357–366.

Zhou, Y., W.Y, Wang, J., Anne Stetler, R., Yang, Q.W., 2014. Inflammation in intracerebral hemorrhage: from mechanisms to clinical translation. Prog. Neurobiol. 115, 25–44.

DECLARATION: This chapter was authored by Wang J, Wang G, Yi J, Xu Y, Duan S, Li T, Sun XG and Dong L published as "The effect of monascin on hematoma clearance and edema after intracerebral hemorrhage in rats" in "Brain Research Bulletin", 2017;134:24-29

CHAPTER 12:

Neuroprotection by Nrf2 via modulating microglial phenotype and phagocytosis after intracerebral hemorrhage

ABSTRACT:

The clearance function is essential for maintaining brain tissue homeostasis, and the glymphatic system is the main pathway for removing brain interstitial solutes. Aquaporin-4 (AQP4) is the most abundantly expressed aquaporin in the central nervous system (CNS) and is an integral component of the glymphatic system. In recent years, many studies have shown that AQP4 affects the morbidity and recovery process of CNS disorders through the glymphatic system, and AQP4 shows notable variability in CNS disorders and is part of the pathogenesis of these diseases. Therefore, there has been considerable interest in AQP4 as a potential and promising target for regulating and improving neurological impairment. This review aims to summarize the pathophysiological role that AQP4 plays in several CNS disorders by affecting the clearance function of the glymphatic system. The findings can contribute to a better understanding of the self-regulatory functions in CNS disorders that AQP4 were involved in and provide new therapeutic alternatives for incurable debilitating neurodegenerative disorders of CNS in the future.

KEY WORDS: Aquaporin 4; Glymphatic system; Central nervous system; Intracerebral hemorrhage; Alzheimer's disease; Traumatic brain injury; Status epilepticus; Migraine; Neuromyelitis optical; Idiopathic normal pressure hydrocephalus

【Introduction】

Central nervous system (CNS) diseases are prevalent in middle-aged and older adults. Several common CNS diseases have become a heavy social burden. Most of the pathogenesis has yet to be elucidated, leading to treatment difficulties. The brain tissue has a high metabolite level, which produces many potential neurotoxic proteins, cell fragments, and other metabolites in metabolism. Iliff et al. (Jeffrey J. Iliff 2012) found that there is a rapid exchange flow system between cerebrospinal fluid and brain tissue fluid widely in the brain, which can promote the clearance of soluble proteins in the brain. This system, one of the ways for the brain to remove metabolites and foreign bodies, has the function of flushing and cleaning brain tissues. In the CNS, Aquaporin-4 (AQP4) is the most critical part of the glymphatic system, the most abundant aquaporin in the brain, spinal cord, and optic nerve, controls cerebral water balance and is highly expressed in astrocyte foot processes around blood vessels (J E Rash 1998;S Nielsen 1997).

Characterization of the glymphatic system clarified the critical role of AQP4 in this clearance network, with AQP4-deficient animals showing astrocytes exhibiting slowed CSF influx through this system and an approximately 70% reduction in interstitial solute clearance, suggesting that the glymphatic system is AQP4-dependent (Jeffrey J. Iliff 2012). The localization of AQP4 also around blood vessels promotes the flow of CSF (Humberto Mestre 2018). Studies have shown that AQP4 activation can enhance interstitial fluid transport from the glial border to the capillaries of the peripapillary membrane (Vincent J Huber 2018). Recent studies have shown that altered AQP4 localization in the brain of aged rodents results in significantly increased retention of adeno-associated viral (AAV) vectors in the brain parenchyma, supporting the importance of AQP4 as an effective promoter of lymphatic transport and clearance (Giridhar Murlidharan 2016). Research has recently focused on AQP4 in the glymphatic system as a hotspot for CNS diseases. Many diseases of the

CNS are associated with AQP4 expression and glymphatic system dysfunction. In this article, we will briefly describe AQP4 and glymphatic function. Then, the relationship between AQP4 and common CNS diseases and their possible mechanism is reviewed.

1. The structure and function of the glymphatic system

The pathway of the glymphatic system is a highly organized fluid transport system and has been well described in animal models(Martin Kaag Rasmussen 2018). The glymphatic fluid exchange and drainage system dependent on astrocytes including the entire perivascular space (PVS) network surrounding the arteries, arterioles, capillaries, venules, and veins in the brain parenchyma. PVS is a network of low-resistance tubes formed by astrocyte foot processes surrounding blood vessels. Specifically, PVS is constructed as a coaxial system in which the inner cylinder is the cerebral vascular wall, and the outer cylinder is the glial boundary that wraps around blood vessels or the ends of astrocytes that penetrate arterioles (Thomas Misje Mathiisen 2010). The flow of cerebrospinal fluid (CSF) into and out of the glymphatic system has been described in detail. At the beginning of the pericapillary pathway, cerebrospinal fluid from the subarachnoid space flows into the brain through the perivascular space of the grand pia meningeal artery. As the vascular tree branches, cerebrospinal fluid enters the brain parenchyma through the perivascular space in the artery (Jeffrey J Iliff 2013; Jeffrey J. Iliff 2012; Qiaoli Ma 2017). Then from the perivascular space, CSF passes through the glial basement membrane and astrocyte terminal processes, wrapping the cerebrovascular system(Jeffrey J. Iliff 2012;Melanie-Jane Hannocks 2018). Furthermore, in brain interstitial fluid, fluid is dispersed by the movement of polarized net fluid toward veins and the space around nerves (Benjamin T Kress 2014; Jeffrey J. Iliff 2012). Eventually, CSF is expelled along the schwannomas, meningeal lymphatics, and arachnoid granulations of cranial and spinal nerves (Jeffrey J. Iliff 2012) (Fig.1). Thus, it can be inferred that under certain conditions, waste products produced by brain tissue can be removed along with cerebrospinal fluid through these pathways.

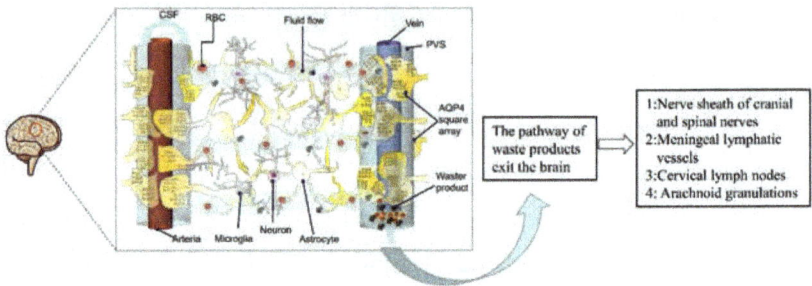

Figure 1. The pathways of the glymphatic system.

The glymphatic system is one of the most important metabolic pathways in the brain, and its normal function depends on the polarization distribution of AQP4 on the astrocyte extremities. This polarized distribution of AQP4 can promote the rapid movement of cerebrospinal fluid (CSF) from the periarterial space to the perivenous space. This process promotes the metabolism of damaged red blood cells (RBC) and metabolic waste from the body, which is beneficial for the recovery of nerve function. Finally, these metabolites are excreted outside the brain from four pathways, including the nerve sheath of cranial and spinal nerves, meningeal lymphatic vessels, cervical lymph node and arachnoid granulations.

The specific mechanisms of solute transport and waste excretion in the glymphatic system remain unclear. There are two ways for solute transport through the brain, including diffusion and convection. Furthermore, the importance of convection in the subarachnoid and perivascular has long been recognized. Iliff et al.(Jeffrey J. Iliff 2012) proposed that the glymphatic system clearance mechanism showed that AQP4 promotes the convective transport of brain parenchyma. Besides, Nedergaard et al.(Nadia Aalling Jessen 2015) proposed that cerebrospinal fluid is spatially transferred from pararenal to paracentral through the extracellular space (ECS), and solute transport in ECS depends on the glymphatic flow. Moreover, ECS consists of the ventricular system and subarachnoid space containing cerebrospinal fluid, parenchyma in grey and white matter, and perivascular space surrounding blood vessels(Stephen B Hladky 2014). Moreover, the glymphatic system is a highly polarized CSF transport system that facilitates the clearance of neurotoxic molecules through a network of perivascular pathways (Anne Sofie Munk 2019). Furthermore, the transport of solutes through brain ECS is essential for transporting nutrients and drugs to brain cells and removing metabolites, neurotransmitters, and toxic macromolecules (Stephen B Hladky 2014).

2. The structure, function and regulation of AQP4

In the brain, it has been found that there are three types of AQPs, including AQP4(K Oshio 2004), AQP1(Daniela Boassa 2005; Kotaro Oshio 2005), and AQP9 (Zelenina 2010). Furthermore, AQP4 was almost expressed in astrocytes and ependymal cells (Zelenina 2010). It has been reported that AQP4 is a homologous tetramer assembled by AQP4 monomer with independent water molecular channels on the cell membrane. There are two subtypes, AQP4-M1 and AQP4-M23, which mainly exist in brain tissues(Thomas Walz 2009). The monomer is about 30 KD, and each monomer crosses the membrane six times to form three extracellular rings (A, C, E) and two intracellular rings (B, D). The free N-terminal and C-terminal are distributed in the cytoplasm, and the B and E ring containing the NPA conserved sequence return to the lipid bilayer of the membrane (Fig.2). In addition, the whole AQP4 monomer is composed of the widely open ends on both sides of the membrane and the constriction part of the NPA conserved sequence in the central of the membrane, forming a three-dimensional "funnel model"(Erlend A Nagelhus 2013). Studies have shown that AQP4 tetramers form orthogonal arrays of particles (OAPs) on astrocyte membranes (Hartwig Wolburg 2011; Manuela de Bellis 2021), mainly composed of AQP4-M1 and AQP4-M23. And the size of OAPs is determined by the proportion of AQP4-M1 and AQP4-M23. Moreover, there is a conclusion that the more AQP4-M23 is, the more stable the OAPs structure will be(Jérôme Badaut 2014) (Jesse A Stokum 2015) (G P Nicchia 2010). In addition, as reported, the M23 isoform exhibits a much stronger water transport capacity than the M1 isoform(Claudia Silberstein 2004). In the case of astrocytes, tetrameric AQP4 is not inserted into the membrane as a supramolecular assembly of water channel molecules independently, and AQP4 molecules form functional complexes with other membrane proteins such as the dystrophin glycoprotein complex (DGC) (T Haenggi 2006). It was found that AQP4 was enriched at three critical locations in astrocytes. Furthermore, it is vital for blood-brain barrier function at the end of perivascular astrocytes. In addition, AQP4 is involved in neurotransmitter clearance in peri-synaptic astrocytes and K+ clearance during contact with Ranvier nodes and unmyelinated axons (Zelenina 2010). It has also been reported that AQP4 is mainly expressed in the cell membrane at the junction of the brain parenchyma and brain fluid components, such as, on the podocytes of astrocytes adjacent to microvascular endothelial cells, on the side of the basement membrane of ependymal cells in the ventricles, and on the cell membrane of astrocytes composing the glial boundary membrane. This polar distribution of AQP4 suggests that AQP4 may be involved in regulating the flow of brain water into and out of the CNS (Hubbard, et al. 2015).

There are mainly two ways of regulating AQP4 expression: short-term and long-term. Conformational alterations or channel gating can affect short-term regulation (E S McCoy 2010; H B Moeller 2009; Monica Carmosino 2007). Besides, because of dynamic regulation, the permeability of AQP channels or the subcellular localization of AQP channels (their abundance in the membrane) may change within seconds or minutes, resulting in an immediate change in membrane permeability (Zelenina 2010).

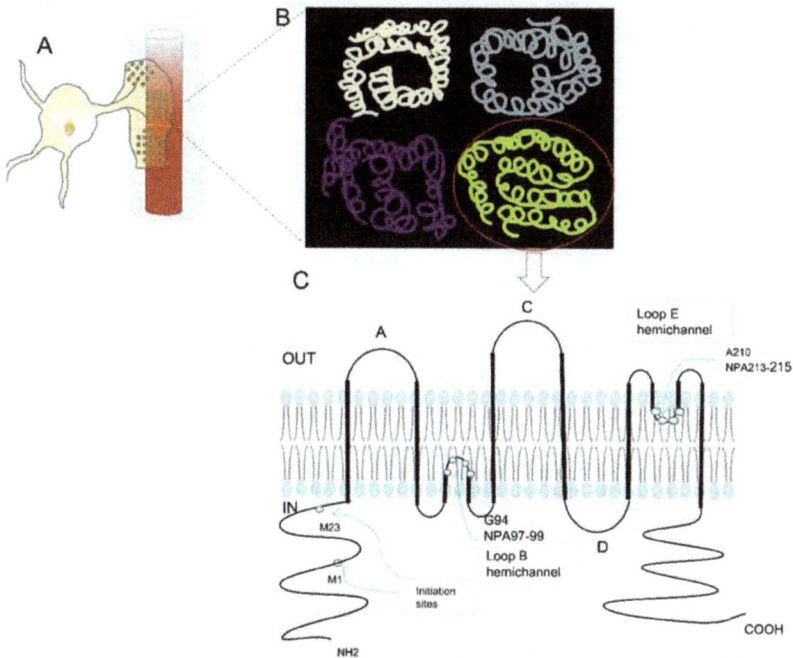

Figure 2. Structure of AQP4 molecule.

 (A) AQP4 was distributed in orthogonal arrays of particles on the astrocyte's end foot. (B) Aquaporins, in general, form tetrameric protein complexes within the membrane plane. (C) The proposed membrane topology of AQP4 comprises six presumed bilayer-spanning domains and five connecting loops. Furthermore, the initiation sites at methionines1 and 23 are shown at the N-terminus.

Unlike short-term adjustment, long-term regulation is mediated by changes in AQP mRNA and protein synthesis or degradation rates. These changes alter the abundance of AQP4 over hours or days, thereby altering the permeability of the AQP4 membrane. As more and more studies have been conducted on AQP4's involvement in nervous system diseases, pharmacological interventions have become more prevalent. Activators and inhibitors of AQP4 are summarized in table1. Therefore, it is reasonable to assume that the regulation of AQP4 is a highly complex process.

The type of drug	Drug' name	The pattern of drugs to regulate the expression of AQP4
Activators of AQP4	Dexamethasone	by inducing small ubiquitin-like modifiers (SUMO) (Xiaoling Zhang 2020).
	Testosterone	Being attenuated by the protein kinase C activator 12-O-tetradecanoylphorbol 13-acetate (Feng Gu 2003).
	Genistein	through the cAMP/PKA/CREB signaling pathway(Haohai Huang 2015).
Inhibitors of AQP4	TGN-020	Direct binding inhibition likely mediated by binding to D69, M70, I73, F77, V145 (rat)/L145 (human), I205, and R216.(Arno Vandebroek 2020;Ionica Pirici 2017)
	Minocycline	by reversing the translocation of AQP4 from astrocyte processes to cell bodies.(Qi Lu 2022)
	Methylene blue	through the ERK1/2 pathway(Zhong-Fang Shi 2021).

Table 1. The regulation of AQP4 through drugs.

AQP4: aquaporin4; TGN-020: N-(1,3,4-thiadiazol-2-yl) pyridine-3-carboxamide

3. The effects of AQP4 in glymphatic system on CNS disorders

3.1 Intracerebral hemorrhage (ICH)

ICH is a subtype of stroke caused by intracerebral vascular rupture, with high mortality and disability rates (Adnan I Qureshi 2009; He Wu 2011). Intracerebral hemorrhage accounts for 10-15% of strokes worldwide and is often associated with inadequate blood pressure control and excessive use of anticoagulants, thrombolytic agents, and antiplatelet drugs (Adnan I Qureshi 2009; C L Sudlow 1997). Several hours after intracerebral hemorrhage, the primary brain injury is mainly caused by the compression and destruction of nearby tissues caused by hematoma. Inflammation, thrombin activation and erythrocyte lysis caused by primary brain injury can promote the formation of brain edema, which has a poor prognosis and can cause more severe and lasting damage (Richard F Keep 2012). Jeon et al. (Hanwool Jeon 2021) found that AQP4 enhancer attenuated peri-hematoma edema by improving the integrity of the blood-brain barrier by up-regulating AQP4 expression on astrocytes with the AQP4 enhancer BQ-788. Besides, Liu et al. (Xichang Liu 2021) used a collagenase-induced rat model of ICH. Ligation and resection of cervical lymph nodes could lead to cerebral lymphatic vessel obstruction. They found that cerebral lymphatic obstruction down-regulated the expression of AQP4, up-regulated the expression of inflammatory TNF-α and inhibited the expression of IL-10, and aggravated brain edema, neuroinflammation and neuronal apoptosis in rats with cerebral hemorrhage, resulting in neurological deficits. Thus, it is concluded that AQP4 is involved in ICH-induced brain edema, BBB destruction and neuronal apoptosis.

Subarachnoid hemorrhage (SAH) is a highly prevalent ICH disorder (Aizawa 1971; Gijn 1992;Jolobe 2007;R Bonita 1985). SAH refers to blood flow into the subarachnoid space due to intracranial vascular rupture, often accompanied by permanent brain damage. Moreover, after SAH, blood components would enter the perivascular space, resulting in varying degrees of coagulation and macrophage chemotaxis, which could impede fluid exchange between cerebrospinal and interstitial fluid (A Jackowski 1990). A report showed that after SAH, for AQP4 knockout rats, CSF flow would significantly reduce through interstitial and parenchyma. The glymphatic system function was also impaired, and there was no improvement in neurological function and neuroinflammation compared with WT rats at seven days. The report indicated that the glymphatic system significantly removes harmful metabolites and excess fluid produced after SAH and plays a positive role in the recovery of neurological function (E Liu 2020). In addition, studies have shown persistent lymphatic and meningeal lymphatic drainage dysfunction and associated neuropathological damage after SAH (Pu, et al. 2019). Therefore, improving the clearance function of the glymphatic system in injured brain tissue after SAH may become a new strategy for treating SAH.

3.2 Ischemic stroke

Ischemic stroke is a disorder of cerebral blood flow caused by vascular obstruction (Wang, et al. 2023). The pathophysiology includes excitotoxicity, free radical release, protein misfolding, mitochondrial response, and inflammatory changes, leading to neuronal death and neurological deficits (George and Steinberg 2015; Jiang, et al. 2022; Li, et al. 2022). In rodent models of acute ischemic stroke, MRI and histological examination showed impaired CSF inflow in the ipsilateral cortex at 3 h after middle cerebral artery occlusion, and glymphatic influx had recovered 24 h after spontaneous arterial recanalization (Gaberel, et al. 2014). Notably, a murine study evaluating clearance of fluorescent tracers from the necrotic infarct core at 7 weeks after a hypoxic middle cerebral artery occlusion showed that solutes trapped in the core leaked through the glial scar and were transported from the brain along perivascular spaces. Otherwise, they also found that the ISF within the core contained elevated levels of proinflammatory cytokines and was toxic to cultured cortical and hippocampal neurons, even at 7 weeks after the middle cerebral artery occlusion, suggesting a beneficial role of glymphatic clearance in disease resolution (Zbesko, et al. 2018). Toh and Siow found that the autoimmune lymphoproliferative syndrome (ALPS) index showed lower values in ischemic stroke suggesting impaired glymphatic function. Following initial impairment, the ALPS index increased with the time since stroke onset, which is suggestive of glymphatic function recovery (Toh and Siow 2021). Cortical spreading depression (mass depolarization of neurons, initiating in the ischemic core, potentially leading to neuronal death in surrounding hypoxic tissue after stroke) has also been implicated in impaired glymphatic flow (Schain, et al. 2017). In mice, cortical spreading depression-induced in the non-hypoxic brain led to a complete transient closure of the perivascular spaces around both arteries and veins lasting up to 10 min, followed by a gradual reopening that did not recover to the baseline calibre within the first 30 min, and resulted in a reduction of interstitial flow (Schain et al. 2017). A mass of studies on astrocytes' roles in ischemic stroke has been conducted. Astrocyte-related structures/proteins play different roles in the activation of astrocytes at different developmental stages of ischemic stroke. In the acute phase of ischemic stroke, the proliferation and hypertrophy of astrocytes in the peri-infarct area are conducive to sealing the site of injury, remodeling the tissue, and controlling the local immune response both spatially and temporally (Wang, et al. 2012). However, in the chronic phase, the formation of glial scarring by excessive astrocyte proliferation may limit the recovery of central nervous function (Daneman and Prat 2015). In addition, many studies have shown the effect of AQP4 on ischemic stroke. For example, a study showed that deletion of AQP4 or TRPV4 channels alone leads to a significant worsening of ischemic brain injury at both time points, whereas their simultaneous deletion results in a smaller brain lesion at day 1 but equal tissue damage at day 2 when compared with controls. The data indicate that the interplay between AQP4 and TRPV4 channels is critical during neuronal and non-neuronal swelling in the acute phase of ischemic injury(Sucha, et al. 2022). Sun and collaborators have found that acutely inhibiting AQP4 using TGN-020 promoted neurological recovery by diminishing brain edema at the early stage and attenuating peri-infarct astrogliosis and AQP4 depolarization at the subacute stage after stroke (Sun, et al. 2022). In addition, oxytocin (OXT) significantly suppresses neuronal damage in the early stage of stroke by inhibiting apoptotic and NF-κB signaling pathways, increasing the expression of VEGF, AQP4 and BDNF proteins and reducing the BBB leakage (Wang et al. 2012). Furthermore, experts concluded that miR-29b could potentially predict stroke outcomes as a novel circulating biomarker, and miR-29b overexpression reduced BBB disruption after ischemic stroke via downregulating AQP-4(Wang, et al. 2015). Now, evidence of the involvement of the glymphatic pathway in stroke, at present, comes from findings in animal research, and the pathway must be investigated in human trials.

3.3 Traumatic brain injury (TBI)

TBI refers to the organic brain tissue lesions caused by trauma, resulting in brain dysfunction (Ann C Mckee 2015; Benjamin L Brett 2022; Hardman 1979;Kara N Corps 2015). TBI patients often perform neurodegenerative features of neurofibrillary tangles composed of Tau aggregates and Aβ amyloid aggregation. By injecting human Tau protein into the brain tissue of a moderate TBI animal model and tracking its clearance path, it was found that human Tau protein was mainly concentrated around the large veins (Jessen, et al. 2015). Studies have shown that TBI significantly inhibited the entry of cerebrospinal fluid tracer (OA-45) in mice, resulting in a glymphatic system function decline of about 60%. Researchers also found that impairing cerebrospinal fluid entry and A β clearance could be observed in the ipsilateral hippocampus one day after the onset of TBI, and the functional inhibition of the glial lymphatic system caused by TBI was still significant 28 days later(Iliff, et al. 2014). Those results suggest that the AQP4-mediated removal of Tau from the glymphatic system is essential for limiting secondary neuronal damage after trauma.

3.4 Alzheimer's disease (AD)

AD is common dementia in the elderly, accounting for about 50-70% of dementia in the elderly (Dhamidhu Eratne 2018; Jose A Soria Lopez 2019; Morgan Robinson 2017). Genetic variants in AQP4 are associated with Aβ accumulation, disease stage progression, and cognitive decline, which may correspond to changes in glymphatic system function and brain Aβ clearance and may be useful biomarkers for predicting the burden of disease in patients with dementia (Chandra, et al. 2021). It has also been shown that loss of perivascular AQP4 localization in neurodegenerative diseases such as AD may be a factor that makes the ageing brain vulnerable to protein mis-aggregation (Zeppenfeld, et al. 2017). Andrea et al. (Arighi, et al. 2019) measured the levels of AQP4 in cerebrospinal fluid (CSF) in 11 AD patients, ten normal pressure hydrocephalus (NPH) patients and nine controls, finding that AQP4 was significantly decreased in AD patients and tended to decrease in NPH patients. Besides, there was also a correlation between AQP4 and the levels of amyloid beta and CSF. This study suggests a potential role of AQP4 and the glymphatic system's pathophysiology of neurodegenerative diseases. The relationship between the glymphatic system and AD is being further studied, and the strategy for treating AD by regulating the glymphatic system is also gradually developing. For example, an experiment found that the β- lactam antibiotics such as ceftriaxone can be efficiently activated by the $NF-\kappa B$ pathway activation of astrocyte glutamate transfer eggs (glutamate transporter, GLT1) express. It alleviated the problems of memory loss and cognitive impairment caused by excessive accumulation of glutamate and glutamatergic N-methyl-d-aspartate (NMDA) receptors, such as Ca2+isorder, massive production of NO, increase of free radicals, activation of proteasome and proliferation of cytotoxic transcription factors (Brhane Teklebrhan Assefa 2018). Now, the most promising drug is the target of AQP4, and its therapeutic effect has been proved by comparison. For example, AQP4 can help regulate the Ca2+ signaling pathway, K+ balance, glutamate transport, astrocyte proliferation and activation, and neuroinflammatory response of astrocytes (Yu-Long Lan 2017).

3.5 Parkinson's disease (PD)

Parkinson's disease (PD) is a multisystem alpha-synucleinopathic neurodegenerative disease and the most prevalent neurodegenerative disorder after Alzheimer's disease, with a high incidence rate in the elderly population (Scott-Massey, et al. 2022). Moreover, its characteristic motor symptoms are tremor, rigidity, bradykinesia/akinesia, and postural stability, but the clinical picture includes other motor and non-motor symptoms (NMSs)(Taylor, et al. 2002). Several studies indicated that extracellular alpha-synuclein might lead to neurotoxic responses by microglia and astrocytes, and deposition and spreading of misfolded proteins (α-synuclein and tau) have been linked to Parkinson's disease cognitive dysfunction. (Han, et al. 2021; Henderson, et al. 2019). Alpha-synucleinopathy is postulated to be central to idiopathic rapid eye movement sleep behavior disorder (iRBD) and Parkinson's disease (PD). And there is an association between the diminished clearance of α-synuclein and glymphatic system dysfunction (Si, et al. 2022). In PD, the impact of dopaminergic deterioration may be crucial in the disruption of sleep and CSF-ISF flow in the glymphatic system, given the significant involvement of dopaminergic contributions to the disease and waste clearance system (Gratwicke, et al. 2015). Recent studies have indicated that aquaporin 4 (AQP4), as a predominant water channel protein in the brain, is involved in the progression of Parkinson's disease (PD) as well. Dopamine has been shown to reduce the proliferation of striatal glial cells and the expression of AQP4 within these cells (Küppers, et al. 2008). Additionally, AQP4 deficiency has been associated with aggravated dopaminergic degeneration and, in particular, enhanced susceptibility to the insult of the dopaminergic neurons between the substantia nigra and ventral tegmental area (Zhang, et al. 2016). Cui and colleagues established a progressive PD model by subjecting AQP4 null (AQP4(+/-)) mice to bilateral intrastriatal injection of α-syn preformed fibrils (PFFs) and investigated the effect of decreased AQP4 expression on the development of PD. Meanwhile, they found that decreased expression of AQP4 accelerated pathologic deposition of α-syn and facilitated the loss of dopamine neurons and behavioral disorders. Draining of macromolecules from the brain via the glymphatic pathway was slowed due to decreased AQP4 expression (Cui, et al. 2021). Additionally, Chi et al. found that AQP4-deficient mice were hypersensitive to stimulations such as 1-methyl-4-phenyl-1,2,3,6-tetrahydropyridine (MPTP) or lipopolysaccharide compared to wild-type (WT) littermates. In a mouse model of MPTP-induced Parkinson's disease (PD), AQP4-deficient animals show more robust microglial inflammatory responses and more severe loss of dopaminergic neurons (DNS) compared with WT mice (Chi, et al. 2011). A study of three-hundred and eighty-two patients with PD and 180 healthy controls with a mean follow-up time of 66.1 months from the Parkinson's Progression Marker Initiative study were analyzed. The result showed that genetic variations of AQP4 and subsequent alterations of glymphatic efficacy might contribute to an altered rate of cognitive decline in PD. AQP4 rs162009 is likely a novel genetic prognostic marker of glymphatic function and cognitive decline in PD (Fang, et al. 2021).

3.6 Vascular dementia (VaD)

Vascular dementia (VaD) is one of the most common causes of dementia after Alzheimer's disease, causing around 15% of cases (O'Brien and Thomas 2015). Furthermore, Vascular and neurodegenerative dementia has emerged as the leading cause of age-related cognitive impairment (Iadecola 2013). Among these cerebrovascular disorders, major stroke, and cerebral small vessel disease (cSVD) constitute the major risk factors for VaD. These conditions alter neurovascular functions leading to blood-brain barrier (BBB) deregulation, neurovascular coupling dysfunction, and inflammation (Lecordier, et al. 2021). The entry of blood-borne macromolecular substances into the brain parenchyma from cerebral vessels is blocked by the blood-brain barrier (BBB) function. Accordingly, increased permeability of the vessels induced by insult noted in patients suffering from vascular dementia likely contributes to cognitive impairment (Ueno, et al. 2019). The glymphatic system plays an essential role in the pathophysiological processes of many cognitive disorders. AQP4 shows noteworthy changes in various cognitive disorders and is part of the pathogenesis of these diseases (Wang, et al. 2022b). Yu and colleagues employed a multiple microinfarction (MMI) model to induce VaD in mice, and investigate VaD-induced cognitive dysfunction, white matter (WM) damage, glymphatic dysfunction and the role of miR-126 in mediating these effects. Results showed that MMI in WT mice decreases synaptic plasticity and dendritic spine density, instigates water channel and glymphatic dysfunction, and decreases serum miR-126 expression. Furthermore, the reduction of endothelial miR-126 expression may mediate cognitive impairment in MMI-induced VaD. (Yu, et al. 2019). Moreover, Venkat's team have investigated the therapeutic effects of human umbilical cord blood cells (HUCBC) treatment on the cognitive outcome, white matter (WM) integrity, and glymphatic system function in rats subject to a multiple microinfarction (MMI) model of VaD. Data indicated that HUCBC treatment of an MMI rat model of VaD promotes WM remodeling and improves glymphatic function, which may aid in improving cognitive function and memory (Venkat, et al. 2020). Therefore, we may infer from the above that a therapeutic strategy to clear brain metabolic waste through the glymphatic pathway may be a promising approach to prevent neurodegenerative diseases.

3.7 Idiopathic normal pressure hydrocephalus (iNPH)

iNPH, one of NPH and with no apparent cause, often occurs in the elderly, and imaging analysis shows normal CSF pressure and ventricular enlargement (Changwu Tan 2021) (Michael A Williams 2016). Moreover, this disease is characterized by progressive ventricular enlargement and the clinical tread of gait ataxia, urinary incontinence, and dementia (Basant R. Nassar and Carol F. Lippa 2016). iNPH presents with similar symptoms to AD, with pathological findings: cortical biopsies of brains with iNPH have shown Aβ deposition, reactive astrocyte proliferation, and AQP4 depolarization (G V Gavrilov 2019). Studies have shown that the inflow and outflow functions of the glymphatic system are impaired in iNPH patients, especially in the entorhinal cortex (ERC) (Per K Eide 2019). ERC is one of the essential bases of hippocampal function, directly affecting memory function. Hasan-Olive et al. (Md Mahdi Hasan-Olive 2019) found that immunohistochemical analysis of AQP4 in cortical brain biopsies from 30 iNPH patients and 12 normal subjects showed decreased AQP4 density at the end arterial end peri-cerebrovascular astrocytes in iNPH compared with control brains. Using intrathecal injection of gadolinium-diethylenetriaminepentacetate (Gd-DTPA), a magnetic resonance imaging (MRI) paramagnetic contrast agent, Ringstad et al.(Per K Eide 2019), and Eide et al. (Geir Ringstad 2018) found that Gd-DTPA extends anteriorly along the great arachnoid artery into the subarachnoid space and then enters the brain parenchyma along the extravascular space. Moreover, compared with ordinary people, the clearance of Gd-DTPA is delayed in patients with idiopathic hydrocephalus, suggesting that the glial lymphatic system is related to the pathogenesis of idiopathic normal pressure hydrocephalus. According to clinical guidelines, patients with iNPH are still advised to undergo early shunt surgery to improve intracranial lymphatic dysfunction (Basant R. Nassar and Carol F. Lippa 2016; Etsuro Mori 2012) and help regulate the rate of cerebrospinal fluid drainage (Albert M Isaacs 2019). In one study, changes in cerebrospinal fluid biomarkers after shunt surgery were found, which suggested that shunt surgery improves the glymphatic system function (Madoka Nakajima 2018). In the end, an in-depth study of the relationship between the glymphatic system and the pathogenesis of iNPH can optimize the current clinical diagnostic methods and prevent the early deterioration of the disease.

3.8 Status epilepticus (SE)

SE is a neurologic emergency characterized by persistent epileptic activity or frequent seizures without return to baseline, with high mortality and morbidity (Bhavpreet S Dham 2014). Moreover, many patients have persistent neurocognitive impairment after completion of SE (Khalil S Husari 2020;Kjersti N Power 2018). In addition to the direct neuronal damage caused by SE, the deposition of hyperphosphorylated tau (p-tau) is thought to contribute to post-SE neurodegeneration (Ali, et al. 2019). In addition, cerebral edema after SE is considered almost inevitable and is associated with a poor prognosis in SE (Amélia Mendes 2016). Liu et al. (Kewei Liu 2021) found that Glymphatic system function was temporarily impaired after SE, and the time course of lymphatic system dysfunction was well matched with the progression of brain edema after SE. In addition, when cerebral edema was relieved by Glibenclamide treatment or Trpm4 gene deletion, the function of the glymphatic system recovered earlier. At the same time, p-tau deposition and neuronal degeneration were reduced, and cognitive function was improved. Furthermore, the results suggest that SE-induced brain edema may lead to lymphatic dysfunction and make the post-SE brain vulnerable to p-tau aggregation and neurocognitive impairment. The cerebellar AQP4 levels in SE were evaluated by constructing pilocarpine-induced SE mouse models. The results showed that the expression of aquaporin decreased from day three after SE and recovered on day 7. In addition, mice showed impaired motor coordination and learning in the acute post-SE phase. Thus, SE is implicated in changes in AQP4 expression and cerebellar injury (Hui Tang 2017). Another study investigated the role of 67-kDa laminin receptor (LR) in SE-induced vasogenic edema formation in rat piriform cortex (PC). SE reduced the expression of 67-kDa LR and SMI-71(a rat BBB barrier marker) in endothelial cells and astrocytes. An additional 67-kDa LR neutralization also reduced dystrophin and aquaporin 4 (AQP4) expression. Therefore, the findings indicate that 67-kDa LR dysfunction may disrupt the dystrophin-AQP4 complex, which would evoke vasogenic edema formation and subsequent laminin over-expression via activating p38 MAPK/VEGF axis (Hana Park 2019). It is concluded that AQP4 is involved in the occurrence and development of SE.

3.9 Migraine and other pathologic pain

Migraine is a common primary headache in clinical practice(Diamond 1991;Elithorn 1969;Michel D Ferrari 2022;Tfelt-Hansen 1994;Walter 2022;William Qubty 2020) . It is characterized by paroxysmal, primarily unilateral, moderate to severe, pulsatile headache, generally lasting 4-72 hours, and can be accompanied by nausea, vomiting, sound stimulation, light stimulation or daily activities, which can aggravate the headache. Furthermore, cortical spreading inhibition (CSD), a cell depolarization autogenous wave, is associated with progressive neuronal damage after migraine (Takano, et al. 2007). Because CSD can be regarded as a neurophysiological precursor of migraine, animal models of migraine are often induced by CSD (Zhang, et al. 2010). Schain et al. (Schain et al. 2017) injected dextran labelled with different fluorescent dyes into the frontal cortex of the cerebral cortex of induced CSD mice and control mice. Through using two-photon imaging technology, the VRS around the arteries and veins on the cerebral cortex of CSD mice were rapidly closed.

The ependyma of VRS is mainly surrounded by astrocyte terminus, and Takano et al. (Schain et al. 2017) previously reported that CSD would cause swelling of neurons and astrocyte terminus. Schain et al. (Nadia Aalling Jessen 2015) suggested that VRS closure was related to this swelling. Moreover, VRS closure was accompanied by a decrease in dye clearance at the injection site, indicating that CSD impeded ISF outflow from brain tissue through the glymphatic system, which would also slow fluid flow in the VRS. This phenomenon is consistent with previous studies on the role of the glymphatic system in the clearance of ISF solutes(Erik N T P Bakker 2016). However, ROSIC et al.(Brana Rosic 2019) used AQP4-/ - and wild-type mice as models to induce CSD and found that the time and volume of astrocyte terminal foot swelling in the two mice were consistent, suggesting that CSD caused astrocyte terminal foot swelling in an AQP4-independent manner. Combined with their previous studies, they hypothesized that astrocyte end foot swelling might be related to abnormal $Ca2+$ signaling of functional molecules assembled in the end foot and that astrocyte end foot swelling may be mediated by membrane proteins such as chloride cotransporters rather than aquaporins. Although the abnormal mechanics of the glymphatic system in migraine is still controversial, the fact that VRS is closed suggests that if the homeostasis of astrocyte terminal foot function is disrupted, this entry point may provide a new therapeutic direction for migraine treatment.

Pain is a common symptom in patients with all types of demyelinating-ON (Ayzenberg, et al. 2021; Kang, et al. 2022) and MOG-IgG-pos (Asseyer, et al. 2018). Moreover, intractable neuropathic pain is a common symptom of neuromyelitis optica spectrum disorder (NMOSD) (Ishikura, et al. 2021). The immune system has long been recognised as important in pain regulation through inflammatory cytokine modulation of peripheral nociceptive fibres (Xu, et al. 2020). However, emerging clinical and experimental evidence demonstrates that neuroinflammation is essential in cognitive impairment associated with neuropathic pain (Mai, et al. 2021). Notably, Lu and collaborators found that Complete Freund's adjuvant-induced chronic inflammatory pain and spared nerve injury-induced neuropathic pain models, AQP4(-/-) mice attenuated pain-related behavioral responses compared with AQP4(+/+) mice, demonstrating that AQP4 deficiency relieved chronic inflammatory pain and neuropathic pain. In the formalin and capsaicin tests, two models of chemical stimuli-induced acute pain, no differences in the durations of licking the injected hind-paw were found between AQP4(+/+) and AQP4(-/-) mice (Lu, et al. 2020). In AQP4-ON, loss of AQP4, impairment of astrocytes and parallel injury in AQP4-coexpressed molecules (such as excitatory amino acid transporter 2, EAAT2), may lead to an excessive accumulation of glutamate in the extracellular space, interrupting the glutamine-glutamate-GABA axis (Kang et al. 2022). In addition, recent studies have found that astrocytes can regulate nociceptive synaptic transmission via neuronal-glial and glial-glial cell interactions and are involved in the modulation of pain signaling and the maintenance of neuropathic pain (Ji, et al. 2019). Many recent studies have shown that the glymphatic system is also associated with other pathologic pain in addition to migraine. The study of Wang and collaborators verified that alterations in glymphatic function are closely related to cancer pain, and the quantification of functional changes reflects pain severity (Wang, et al. 2022a). Goldman and his partners' study showed that the glymphatic system is regulated by sleep and norepinephrine, with increased levels of norepinephrine during wakefulness inhibiting fluid movement. Norepinephrine is also essential for transitioning from acute to chronic pain, and sufferers of chronic neuropathic pain frequently present with sleep disruption (Goldman, et al.

2020). However, it remains unclear how AQP4 mediates the glymphatic system specifically to affect the pathophysiology of pathologic pain.

3.10 Neuromyelitis optical (NMO)

NMO is a chronic inflammatory autoimmune disease of the CNS associated with a characteristic pattern of astrocyte dysfunction and loss, leading to secondary demyelination and neurodegeneration (Izumi Kawachi and Lassmann 2017). In most patients, NMO is caused by pathogenic serum IgG antibodies against AQP4(Carnero Contentti and Correale 2021). In most patients, NMO is caused by pathogenic serum IgG antibodies against AQP4[87]. The binding of AQP4-antibody (AQP4-ab) to AQP4 expressed by astrocytes triggers activation of a classical complement cascade, followed by granulocyte, eosinophil, and lymphocyte infiltration. Eventually, astrocytes are injured first, followed by oligodendrocytes, demyelination, neuronal loss, and neurodegeneration (Carnero Contentti and Correale 2021). However, how AQP4-IgG enters the brain from the periphery must be clarified. It has been suggested that the blood-brain barrier may not be fully developed in the anterior lamina part of the optic nerve and the root entrance area of the spinal cord, making IgG more likely to enter the circulation than elsewhere in the CNS (Hofman, et al. 2001; Iorio, et al. 2011). Here somebody also hypothesized that infection temporarily preferentially destroys the blood-brain barrier in the optic nerve or spinal cord, allowing AQP4-IgG entry (Koga, et al. 2011). There are many methods to treat NMO, currently available methylprednisolone and maintenance plasmapheresis in resistant cases, including corticosteroids, azathioprine, rituximab, mitoxantrone, cyclophosphamide, and mycophenolate salts (Collongues and Seze 2011). Besides, an emerging approach to targeted therapy that prevents AQP4-IgG from binding to AQP4 has recently been proposed (Verkman, et al. 2012).

In brain tissue, AQP4 is mainly expressed in the astrocyte terminus, and both AQP4 and astrocytes are related to the pathogenesis of NMO. Therefore, we might hypothesize that the glymphatic system influences NMO, but further research is required.

Disease	The effects of AQP4 in CNS disorders
ICH	• AQP4 might improve the integrity of the blood-brain barrier • AQP4 up-regulated the expression of inflammatory cytokines, such as TNF-α and IL-10
Ischemic stroke	•AQP4 expression is altered in a stage-specific manner •AQP4 expression may be regulated by oxytocin and miR-29b
TBI	•AQP4 mediated removal of Tau from the glymphatic system
AD	•The loss of perivascular AQP4 localization may be a factor to make protein mis-aggregation •AQP4 could help regulate the Ca2+ signaling pathway, K+ balance, glutamate transport, astrocyte proliferation and activation, and neuroinflammatory response of astrocytes
PD	• AQP4 deficiency was associated with aggravated dopaminergic degeneration • Decreased expression of AQP4 accelerated pathologic deposition of α-syn and facilitated the loss of dopamine neurons and behavioral disorders. •The genetic variations of AQP4 might contribute to an altered rate of cognitive decline in PD
VaD	•AQP4 showed noteworthy changes in various cognitive disorders and is part of the pathogenesis of these diseases
iNPH	•AQP4 depolarization may help regulate the rate of cerebrospinal fluid drainage
SE	•The changes in AQP4 expression •67-kDa laminin receptor (LR) dysfunction may disrupt the dystrophin-AQP4 complex
Migraine	•AQP4 may be not participate in the process of astrocyte end foot swelling
pathologic pain	•AQP4 deficiency relieved chronic inflammatory pain and neuropathic pain •The AQP4-coexpressed molecules may lead to an excessive accumulation of glutamate in the extracellular space, interrupting the glutamine-glutamate-GABA axis
NMO	•Often defined by the presence of anti-AQP IgGs •The binding of AQP4-antibody (AQP4-ab) to AQP4 expressed by astrocytes triggers activation of a classical complement cascade

Table.2 Summary of AQP4 regulation in various neurological disorders.

Summary

As the most abundantly expressed aquaporin in the CNS, AQP4 has always been the focus of research on related CNS disorders. The glymphatic system has emerged as a major clearance pathway for brain metabolic waste, with AQP4 being an essential component. As a result, AQP4 provides a new avenue for research in various disorders of the CNS.

There is a brief review of the mechanisms and effects of AQP4 in several common disorders of the central nervous system (Table.2). In ICH diseases, AQP4 and the glymphatic system play a critical role in maintaining the integrity of the blood-brain barrier, removing hematoma and reducing edema. In the case of AD is to clear away the deposits of Aβ and tau, and in PD, AQP4 is a significant effect on the accumulation of α-Synuclein and dopamine secretion. But as for the VaD, it is not clear about the role of AQP4. In iNPH may be caused by insufficient drainage of the glymphatic system and AQP4 depolarization. In SE, it is likely that the integrity of the BBB and the dystrophin-AQP4 complex are disrupted. In migraine, AQP4 may affect the homeostasis of astrocyte foot processes. In other pathologic pain, AQP4 is associated with interrupting the glutamine-glutamate-GABA axis and synaptic transmission. Moreover, triggering the closure of the VRS. And the pathogenesis of NMO is correlated with pathogenic serum IgG antibodies to AQP4.

In summary, the pathogenesis of the central nervous system is challenging to elucidate. Usually, it results from multiple factors, which undoubtedly increases the difficulty and complexity of patient treatment. This review indicates that AQP4 plays a non-negligible role in neurological disorders due to its location in the glymphatic system, which means that AQP4 is a promising therapeutic target. It has been shown that regulating the expression of AQP4 in the glymphatic system can delay or improve the occurrence and development of disorders related to the central nervous system. Although research on AQP4 and the glymphatic system has increased in recent years, the field is still in its infancy. As a result of the pathway's distribution throughout the brain, it is difficult to pinpoint the exact routes of glymphatic system in brain. More researches should be conducted to strengthen the function of the waste clearance system in brain by regulating phagocytosis and AQP4 in order to treat CNS diseases precisely, which provides new possibilities for incurable debilitating neurodegenerative disorders of CNS in the future.

Author Contributions Statement

All authors listed have made a substantial, direct and intellectual contribution to the work, and approved it for publication.

Conflict of Interest Statement

The authors declare that the research was conducted in the absence of any commercial or financial relationships that could be construed as a potential conflict of interest.

Acknowledgments:

This work was supported by Hainan Province Clinical Medical Center, National Natural Science Foundation of China (No.81771294; 82160237) and Shenzhen Municipal Science, Technology and Innovation Commission (No. JCYJ20190808161013492).

REFERENCE:

A Jackowski AC, G Burnstock,R R Russell,F Kristek. 1990.The Time Course of Intracranial Pathophysiological Changes Following Experimental Subarachnoid Haemorrhage in the Rat. J Cereb Blood Flow Metab.10(6),835-849 https://doi.org /10.1038/jcbfm.1990.140

Adnan I Qureshi ADM, Daniel F Hanley. 2009.Intracerebral Haemorrhage. Lancet.373(9675),1632-1644 https://doi.org/10.1016/S0140-6736(09)60371-8

Aizawa T. 1971.Subarachnoid Hemorrhage. Nihon Ishikai Zasshi.66(12),1423-1428

Albert M Isaacs MAW, Mark G Hamilton. 2019.Current Update on Treatment Strategies for Idiopathic Normal Pressure Hydrocephalus. Curr Treat Options Neurol.21(12),65 https://doi.org/10.1007/s11940-019-0604-z

Ali I, Silva JC, Liu S, Shultz SR, Kwan P, Jones NC, O'Brien TJ. 2019.Targeting

Neurodegeneration to Prevent Post-Traumatic Epilepsy. Neurobiology of Disease.123,100-109 https://doi.org/10.1016/j.nbd.2018.08.006

Amélia Mendes LS. 2016.Brain Magnetic Resonance in Status Epilepticus: A Focused Review. Seizure.38,63-67 https://doi.org/10.1016/j.seizure.2016.04.007

Ann C Mckee DHD. 2015.The Neuropathology of Traumatic Brain Injury. Handb Clin Neurol.127,45-66 https://doi.org/10.1016/B978-0-444-52892-6.00004-0

Anne Sofie Munk WW, Nicholas Burdon Bèchet,Ahmed M Eltanahy,Anne Xiaoan Cheng,Björn Sigurdsson,Abdellatif Benraiss,Maarja A Mäe,Benjamin Travis Kress,Douglas H Kelley,Christer Betsholtz,Kjeld Møllgård,Anja Meissner,Maiken Nedergaard,Iben Lundgaard. 2019.Pdgf-B Is Required for Development of the Glymphatic System. Cell Rep.26(11),2955-2969.e2953 https://doi.org/10.1016/j.celrep. 2019.02.050

Arighi A, Di Cristofori A, Fenoglio C, Borsa S, D'Anca M, Fumagalli GG, Locatelli M, Carrabba G, Pietroboni AM, Ghezzi L, Carandini T, Colombi A, Scarioni M, De Riz MA, Serpente M, Rampini PM, Scarpini E, Galimberti D, Bozzali M. 2019.Cerebrospinal Fluid Level of Aquaporin4: A New Window on Glymphatic System Involvement in Neurodegenerative Disease? Journal of Alzheimer's Disease.69(No.3), 663-669 https://doi.org/10.3233/JAD-190119

Arno Vandebroek MY. 2020.Regulation of Aqp4 in the Central Nervous System. Int J Mol Sci.21(5),1603 https://doi.org/10.3390/ijms21051603

Asseyer S, Schmidt F, Chien C, Scheel M, Ruprecht K, Bellmann-Strobl J, Brandt AU, Paul F. 2018.Pain in Aqp4-Igg-Positive and Mog-Igg-Positive Neuromyelitis Optica Spectrum Disorders. Mult Scler J Exp Transl Clin.4(3),2055217318796684 https:// doi.org/10.1177/2055217318796684

Ayzenberg I, Richter D, Henke E, Asseyer S, Paul F, Trebst C, Hümmert MW, Havla J, Kümpfel T, Ringelstein M, Aktas O, Wildemann B, Jarius S, Häußler V, Stellmann JP, Senel M, Klotz L, Pellkofer HL, Weber MS, Pawlitzki M, Rommer PS, Berthele A, Wernecke KD, Hellwig K, Gold R, Kleiter I. 2021.Pain, Depression, and Quality of Life in Neuromyelitis Optica Spectrum Disorder: A Cross-Sectional Study of 166 Aqp4 Antibody-Seropositive Patients. Neurol Neuroimmunol Neuroinflamm.8(3) https:// doi.org/10.1212/nxi.0000000000000985

Basant R. Nassar B, Carol F. Lippa M. 2016.Idiopathic Normal Pressure Hydrocephalus: A Review for General Practitioners. Gerontology and Geriatric Medicine (3) https://doi.org/10.1177/2333721416643702

Benjamin L Brett RCG, Jonathan Godbout,Kristen Dams-O'Connor,C Dirk Keene. 2022.Traumatic Brain Injury and Risk of Neurodegenerative Disorder. Biol Psychiatry. 91(5),498-507 https://doi.org/10.1016/j.biopsych.2021.05.025

Benjamin T Kress JJI, Maosheng Xia,Minghuan Wang,Helen S Wei,Douglas Zeppenfeld,Lulu Xie,Hongyi Kang,Qiwu Xu,Jason A Liew,Benjamin A Plog,Fengfei Ding,Rashid Deane,Maiken Nedergaard. 2014.Impairment of Paravascular Clearance

Pathways in the Aging Brain. Ann Neurol.76(6),845-861 https://doi.org/10.1002/ana.
24271

Bhavpreet S Dham KH, Fred Rincon. 2014.The Epidemiology of Status Epilepticus in the United States. Neurocrit Care.20(3),476-483 https://doi.org/10.1007/s12028-013-9935-x

Brana Rosic DBD, Knut Sindre Åbjørsbråten,Wannan Tang,Vidar Jensen,Ole Petter Ottersen,Rune Enger,Erlend A Nagelhus. 2019.Aquaporin-4-Independent Volume Dynamics of Astroglial Endfeet During Cortical Spreading Depression. Glia.67(6),1113-1121 https://doi.org/10.1002/glia.23604

Brhane Teklebrhan Assefa AKG, Birhanetensay Masresha Altaye. 2018.Reactive Astrocytes as Drug Target in Alzheimer's Disease. Biomed Res Int.2018,4160247 https://doi.org/10.1155/2018/4160247

C L Sudlow CPW. 1997.Comparable Studies of the Incidence of Stroke and Its Pathological Types: Results from an International Collaboration. International Stroke Incidence Collaboration. Stroke.28(3),491-499 https://doi.org/10.1161/01.str.28.3.491

Carnero Contentti E, Correale JD. 2021.Neuromyelitis Optica Spectrum Disorders: From Pathophysiology to Therapeutic Strategies. Journal of Neuroinflammation. 18 (No.1),208 https://doi.org/10.1186/s12974-021-02249-1

Chandra A, Farrell C, Wilson H, b, Dervenoulas G, c, de Natale ER, b, Politis M, b, Initiative AsDN. 2021.Aquaporin-4 Polymorphisms Predict Amyloid Burden and Clinical Outcome in the Alzheimer's Disease Spectrum. Neurobiology of aging.97,1-9 https://doi.org/10.1016/j.neurobiolaging.2020.06.007

Changwu Tan XW, Yuchang Wang,Chuansen Wang,Zhi Tang,Zhiping Zhang, Jingping Liu,Gelei Xiao. 2021.The Pathogenesis Based on the Glymphatic System, Diagnosis, and Treatment of Idiopathic Normal Pressure Hydrocephalus. Clin Interv Aging.16,139-153 https://doi.org/10.2147/CIA.S290709

Chi Y, Fan Y, He L, Liu W, Wen X, Zhou S, Wang X, Zhang C, Kong H, Sonoda L, Tripathi P, Li CJ, Yu MS, Su C, Hu G. 2011.Novel Role of Aquaporin-4 in Cd4+ Cd25+ T Regulatory Cell Development and Severity of Parkinson's Disease. Aging Cell.10(3),368-382 https://doi.org/10.1111/j.1474-9726.2011.00677.x

Claudia Silberstein RB, Yan Huang,Pingke Fang,Nuria Pastor-Soler,Dennis Brown,Alfred N Van Hoek. 2004.Membrane Organization and Function of M1 and M23 Isoforms of Aquaporin-4 in Epithelial Cells. Am J Physiol Renal Physiol.287(3),F501-511 https://doi.org/10.1152/ajprenal.00439.2003

Collongues N, Seze Jd. 2011.Current and Future Treatment Approaches for Neuromyelitis Optica. Therapeutic advances in neurological disorders.4(No.2),111-121 https://doi.org/10.1177/1756285611398939

Cui H, Wang W, Zheng X, Xia D, Liu H, Qin C, Tian H, Teng J. 2021.Decreased Aqp4 Expression Aggravates ɑ-Synuclein Pathology in Parkinson's Disease Mice,

Possibly Via Impaired Glymphatic Clearance. J Mol Neurosci.71(12),2500-2513 https://doi.org/10.1007/s12031-021-01836-4

Daneman R, Prat A. 2015.The Blood-Brain Barrier. Cold Spring Harb Perspect Biol.7(1),a020412 https://doi.org/10.1101/cshperspect.a020412

Daniela Boassa AJY. 2005.Physiological Roles of Aquaporins in the Choroid Plexus. Curr Top Dev Biol.67,181-206 https://doi.org/10.1016/S0070-2153(05)67005-6

Dhamidhu Eratne SML, Sarah Farrand,Wendy Kelso,Dennis Velakoulis,Jeffrey Cl Looi. 2018.Alzheimer's Disease: Clinical Update on Epidemiology, Pathophysiology and Diagnosis. Australas Psychiatry.26(4),347-357 https://doi.org/10.1177/ 1039856218 762308

Diamond S. 1991.Migraine Headaches. Med Clin North Am.75(3),545-566 https://doi.org/10.1016/S0025-7125(16)30432-1

E Liu XP, Haowen Ma,Yan Zhang, Xiaomei Yang,Yixuan Zhang,Linlin Sun,Junhao Yan. 2020.The Involvement of Aquaporin-4 in the Interstitial Fluid Drainage Impairment Following Subarachnoid Hemorrhage. Front Aging Neurosci.12,611494 https://doi.org/10.3389/fnagi.2020.611494

E S McCoy BRH, H Sontheimer. 2010.Water Permeability through Aquaporin-4 Is Regulated by Protein Kinase C and Becomes Rate-Limiting for Glioma Invasion. Neuroscience.168(4),971-981 https://doi.org/10.1016/j.neuroscience.2009.09.020

Elithorn A. 1969.Migraine. Br Med J.4(5680),411-413 https://doi.org/10.1136/ bmj.4.5680.411

Erik N T P Bakker BJB, Michal Arbel-Ornath,Roxana Aldea,Beatrice Bedussi,Alan W J Morris,Roy O Weller,Roxana O Carare. 2016.Lymphatic Clearance of the Brain: Perivascular, Paravascular and Significance for Neurodegenerative Diseases. Cell Mol Neurobiol.36(2),181-194 https://doi.org/10.1007/s10571-015-0273-8

Erlend A Nagelhus OPO. 2013.Physiological Roles of Aquaporin-4 in Brain. Physiol Rev.93(4),1543-1562 https://doi.org/10.1152/physrev.00011.2013

Etsuro Mori MI, Takeo Kato,Hiroaki Kazui,Hiroji Miyake,Masakazu Miyajima, Madoka Nakajima, Masaaki Hashimoto,Nagato Kuriyama,Takahiko Tokuda,Kazunari Ishii, Mitsunobu Kaijima,Yoshihumi Hirata,Makoto Saito,Hajime Arai,. 2012.Guidelines for Management of Idiopathic Normal Pressure Hydrocephalus: Second Edition. Neurol Med Chir (Tokyo).52(11),775-809 https://doi.org/10.2176/nmc.52.775

Fang Y, Dai S, Jin C, Si X, Gu L, Song Z, Gao T, Chen Y, Yan Y, Yin X, Pu J, Zhang B. 2021.Aquaporin-4 Polymorphisms Are Associated with Cognitive Performance in Parkinson's Disease. Front Aging Neurosci.13,740491 https://doi.org/10.3389/fnagi. 2021.740491

Feng Gu RH, Kazuko Toku,Lihua Yang,Yong-Jie Ma,Nobuji Maeda,Masahiro Sakanaka,Junya Tanaka. 2003.Testosterone up-Regulates Aquaporin-4 Expression in Cultured Astrocytes. J Neurosci Res.72(6),709-715 https://doi.org/10.1002/jnr.10603

G P Nicchia AR, M G Mola,F Pisani,C Stigliano,D Basco,M Mastrototaro,M Svelto,A Frigeri. 2010.Higher Order Structure of Aquaporin-4. Neuroscience.168(4), 903-914 https://doi.org/10.1016/j.neuroscience.2010.02.008

G V Gavrilov AVS, B V Gaydar,N M Paramonova,O N Gaykova,D V Svistov. 2019.Pathological Changes in Human Brain Biopsies from Patients with Idiopathic Normal Pressure Hydrocephalus. Zh Nevrol Psikhiatr Im S S Korsakova.119(3),50-54 https://doi.org/10.17116/jnevro201911903150

Gaberel T, Gakuba C, Goulay R, Martinez De Lizarrondo S, Hanouz JL, Emery E, Touze E, Vivien D, Gauberti M. 2014.Impaired Glymphatic Perfusion after Strokes Revealed by Contrast-Enhanced Mri: A New Target for Fibrinolysis? Stroke. 45(10),3092-3096 https://doi.org/10.1161/strokeaha.114.006617

Geir Ringstad LMV, Anders M Dale,Are H Pripp,Svein-Are S Vatnehol,Kyrre E Emblem,Kent-Andre Mardal,Per K Eide. 2018.Brain-Wide Glymphatic Enhancement and Clearance in Humans Assessed with Mri. JCI Insight.3(13),M 29997300 https://doi.org/10.1172/jci.insight.121537

George PM, Steinberg GK. 2015.Novel Stroke Therapeutics: Unraveling Stroke Pathophysiology and Its Impact on Clinical Treatments. Neuron.87(2),297-309 https://doi.org/10.1016/j.neuron.2015.05.041

Gijn Jv. 1992.Subarachnoid Haemorrhage. Lancet.339(8794),653-655 https://doi.org /10.1016/0140-6736(92)90803-B

Giridhar Murlidharan AC, Rebecca A Reardon,Juan Song,Aravind Asokan. 2016.Glymphatic Fluid Transport Controls Paravascular Clearance of Aav Vectors from the Brain. JCI Insight.1(14),e88034 https://doi.org/10.1172/jci.insight.88034

Goldman N, Hablitz LM, Mori Y, Nedergaard M. 2020.The Glymphatic System and Pain. Med Acupunct.32(6),373-376 https://doi.org/10.1089/acu.2020.1489

Gratwicke J, Jahanshahi M, Foltynie T. 2015.Parkinson's Disease Dementia: A Neural Networks Perspective. Brain.138(Pt 6),1454-1476 https://doi.org/10.1093/brain/awv104

H B Moeller RAF, T Zeuthen,N Macaulay. 2009.Vasopressin-Dependent Short-Term Regulation of Aquaporin 4 Expressed in Xenopus Oocytes. Neuroscience.164(4),1674-1684 https://doi.org/10.1016/j.neuroscience.2009.09.072

Han F, Brown GL, Zhu Y, Belkin-Rosen AE, Lewis MM, Du G, Gu Y, Eslinger PJ, Mailman RB, Huang X, Liu X. 2021.Decoupling of Global Brain Activity and Cerebrospinal Fluid Flow in Parkinson's Disease Cognitive Decline. Mov Disord.36(9),2066-2076 https://doi.org/10.1002/mds.28643

Hana Park S-HC, Min-Jeong Kong,Tae-Cheon Kang. 2019.Dysfunction of 67-Kda

Laminin Receptor Disrupts Bbb Integrity Via Impaired Dystrophin/Aqp4 Complex and P38 Mapk/Vegf Activation Following Status Epilepticus. Front Cell Neurosci.13,236 https://doi.org/10.3389/fncel.2019.00236

Hanwool Jeon MK, Wonhyoung Park,Joon Seo Lim,Eunyeup Lee,Hyeuk Cha,Jae Sung Ahn,Jeong Hoon Kim,Seok Ho Hong,Ji Eun Park,Eun-Jae Lee,Chul-Woong Woo,Seungjoo Lee. 2021.Upregulation of Aqp4 Improves Blood-Brain Barrier Integrity and Perihematomal Edema Following Intracerebral Hemorrhage. Neurotherapeutics. 18(4),2692-2706 https://doi.org/10.1007/s13311-021-01126-2

Haohai Huang DL, Liping Liang,Lijun Song,Wenchang Zhao. 2015.Genistein Inhibits Rotavirus Replication and Upregulates Aqp4 Expression in Rotavirus-Infected Caco-2 Cells. Arch Virol.160(6),1421-1433 https://doi.org/10.1007/s00705-015-2404-4

Hardman JM. 1979.The Pathology of Traumatic Brain Injuries. Adv Neurol.22,15-50

Hartwig Wolburg KW-B, Petra Fallier-Becker,Susan Noell,Andreas F Mack. 2011.Structure and Functions of Aquaporin-4-Based Orthogonal Arrays of Particles. Int Rev Cell Mol Biol.287,1-41 https://doi.org/10.1016/B978-0-12-386043-9.00001-3

He Wu TW, Xueying Xu,Jessica Wang,Jian Wang. 2011.Iron Toxicity in Mice with Collagenase-Induced Intracerebral Hemorrhage. J Cereb Blood Flow Metab.31(5),1243-1250 https://doi.org/10.1038/jcbfm.2010.209

Henderson MX, Trojanowski JQ, Lee VM. 2019.A-Synuclein Pathology in Parkinson's Disease and Related A-Synucleinopathies. Neurosci Lett.709,134316 https:// doi.org/10.1016/j.neulet.2019.134316

Hofman P, Hoyng P, vanderWerf F, Vrensen GF, Schlingemann RO. 2001.Lack of Blood-Brain Barrier Properties in Microvessels of the Prelaminar Optic Nerve Head. Investigative ophthalmology & visual science.42(No.5),895-901

Hubbard J, Hsu M, Seldin M, Binder D. 2015.Expression of the Astrocyte Water Channel Aquaporin-4 in the Mouse Brain. ASN Neuro.7(No.5) https://doi.org/10.1177/1759091415605486

Hui Tang CS, Jiaquan He. 2017.Down-Regulated Expression of Aquaporin-4 in the Cerebellum after Status Epilepticus. Cogn Neurodyn.11(2),183-188 https://doi.org/10.1007/s11571-016-9420-2

Humberto Mestre LMH, Anna Lr Xavier,Weixi Feng,Wenyan Zou,Tinglin Pu,Hiromu Monai,Giridhar Murlidharan,Ruth M Castellanos Rivera,Matthew J Simon,Martin M Pike,Virginia Plá,Ting Du,Benjamin T Kress,Xiaowen Wang,Benjamin A Plog,Alexander S Thrane,Iben Lundgaard,Yoichiro Abe,Masato Yasui,John H Thomas,Ming Xiao,Hajime Hirase,Aravind Asokan,Jeffrey J Iliff,Maiken Nedergaard. 2018.Aquaporin-4-Dependent Glymphatic Solute Transport in the Rodent Brain. Elife.7,M 30561329 https://doi.org/10.7554/eLife.40070

Iadecola C. 2013.The Pathobiology of Vascular Dementia. Neuron.80(4),844-866 https://doi.org/10.1016/j.neuron.2013.10.008

Iliff JJDoGD, Therapeutics CfTN, Department of Neurosurgery, University of Rochester Medical Center, Rochester, NY, US, iliffj@ohsu.edu, Chen MJDoGD, Therapeutics CfTN, Department of Neurosurgery, University of Rochester Medical Center, Rochester, NY, US, Plog BADoGD, Therapeutics CfTN, Department of Neurosurgery, University of Rochester Medical Center, Rochester, NY, US, Zeppenfeld DMDoA, Peri-Operative Medicine OH, Science University P, OR, US, Soltero MDoA, Peri-Operative Medicine OH, Science University P, OR, US, Yang LDoGD, Therapeutics CfTN, Department of Neurosurgery, University of Rochester Medical Center, Rochester, NY, US, Singh IDoGD, Therapeutics CfTN, Department of Neurosurgery, University of Rochester Medical Center, Rochester, NY, US, Deane RDoGD, Therapeutics CfTN, Department of Neurosurgery, University of Rochester Medical Center, Rochester, NY, US, Nedergaard MDoGD, Therapeutics CfTN, Department of Neurosurgery, University of Rochester Medical Center, Rochester, NY, US. 2014.Impairment of Glymphatic Pathway Function Promotes Tau Pathology after Traumatic Brain Injury. The Journal of Neuroscience.Vol.34(No.49),16180-16193 https://doi.org/10.1523/JNEUROSCI.3020-14.2014

Ionica Pirici TAB, Catalin Bogdan,Claudiu Margaritescu,Tamir Divan,Vacaras Vitalie,Laurentiu Mogoanta,Daniel Pirici,Roxana Octavia Carare,Dafin Fior Muresanu. 2017.Inhibition of Aquaporin-4 Improves the Outcome of Ischaemic Stroke and Modulates Brain Paravascular Drainage Pathways. Int J Mol Sci.19(1),M 29295526 https://doi.org/10.3390/ijms19010046

Iorio RDoLM, Mayo Clinic College of Medicine, Rochester, MN, US, Lucchinetti CFDoN, Mayo Clinic College of Medicine, Rochester, MN, US, Lennon VADoN, Mayo Clinic College of Medicine, Rochester, MN, US, Costanzi CDoN, Mayo Clinic College of Medicine, Rochester, MN, US, Hinson SDoLM, Mayo Clinic College of Medicine, Rochester, MN, US, Weinshenker BGDoN, Mayo Clinic College of Medicine, Rochester, MN, US, Pittock SJDoLM, Mayo Clinic College of Medicine, Rochester, MN, US, pittock.sean@mayo.edu. 2011.Syndrome of Inappropriate Antidiuresis May Herald or Accompany Neuromyelitis Optica. Neurology.Vol.77(No.17),1644-1646   https://doi.org/ 10.1212/WNL.0b013e3182343377

Ishikura T, Kinoshita M, Shimizu M, Yasumizu Y, Motooka D, Okuzaki D, Yamashita K, Murata H, Beppu S, Koda T, Tada S, Shiraishi N, Sugiyama Y, Miyamoto K, Kusunoki S, Sugimoto T, Kumanogoh A, Okuno T, Mochizuki H. 2021.Anti-Aqp4 Autoantibodies Promote Atp Release from Astrocytes and Induce Mechanical Pain in Rats. J Neuroinflammation.18(1),181 https://doi.org/10.1186/s12974-021-02232-w

Izumi Kawachi, Lassmann H. 2017.Neurodegeneration in Multiple Sclerosis and Neuromyelitis Optica. Journal of Neurology, Neurosurgery & Psychiatry. Vol.88(No.2), 137-145 https://doi.org/10.1136/jnnp-2016-313300

J E Rash TY, C S Hudson,P Agre,S Nielsen. 1998.Direct Immunogold Labeling of Aquaporin-4 in Square Arrays of Astrocyte and Ependymocyte Plasma Membranes in Rat Brain and Spinal Cord. Proc Natl Acad Sci U S A.95(20),11981-11986 https://doi.org/10.1073/pnas.95.20.11981

Jeffrey J Iliff HL, Mei Yu,Tian Feng,Jean Logan,Maiken Nedergaard,Helene Benveniste. 2013.Brain-Wide Pathway for Waste Clearance Captured by Contrast-Enhanced Mri. J Clin Invest.123(3),1299-1309 https://doi.org/10.1172/JCI67677

Jeffrey J. Iliff MW, 1,2 Yonghong Liao,1 2012.A Paravascular Pathway Facilitates Csf Flow through the Brain Parenchyma and the Clearance of Interstitial Solutes, Including Amyloid B. CEREBROSPINAL FLUID C I RCULATION.4(No.147), 147ra111 https://doi.org/10.1126/scitranslmed.3003748

Jérôme Badaut AMF, Amandine Jullienne,Klaus G Petry. 2014.Aquaporin and Brain Diseases. Biochim Biophys Acta.1840(5),1554-1565 https://doi.org/10.1016/ j.bbagen. 2013.10.032

Jesse A Stokum DBK, Volodymyr Gerzanich,J Marc Simard. 2015.Mechanisms of Astrocyte-Mediated Cerebral Edema. Neurochem Res.40(2),317-328 https://doi.org/ 10.1007/s11064-014-1374-3

Jessen NA, Munk ASF, Lundgaard I, Nedergaard M. 2015.The Glymphatic System: A Beginner's Guide(Article). Neurochemical Research (No.12),2583-2599 https:// doi. org/10.1007/s11064-015-1581-6

Ji RR, Donnelly CR, Nedergaard M. 2019.Astrocytes in Chronic Pain and Itch. Nat Rev Neurosci.20(11),667-685 https://doi.org/10.1038/s41583-019-0218-1

Jiang C, Wang ZN, Kang YC, Chen Y, Lu WX, Ren HJ, Hou BR. 2022.Ki20227 Aggravates Apoptosis, Inflammatory Response, and Oxidative Stress after Focal Cerebral Ischemia Injury. Neural Regen Res.17(1),137-143 https://doi.org/10.4103/ 1673-5374.314318

Jolobe OM, 2007. Subarachnoid Haemorrhage, Vol 369, 904 p.

Jose A Soria Lopez HMG, Gabriel C Léger. 2019.Alzheimer's Disease. Handb Clin Neurol.167,231-255 https://doi.org/10.1016/B978-0-12-804766-8.00013-3

K Oshio DKB, B Yang,S Schecter,A S Verkman,G T Manley. 2004.Expression of Aquaporin Water Channels in Mouse Spinal Cord. Neuroscience.127(3),685-693 https://doi.org/10.1016/j.neuroscience.2004.03.016

Kang H, Qiu H, Hu X, Wei S, Tao Y. 2022.Differences in Neuropathic Pain and Radiological Features between Aqp4-on, Mog-on, and Idon. Front Pain Res (Lausanne).3,870211 https://doi.org/10.3389/fpain.2022.870211

Kara N Corps TLR, Dorian B McGavern. 2015.Inflammation and Neuroprotection in Traumatic Brain Injury. JAMA Neurol.72(3),355-362 https://doi.org/10.1001/ jamaneurol.2014.3558

Kewei Liu JZ, Yuan Chang,Zhenzhou Lin,Zhu Shi,Xing Li,Xing Chen,Chuman

Lin,Suyue Pan,Kaibin Huang. 2021.Attenuation of Cerebral Edema Facilitates Recovery of Glymphatic System Function after Status Epilepticus. JCI Insight.6(17),M 34494549 https://doi.org/10.1172/jci.insight.151835

Khalil S Husari KL, Rong Huang,Rana R Said. 2020.New-Onset Refractory Status Epilepticus in Children: Etiologies, Treatments, and Outcomes. Pediatr Crit Care Med.21(1),59-66 https://doi.org/10.1097/PCC.0000000000002108

Kjersti N Power AG, Nils Erik Gilhus,Karl Ove Hufthammer,Bernt A Engelsen. 2018.Cognitive Function after Status Epilepticus Versus after Multiple Generalized Tonic-Clonic Seizures. Epilepsy Res.140,39-45 https://doi.org/10.1016/j.eplepsyres. 2017.11.014

Koga M, Takahashi T, Kawai M, Fujihara K, Kanda T. 2011.A Serological Analysis of Viral and Bacterial Infections Associated with Neuromyelitis Optica. Journal of the neurological sciences.Vol.300(No.1-2),19-22 https://doi.org/10.1016/j.jns.2010.10.013

Kotaro Oshio HW, Yaunlin Song,A S Verkman,Geoffrey T Manley. 2005.Reduced Cerebrospinal Fluid Production and Intracranial Pressure in Mice Lacking Choroid Plexus Water Channel Aquaporin-1. FASEB J.19(1),76-78 https://doi.org/10.1096/fj.04-1711fje

Küppers E, Gleiser C, Brito V, Wachter B, Pauly T, Hirt B, Grissmer S. 2008.Aqp4 Expression in Striatal Primary Cultures Is Regulated by Dopamine--Implications for Proliferation of Astrocytes. Eur J Neurosci.28(11),2173-2182 https://doi.org/10.1111/ j.1460-9568.2008.06531.x

Lecordier S, Manrique-Castano D, El Moghrabi Y, ElAli A. 2021.Neurovascular Alterations in Vascular Dementia: Emphasis on Risk Factors. Front Aging Neurosci.13,727590 https://doi.org/10.3389/fnagi.2021.727590

Li TT, Wan Q, Zhang X, Xiao Y, Sun LY, Zhang YR, Liu XN, Yang WC. 2022.Stellate Ganglion Block Reduces Inflammation and Improves Neurological Function in Diabetic Rats During Ischemic Stroke. Neural Regen Res.17(9),1991-1997 https://doi.org/10.4103/1673-5374.335162

Lu G, Pang C, Chen Y, Wu N, Li J. 2020.Aquaporin 4 Is Involved in Chronic Pain but Not Acute Pain. Behav Brain Res.393,112810 https://doi.org/10.1016/j.bbr. 2020.112810

Madoka Nakajima MM, Ikuko Ogino,Chihiro Akiba,Kaito Kawamura,Chihiro Kamohara,Keiko Fusegi,Yoshinao Harada,Takeshi Hara,Hidenori Sugano,Yuichi Tange,Kostadin Karagiozov,Kensaku Kasuga,Takeshi Ikeuchi,Takahiko Tokuda,Hajime Arai. 2018.Preoperative Phosphorylated Tau Concentration in the Cerebrospinal Fluid Can Predict Cognitive Function Three Years after Shunt Surgery in Patients with Idiopathic Normal Pressure Hydrocephalus. J Alzheimers Dis.66(1),319-331 https://doi. org/10.3233/JAD-180557

Mai CL, Tan Z, Xu YN, Zhang JJ, Huang ZH, Wang D, Zhang H, Gui WS, Zhang J, Lin ZJ, Meng YT, Wei X, Jie YT, Grace PM, Wu LJ, Zhou LJ, Liu XG. 2021.Cxcl12-

Mediated Monocyte Transmigration into Brain Perivascular Space Leads to Neuroinflammation and Memory Deficit in Neuropathic Pain. Theranostics.11(3),1059-1078 https://doi.org/10.7150/thno.44364

Manuela de Bellis AC, Maria Grazia Mola,Francesco Pisani,Barbara Barile,Maria Mastrodonato,Shervin Banitalebi,Mahmood Amiry-Moghaddam,Pasqua Abbrescia, Antonio Frigeri,Maria Svelto,Grazia Paola Nicchia. 2021.Orthogonal Arrays of Particle Assembly Are Essential for Normal Aquaporin-4 Expression Level in the Brain. Glia.69(2),473-488 https://doi.org/10.1002/glia.23909

Martin Kaag Rasmussen HM, Maiken Nedergaard. 2018.The Glymphatic Pathway in Neurological Disorders. Lancet Neurol.17(11),1016-1024 https://doi.org/10.1016/S1474-4422 (18)30318-1

Md Mahdi Hasan-Olive RE, Hans-Arne Hansson,Erlend A Nagelhus,Per Kristian Eide. 2019.Loss of Perivascular Aquaporin-4 in Idiopathic Normal Pressure Hydrocephalus. Glia.67(1),91-100 https://doi.org/10.1002/glia.23528

Melanie-Jane Hannocks MEP, Jula Huppert,Tushar Deshpande,N Joan Abbott, Robert G Thorne,Lydia Sorokin. 2018.Molecular Characterization of Perivascular Drainage Pathways in the Murine Brain. J Cereb Blood Flow Metab.38(4),669-686 https://doi.org/10.1177/0271678X17749689

Michael A Williams JM. 2016.Diagnosis and Treatment of Idiopathic Normal Pressure Hydrocephalus. Continuum (Minneap Minn).Vol.22(No.2),579-599 https://doi.org/10.1212/CON.0000000000000305

Michel D Ferrari PJG, Rami Burstein,Tobias Kurth,Cenk Ayata,Andrew Charles, Messoud Ashina,Arn M J M van den Maagdenberg,David W Dodick. 2022.Migraine. Nat Rev Dis Primers.8(1),2 https://doi.org/10.1038/s41572-022-00335-z

Monica Carmosino GP, Grazia Tamma,Roberta Mannucci,Maria Svelto,Giovanna Valenti. 2007.Trafficking and Phosphorylation Dynamics of Aqp4 in Histamine-Treated Human Gastric Cells. Biol Cell.99(1),25-36 https://doi.org/10.1042/BC20060068

Morgan Robinson BYL, Francis T Hane. 2017.Recent Progress in Alzheimer's Disease Research, Part 2: Genetics and Epidemiology. J Alzheimers Dis.57(2),317-330 https://doi.org/10.3233/JAD-161149

Nadia Aalling Jessen ASFM, Iben Lundgaard,Maiken Nedergaard. 2015.The Glymphatic System: A Beginner's Guide. Neurochem Res.40(12),2583-2599 https://doi.org/10.1007/s11064-015-1581-6

O'Brien JT, Thomas A. 2015.Vascular Dementia. Lancet.386(10004),1698-1706 https://doi.org/10.1016/s0140-6736(15)00463-8

Per K Eide GR. 2019.Delayed Clearance of Cerebrospinal Fluid Tracer from Entorhinal Cortex in Idiopathic Normal Pressure Hydrocephalus: A Glymphatic Magnetic Resonance Imaging Study. J Cereb Blood Flow Metab.39(7),1355-1368 https://doi.org/10.1177/0271678X18760974

Pu T, Zou W, Feng W, Zhang Y, Wang L, Wang H, Xiao M. 2019.Persistent Malfunction of Glymphatic and Meningeal Lymphatic Drainage in a Mouse Model of Subarachnoid Hemorrhage. EXPERIMENTAL NEUROBIOLOGY.Vol.28(No.1),104-118 https://doi.org/10.5607/en.2019.28.1.104

Qi Lu JX, Yuan Yuan,Zhanwei Ruan,Yu Zhang,Bo Chai,Lei Li,Shufang Cai,Jian Xiao,Yanqing Wu,Peng Huang,Hongyu Zhang. 2022.Minocycline Improves the Functional Recovery after Traumatic Brain Injury Via Inhibition of Aquaporin-4. Int J Biol Sci.18(1),441-458 https://doi.org/10.7150/ijbs.64187

Qiaoli Ma BVI, Michael Detmar,Steven T Proulx. 2017.Outflow of Cerebrospinal Fluid Is Predominantly through Lymphatic Vessels and Is Reduced in Aged Mice. Nat Commun.8(1),1434 https://doi.org/10.1038/s41467-017-01484-6

R Bonita ST. 1985.Subarachnoid Hemorrhage: Epidemiology, Diagnosis, Management, and Outcome. Stroke.16(4),591-594 https://doi.org/10.1161/01.STR.16.4.591

Richard F Keep YH, Guohua Xi. 2012.Intracerebral Haemorrhage: Mechanisms of Injury and Therapeutic Targets. Lancet Neurol.11(8),720-731 https://doi.org/10.1016/S1474-4422(12)70104-7

S Nielsen EAN, M Amiry-Moghaddam,C Bourque,P Agre,O P Ottersen. 1997.Specialized Membrane Domains for Water Transport in Glial Cells: High-Resolution Immunogold Cytochemistry of Aquaporin-4 in Rat Brain. J Neurosci.17(1),171-180 https://doi.org/10.1523/jneurosci.17-01-00171.1997

Schain AJ, Melo-Carrillo A, Strassman AM, Burstein R. 2017.Cortical Spreading Depression Closes Paravascular Space and Impairs Glymphatic Flow: Implications for Migraine Headache. J Neurosci.37(11),2904-2915 https://doi.org/10.1523/jneurosci.3390-16.2017

Scott-Massey A, Boag MK, Magnier A, Bispo D, Khoo TK, Pountney DL. 2022.Glymphatic System Dysfunction and Sleep Disturbance May Contribute to the Pathogenesis and Progression of Parkinson's Disease. Int J Mol Sci.23(21) https://doi.org/10.3390/ijms232112928

Si X, Guo T, Wang Z, Fang Y, Gu L, Cao L, Yang W, Gao T, Song Z, Tian J, Yin X, Guan X, Zhou C, Wu J, Bai X, Liu X, Zhao G, Zhang M, Pu J, Zhang B. 2022.Neuroimaging Evidence of Glymphatic System Dysfunction in Possible Rem Sleep Behavior Disorder and Parkinson's Disease. NPJ Parkinsons Dis.8(1),54 https://doi.org/10.1038/s41531-022-00316-9

Stephen B Hladky MAB. 2014.Mechanisms of Fluid Movement into, through and out of the Brain: Evaluation of the Evidence. Fluids Barriers CNS.11(1),26 https://doi.org/10.1186/2045-8118-11-26

Sucha P, Hermanova Z, Chmelova M, Kirdajova D, Camacho Garcia S, Marchetti

V, Vorisek I, Tureckova J, Shany E, Jirak D, Anderova M, Vargova L. 2022.The Absence of Aqp4/Trpv4 Complex Substantially Reduces Acute Cytotoxic Edema Following Ischemic Injury. Front Cell Neurosci.16,1054919 https://doi.org/10.3389/fncel. 2022.1054919

Sun C, Lin L, Yin L, Hao X, Tian J, Zhang X, Ren Y, Li C, Yang Y. 2022.Acutely Inhibiting Aqp4 with Tgn-020 Improves Functional Outcome by Attenuating Edema and Peri-Infarct Astrogliosis after Cerebral Ischemia. Front Immunol.13,870029 https://doi. org/10.3389/fimmu.2022.870029

T Haenggi J-MF. 2006.Role of Dystrophin and Utrophin for Assembly and Function of the Dystrophin Glycoprotein Complex in Non-Muscle Tissue. Cell Mol Life Sci.63(14),1614-1631 https://doi.org/10.1007/s00018-005-5461-0

Takano T, Tian GF, Peng W, Lou N, Lovatt D, Hansen AJ, Kasischke KA, Nedergaard M. 2007.Cortical Spreading Depression Causes and Coincides with Tissue Hypoxia. Nat Neurosci.10(6),754-762 https://doi.org/10.1038/nn1902

Taylor JP, Hardy J, Fischbeck KH. 2002.Toxic Proteins in Neurodegenerative Disease. Science.296(5575),1991-1995 https://doi.org/10.1126/science.1067122

Tfelt-Hansen P. 1994.Migraine--Diagnosis and Pathophysiology. Pharmacol Toxicol.75 Suppl 2,72-75 https://doi.org/10.1111/j.1600-0773.1994.tb02003.x

Thomas Misje Mathiisen KPL, Niels Christian Danbolt,Ole Petter Ottersen. 2010.The Perivascular Astroglial Sheath Provides a Complete Covering of the Brain Microvessels: An Electron Microscopic 3d Reconstruction. Glia.58(9),1094-1103

Thomas Walz YF, Andreas Engel. 2009.The Aqp Structure and Functional Implications. Handb Exp Pharmacol (190),31-56

Toh CH, Siow TY. 2021.Glymphatic Dysfunction in Patients with Ischemic Stroke. Front Aging Neurosci.13,756249 https://doi.org/10.3389/fnagi.2021.756249

Ueno M, Chiba Y, Murakami R, Matsumoto K, Fujihara R, Uemura N, Yanase K, Kamada M. 2019.Disturbance of Intracerebral Fluid Clearance and Blood-Brain Barrier in Vascular Cognitive Impairment. Int J Mol Sci.20(10)https://doi.org/10.3390/ijms20102600

Venkat P, Culmone L, Chopp M, Landschoot-Ward J, Wang F, Zacharek A, Chen J. 2020.Hucbc Treatment Improves Cognitive Outcome in Rats with Vascular Dementia. Front Aging Neurosci.12,258 https://doi.org/10.3389/fnagi.2020.00258

Verkman AS, Phuan P-W, Zhang H, Papadopoulos MC, Lam C, Bennett JL, Saadoun S, Tradtrantip L. 2012.Anti–Aquaporin-4 Monoclonal Antibody Blocker Therapy for Neuromyelitis Optica. Annals of Neurology.Vol.71(No.3),314-322 https://doi.org/10. 1002/ana.22657

Vincent J Huber HI, Satoshi Ueki,Ingrid L Kwee,Tsutomu Nakada. 2018.Aquaporin-4 Facilitator Tgn-073 Promotes Interstitial Fluid Circulation within the Blood-Brain Barrier: [17o]H2o Jjvcpe Mri Study. Neuroreport.29(9),697-703 https://doi.org/10.1097/ WNR.0000000000000990

Walter K, 2022. What Is Migraine?, Vol 327, 93 p.

Wang A, Chen L, Tian C, Yin X, Wang X, Zhao Y, Zhang M, Yang L, Ye Z. 2022a.Evaluation of the Glymphatic System with Diffusion Tensor Imaging-Along the Perivascular Space in Cancer Pain. Front Neurosci.16,823701 https://doi.org/10.3389 /fnins.2022.823701

Wang R, Zhang X, Zhang J, Fan Y, Shen Y, Hu W, Chen Z. 2012.Oxygen-Glucose Deprivation Induced Glial Scar-Like Change in Astrocytes. PLoS One.7(5),e37574 https://doi.org/10.1371/journal.pone.0037574

Wang Y, Huang C, Guo Q, Chu H. 2022b.Aquaporin-4 and Cognitive Disorders. Aging Dis.13(1),61-72 https://doi.org/10.14336/ad.2021.0731

Wang Y, Huang J, Ma Y, Tang G, Liu Y, Chen X, Zhang Z, Zeng L, Wang Y, Ouyang YB, Yang GY. 2015.Microrna-29b Is a Therapeutic Target in Cerebral Ischemia Associated with Aquaporin 4. J Cereb Blood Flow Metab.35(12),1977-1984 https://doi.org/10.1038/jcbfm.2015.156

Wang YJ, Sun YR, Pei YH, Ma HW, Mu YK, Qin LH, Yan JH. 2023.The Lymphatic Drainage Systems in the Brain: A Novel Target for Ischemic Stroke? Neural Regen Res.18(3),485-491 https://doi.org/10.4103/1673-5374.346484

William Qubty IP. 2020.Migraine Pathophysiology. Pediatr Neurol.107,1-6 https:// doi.org/10.1016/j.pediatrneurol.2019.12.014

Xiaoling Zhang XM, Yanxia Li,Weiheng Yan,Quan Zheng,Lili Li,Yulan Yan,Xiaozhi Liu,Jun Zheng. 2020.Dexamethasone Upregulates the Expression of Aquaporin4 by Increasing Sumoylation in A549 Cells. Inflammation.43(5),1925-1935 https://doi.org/ 10.1007/s10753-020-01267-0

Xichang Liu GW, Na Tang,Li Li,Cuimin Liu,Feng Wang,Shaofa Ke. 2021.Glymphatic Drainage Blocking Aggravates Brain Edema, Neuroinflammation Via Modulating Tnf-A, Il-10, and Aqp4 after Intracerebral Hemorrhage in Rats. Front Cell Neurosci.15,784154 https://doi.org/10.3389/fncel.2021.784154

Xu M, Bennett DLH, Querol LA, Wu LJ, Irani SR, Watson JC, Pittock SJ, Klein CJ. 2020.Pain and the Immune System: Emerging Concepts of Igg-Mediated Autoimmune Pain and Immunotherapies. J Neurol Neurosurg Psychiatry.91(2),177-188 https://doi.org/10.1136/jnnp-2018-318556

Yu-Long Lan J-JC, Gang Hu,Jun Xu,Ming Xiao,Shao Li. 2017.Aquaporin 4 in Astrocytes Is a Target for Therapy in Alzheimer's Disease. Curr Pharm Des.23(33),4948-4957 https://doi.org/10.2174/1381612823666170714144844

Yu P, Venkat P, Chopp M, Zacharek A, Shen Y, Ning R, Liang L, Li W, Zhang L, Landschoot-Ward J, Jiang R, Chen J. 2019.Role of Microrna-126 in Vascular Cognitive Impairment in Mice. J Cereb Blood Flow Metab.39(12),2497-2511 https://doi.org/ 10.1177/0271678x18800593

Zbesko JC, Nguyen TV, Yang T, Frye JB, Hussain O, Hayes M, Chung A, Day WA, Stepanovic K, Krumberger M, Mona J, Longo FM, Doyle KP. 2018.Glial Scars Are Permeable to the Neurotoxic Environment of Chronic Stroke Infarcts. Neurobiol Dis.112,63-78 https://doi.org/10.1016/j.nbd.2018.01.007

Zelenina M. 2010.Regulation of Brain Aquaporins. Neurochem Int.57(4),468-488 https://doi.org/10.1016/j.neuint.2010.03.022

Zeppenfeld DMB, Simon MB, Haswell JDB, DAbreo D, Murchison CM, Quinn JFM, Grafe MRM, PhD, Woltjer RLM, PhD, Kaye JM, Iliff JJP. 2017.Association of Perivascular Localization of Aquaporin-4 with Cognition and Alzheimer Disease in Aging Brains. JAMA Neurology.Vol.74(No.1),91-99 https://doi.org/10.1001/jamaneurol. 2016.4370

Zhang J, Yang B, Sun H, Zhou Y, Liu M, Ding J, Fang F, Fan Y, Hu G. 2016.Aquaporin-4 Deficiency Diminishes the Differential Degeneration of Midbrain Dopaminergic Neurons in Experimental Parkinson's Disease. Neurosci Lett.614,7-15 https://doi.org/10.1016/j.neulet.2015.12.057

Zhang X, Levy D, Noseda R, Kainz V, Jakubowski M, Burstein R. 2010.Activation of Meningeal Nociceptors by Cortical Spreading Depression: Implications for Migraine with Aura. J Neurosci.30(26),8807-8814 https://doi.org/10.1523/JNEUROSCI.0511-10.2010

Zhong-Fang Shi QF, Ye Chen,Li-Xin Xu,Min Wu,Mei Jia,Yi Lu,Xiao-Xuan Wang,Yu-Jiao Wang,Xu Yan,Li-Ping Dong,Fang Yuan. 2021.Methylene Blue Ameliorates Brain Edema in Rats with Experimental Ischemic Stroke Via Inhibiting Aquaporin 4 Expression. Acta Pharmacol Sin.42(3),382-392 https://doi.org/10.1038/s41401-020-0468-5

DECLARATION: This chapter was authored by Chuntian Liang, Lirong Liu, Shuangjin Bao, Zhenjia Yao, Qinqin Bai, Pengcheng Fu, Xiangyu Liu, John H Zhang and Gaiqing Wang published as "Neuroprotection by Nrf2 via modulating microglial phenotype and phagocytosis after intracerebral hemorrhage" in "Heliyon", 2023; 9(2): e13777

CHAPTER 13:

Hematoma scavenging in intracerebral hemorrhage: From mechanisms to the clinic

ABSTRACT:

The products of erythrocyte lyses, haemoglobin (Hb) and haem, are recognized as neurotoxins and the main contributors to delayed cerebral oedema and tissue damage after intracerebral haemorrhage (ICH). Finding a means to efficiently promote absorption of the haemolytic products (Hb and haem) around the bleeding area in the brain through stimulating the function of the body's own garbage cleaning system is a novel clinical challenge and critical for functional recovery after ICH. In this review, available information of the brain injury mechanisms underlying ICH and endogenous haematoma scavenging system is provided. Meanwhile, potential intervention strategies are discussed. Intracerebral blood itself has 'toxic' effects beyond its volume effect after ICH. Haptoglobin–Hb–CD163 as well as haemopexin–haem–LRP1 is believed to be the most important endogenous scavenging pathway which participates in blood components resolution following ICH. PPARγ–Nrf2 activates the aforementioned clearance pathway and then accelerates haematoma clearance. Meanwhile, the scavenger receptors as novel targets for therapeutic interventions to treat ICH are also highlighted.

KEY WORDS: Haematoma resolution; Haematoma scavenge; Scavenger receptors; Intracerebral haemorrhage; Neural recovery

Introduction

Extravasated blood and subsequent intrahaematoma haemolytic products trigger a series of adverse events after intracerebral haemorrhage (ICH), leading to secondary brain injury, oedema and severe neurological deficits or death. Haematomas are the primary cause of neurological deficits associated with ICH. Although the haematoma in human's brain gradually resolves within months, full restoration of neurological function can be slow and often incomplete, leaving survivors with devastating neurological deficits. Unless haematoma is cleared, the reservoirs of blood continue to inflict injury to neurovascular structures and blunt the brain repair processes [1]. However, only a few evidence-based targeted treatments are used for ICH management, and interventions focus primarily on supportive care and comorbidity prevention. Effective haematoma clearance and/or facilitating haematoma absorption result in the removal of all the toxic components, which is a goal and a novel therapeutic strategy for ICH, as haematoma removal/resolution can relieve mechanical compression, limit inflammatory injury and promote the recovery of neuronal function [2–4].

Endogenous garbage cleaning system also known as scavenger receptors plays important roles in the regulation of haematoma resolution in ICH [5]. This review seeks to understand how the endogenous garbage cleaning system or scavenger receptor system in the brain works together to remove blood from the brain and reduce brain damage, then find a medical measure to speed up this process.

Current understanding of the mechanisms underlying ICH-induced brain injury

Brain injury due to ICH initially occurs within the first few hours as a result of mass effect due to haematoma formation. But many patients continue to deteriorate clinically despite no signs of rehaemorrhage or haematoma expansion. This continued insult after primary haemorrhage is believed to be mediated by direct toxicity and inflammatory responses induced by the components and metabolic products of late-stage haematomas and aggravates neurological deficits [6]. In other words, intracerebral blood itself has 'toxic' effects beyond its mass effect [7]. Oxidative stress caused by components of the lysed erythrocytes contributes to the brain injury after ICH [8]. Hb, haem and iron released after red blood cell lysis aggravate ICH-induced severe brain oedema and direct neuronal damage (Fig. 1). To offset this process, phagocytic cells, including the brain's microglia and haematogenous macrophages, phagocytose and then remove extravasated erythrocytes before lysis and subsequent toxicity occurs [3]. So the better understanding of phagocytosis through corresponding scavenger receptors is beneficial to explore removal of blood from the

ICH-affected brain, thus limiting/preventing haemolysis from occurring [5]. The potential endogenous scavenger receptors following ICH were illustrated in Figure 2.

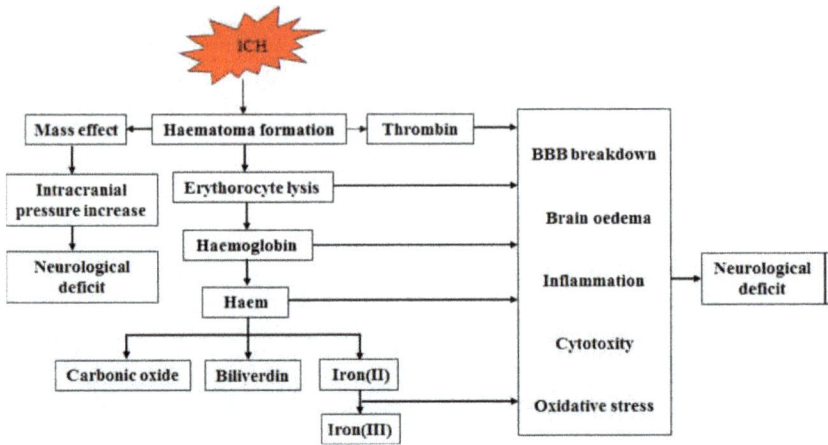

Fig. 1 The major factors contributing to brain injury after ICH (including mass effect, thrombin and blood components).

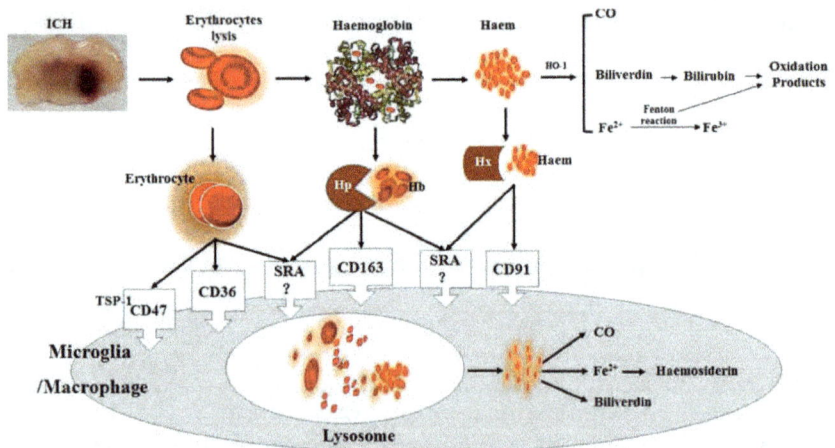

Fig. 2 The potential endogenous scavenger receptors (such as CD36, CD47, SRA, Hp–Hb–CD163 and Hx–haem–CD91) following ICH.

Phagocytosis in haematoma resolution

Microglia/macrophages (MMΦ) represent the primary phagocytic system and the first line of defence against brain injuries that mediates the clean-up of haematoma. Thus, the efficacy of phagocytic function by microglia/MMΦ is an essential step in limiting ICH mediated damage [1]. The resident microglia and peripheral macrophages are rapidly mobilized to the lesions and initiate the release of mediators and recruitment of other immune cells [9].

Microglia is a key factor to remove the haematoma and clear debris, but it is a source of ongoing inflammation. Activated microglia/MMΦ may play a potentially detrimental neurotoxic role by eliciting the expression of pro-inflammatory and initiating neuroprotective properties. Although overactivation of microglia/MMΦ amplifies inflammatory neuronal damage, anti-inflammatory agents have failed to show clinical benefits in many stroke trials so far. The undesired effects may result from a broad suppression of microglia/MMΦ which deprive the normal defensive functions of brain.

It is worth noting that acute inflammation serves many protective functions, whereas chronic inflammation is more likely to exacerbate injury. So experimental stroke therapies should be shifted from blanketed microglia/MMΦ suppression towards a more nuanced adjustment of the balance between protective and toxic microglia/MMΦ phenotypes [10]. Phagocyte activation inevitably release pro-inflammatory mediators and free radicals during haematoma resolution which is toxic to neighbouring cells, leading to secondary brain injury, but promotion of phagocytosis in a timely and efficient manner which may limit the toxic effects of persistent blood products on surrounding tissue and this manner may be important for recovery after ICH [2]. The process of the haematoma resolution probably be related to the concomitant acute brain swelling. Recent studies found that enhancing microglia/MMΦ-mediated phagocytosis speeds up haematoma clearance and then improves functional outcome after ICH [1]. Scavenger receptors, expressed on microglia/astrocytes or endothelial cells, play important roles in the regulation of phagocytosis in microglia/MMΦ.

Potential endogenous haematoma scavenger receptors after ICH

As shown in Figure 2, potential endogenous scavenger receptors, as a major subset of innate pattern recognition receptors, are mainly functioned in endocytosis and exogenous invaders [11]. They play a crucial role in maintenance of cerebral homeostasis and phagocytic regulation. This section summarizes the newly recognized functions of scavenger receptors in haematoma clearance following ICH.

CD36

CD36 is a well-recognized integral microglia/macrophage cell membrane protein and a type II scavenger receptor which is expressed on the surface of macrophages and monocytes and plays an important role in mediating the recognition and phagocytosis. Cells lacking phagocytic abilities acquire phagocytic functions following transfection with CD36 [12]. The low levels of CD36 present may control adhesion of erythrocytes and may have a signal transduction role in platelets and monocytes. CD36 and thrombospondin (TSP) appear to be involved in several cell adhesion processes, including thrombin-induced platelet aggregation, adhesion of platelets to monocytes and so on [13].

CD47

CD47 is an integrin-associated transmembrane protein expressed in a variety of cells types including microglia/ MMΦ, oligodendrocytes and erythrocytes. CD47, a well-known 'don't eat me' signal, controls erythrocyte lifespan positively through inhibition of phagocytosis via signal regulatory protein (SIRPa) on normal/healthy erythrocytes, and it revealed an important role in the clearance of aged erythrocytes[14]. CD47 on erythrocytes and other cells can function as a regulator of target cell phagocytosis [15]. As a switch for erythrophagocytosis, CD47 undergoes a conformational change during ageing, which causes thrombospondin (TSP-1) binding and recognition of CD47 as an 'eat me' signal by SIRPa. The conformational status of CD47 can be changed through oxidative stress, and binding of TSP-1 to apoptotic cells enhanced phagocytosis without inducing the secretion of pro-inflammatory cytokines [14]. CD47 expression was increased in the perihaematomal white and grey matter after ICH, and deferoxamine treatment attenuated brain CD47 expression after ICH [16]. Higher microglial activation at day 3 after experimental ICH was found after CD47 knockout blood injection, and CD47 has a key role in haematoma clearance after ICH [17]. The present results of CD47 in ICH are confusing and are contradictory to its phagocytic property in pathological conditions, and the exact role of CD47 in erythrocyte clearance after ICH still needs to be further study.

SRA

Scavenger receptor A (SRA), also known as the macrophage scavenger receptor and cluster of differentiation 204 (CD204), plays roles in lipid metabolism, atherogenesis and a number of metabolic processes. SRA is reported to be host protective in some disease states, but there is also compelling evidence that SRA plays a role in the pathophysiology of other diseases [18, 19]. On the one hand, SRA is clearly beneficial and host protective in some models of disease. SRA on microglial cells mediates the binding of b amyloid fibrils and is responsible for preventing the accumulation of amyloid in the brain. The decrease in SRA activity could contribute to the progression of neurodegeneration [20]. SRA was highly expressed in erythrocyte lysate-treated microglia. Genetic SRA ablation increased microglia activation and cytokine production, and sensitized mice to ICH-induced neuron injury [21]. SRA down-regulated inflammatory response expression in microglia by suppressing TLR4-induced activation [22]. SRA mediates activation of inflammatory signaling and apoptosis in ischaemic stroke, both of which contribute to cerebral injury. The published data have given rise to an intriguing dilemma. As well as the other markers of microglia/MMΦ activation, SRA is a two-edged sword in health and disease [18,19]. Oxidized erythrocytes were internalized via SRA on macrophages and then sent to lysosomes for scavenging. The exact role of SRA in ICH is dramatic and unclear, as a scavenger receptor, and it should participate in haematoma resolution through microglia activation and maybe produce undesirable inflammatory response, but the results of SRA in ICH are confusing [21, 22].

Hp–Hb–CD163

CD163 is a phagocytic marker and a haemoglobin scavenger receptor, of which expression is thought to be exclusive to perivascular (PVM) and monocyte—macrophage system. It is a glycoprotein belonging to class B of the scavenger receptor cysteine-rich superfamily. It functions as a membrane-bound scavenger receptor for clearing extracellular haptoglobin–haemoglobin (Hp-Hb) complexes [23]. Both in vitro and in vivo investigations have shown that ROS is highly produced after exposing Hb to cell culture or injecting Hb into mouse striatum [24, 25]. Haptoglobin (Hp) is the primary Hb-binding protein in human plasma, which attenuates the adverse biochemical and physiological effects of extracellular Hb. The cellular receptor target of Hp is the monocyte/MMΦ scavenger receptor, CD163. Excessive Hb up-regulated expression of Hp and the Hb–Hp receptor CD163 in neurons in vivo and in vitro [26]. Free Hb binds to Hp and once Hp-Hb complex is endocytosed by CD163, which mediated delivery of Hb to the macrophage may fuel an anti-inflammatory response because haem metabolites have potent anti-inflammatory effects [27].

Hx–Haem–LRP1

With chronic haemolysis following ICH, Hp is depleted and Hb readily distributes to tissues where it might be exposed to oxidative conditions. In such conditions, haem can be released from ferric Hb. The free haem is highly toxic which can accelerate tissue damage by promoting peroxidative reactions and activation of inflammatory cascades [28]. The haem scavenger protein–haemopexin (Hx) contributes to haematoma removal as well as Hp-Hb after ICH [29], and Hx is another plasma glycoprotein able to bind haem with high affinity. Hx sequesters haem in an inert, non-toxic form and transports it to the liver for catabolism and excretion [30]. Hp and Hx have been characterized as a sequential defence system with Hp as the primary protector and Hx as a backup when Hp has been depleted during severe ICH. The linear relationship between Hx concentration and protection defined a highly efficient backup scavenger system during conditions of large excess of free Hb [31]. The haem–Hx complex is endocytosed by cells expressing the low-density lipoprotein receptor related protein-1 (LRP1)/CD91 receptor [32, 33]. LRP1 is a transmembrane receptor expressed on several cell types including macrophages, hepatocytes, neurons, vascular endothelial cells, pericytes, smooth muscle cells and astrocytes. Half of the BBB clearance is mediated by brain endothelial LRP1 in various model systems [34]. As the only known endocytic receptor for Hx–haem complexes, LRP1 combined function of Hx may mediate localized haem clearance in the brain during cerebral haemorrhage. Upon binding of haem–Hx to LRP1, the complex becomes internalized via endocytosis into cells, and inside the cell, the haem–Hx complex is dissociated by lysosomal activity. Haem is catabolized by haem oxygenases into biliverdin, carbon monoxide and iron. Activation of LRP1 scavenging system in humans has favourable effects after subarachnoid haemorrhage (SAH) [35]. Recently, it is confirmed that the activation of the LRP1 system is beneficial in experimental ICH [33]. It should be proved in clinic through above-mentioned findings.

The upstream regulatory mechanism and intervention strategy for scavenger receptors after ICH

Nuclear factor erythroid 2-related factor 2 (Nrf2)

Nrf2 itself is a ubiquitous pleiotropic transcription factor and a pivotal mediator in redox homeostasis and inflammatory disorders, within the regulated region of many cytoprotective and antioxidant target genes which encode for critical mediators of cellular defence functions [36]. In unstressed conditions, Nrf2 is retained in the cytoplasm by its inhibitor kelch-like ECH-associated protein 1 (Keap1), upon activation by oxidative and electrophilic stress, and Nrf2 disassociates from Keap1, transactivates the antioxidant response element (ARE) and then promotes the related cytoprotective pathways. So Nrf2 is a key regulator of cellular resistance against oxidants [37]. In addition, the transcriptional activity of Nrf2 is essential for the clearance of phosphorylated tau via the selective autophagy [38]. Also, knockout of Nrf2 reduced the efficiency of macrophage accumulation and impaired clearance of myelin debris and phosphorylated tau [39]. Nrf2 controls the expression of CD36, which may represent a key component in attaining brain clean-up after stroke or ICH. Removal of RBC by microglia and/or MMΦ may have a multiple indirect effect on oxidative stress, as it could reduce the accumulation of haemoglobin–haem–free iron and consequently the formation of free radicals. Furthermore, activated Nrf2 up-regulated the levels of Hp in blood plasma and in ICH-affected brain in animals as well as the expression of CD163 [40]. In conclusion, Nrf2 in microglia/ MMΦ plays a pivotal role in regulating the phagocytic functions of these cells, and that in an experimental model of ICH, Nrf2 appears to be essential to haematoma clearance [1]. The potential role of Nrf2 following ICH is illustrated in Figure 3.

Peroxisome proliferator-activated receptor-γ (PPAR-γ)

The peroxisome proliferator-activated receptor-c (PPAR-γ) is a ligand-activated transcription factor belonging to the nuclear hormone receptor superfamily and controlling reproduction, metabolism, development and immune response. PPAR-γ expressed not only in adipocytes, but also in vascular tissues, such as vascular smooth muscle cells (VSMCs) and endothelial cells, and in macrophages [41]. PPAR-γ and its agonists have a protective role in several neurological diseases via reducing inflammation, decreasing oxidative damage and attenuating cell death [42]. PPAR-γ is protective not only to neurons, astrocytes, oligodendrocytes, endothelia, but also to microglia/MMΦ both in vitro and in vivo. PPAR-γ agonists reduce the ability of inflammatory stimuli to activate the alveolar macrophage while simultaneously stimulating phagocytosis of both opsonized and unopsonized particles, via the Fc-γ and CD36 receptors, respectively [43]. PPAR-γ ligands have also been shown to up-regulate the

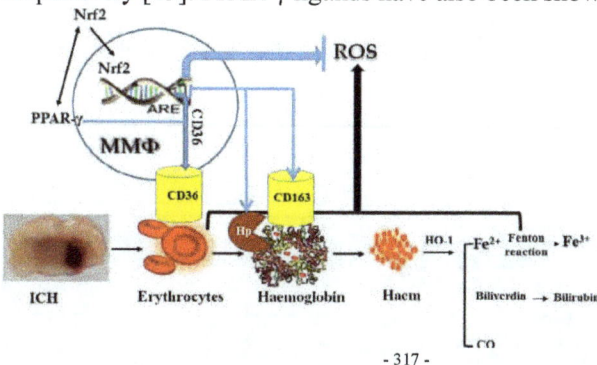

Fig.3
The potential role of Nrf2 and the interaction of PPAR-γ with Nrf2 following ICH.

expression of

CD36 and then promote microglia/MMΦ-mediated clearance of toxic cellular debris [44]. PPAR-γ agonists not only increased microglia-mediated phagocytosis of RBC, but also reduced the production of H2O2 during the process of engulfment [2, 44]. So enhancement of phagocytosis by PPAR-γ agonists inevitably results in the inflammatory response and the dose-dependent neurotoxicity.

Some studies showed PPAR-γ had an interaction with Nrf2. Endogenous PPAR-γ ligands activate Nrf2 expression, meanwhile Nrf2 regulated PPAR-γ expression [45]. Nrf2 controls CD36 expression independently of PPAR-γ. Expression of Nrf2 was reduced by knockdown of PPAR-γ, whereas PPAR-γ was reduced by knockdown of Nrf2, thereby demonstrating two-way positive interactions. PPARγ agonists up-regulate Nrf2, and knockdown of PPAR-γ reduced the mRNA expression for Nrf2 [46]. This indicates a tight, positive, two way reinforcing transcriptional interaction between PPAR-γ and Nrf2 that may improve endothelial function [46]. The interaction of PPARγ with Nrf2 following ICH was illustrated in Figure 3. exogenous pharmacological/molecular manipulations direct at haematoma resolution after ICH (as illustrated in Fig. 4).

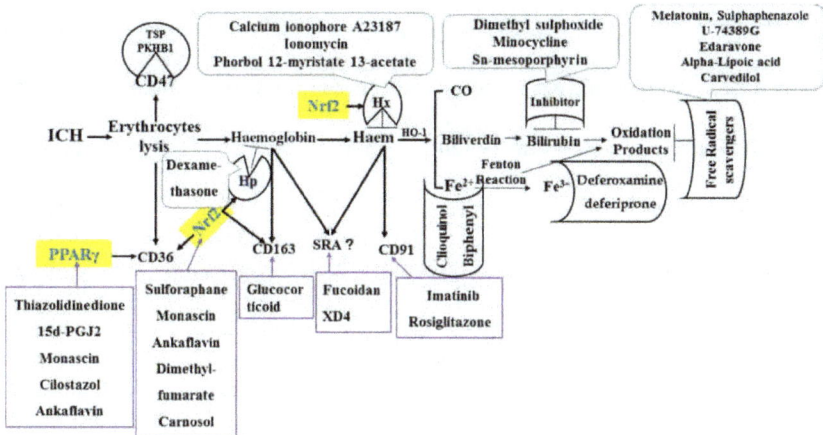

Fig.4 Summary of current potential exogenous pharmacological/molecular manipulations direct at haematoma resolution after ICH.

Potential treatment options/strategies for haematoma resolution via CD36

PPAR-γ agonists

PPAR-γ agonist-induced up-regulation of CD36 in macrophages enhances the ability of microglia to phagocytose red blood cells (in vitro assay), helps to improve haematoma resolution and reduces a mouse ICH-induced deficit. In rat primary microglia in culture, PPAR-γ agonists not only increased microglia-mediated phagocytosis of RBC, but also reduced the production of H2O2 during the process of engulfment [2]. PPAR-γ agonists could represent a potential treatment strategy for ICH [3].

Thiazolidinediones are potent and selective activators of PPAR-γ [47]. The derivatives of the parent compound thiazolidinedione such as rosiglitazone and pioglitazone are generally well tolerated in AD and aMCI patients [48]. The Safety of Pioglitazone for Hematoma Resolution In ICH (SHRINC)

Study [49], a prospective, randomized, blinded, placebo-controlled, dose-escalation safety trial, was recently completed, and its results showed that pioglitazone should be a potential therapy for ICH in future. The cyclopentanone prostaglandins (e.g. 15d–PGJ2) and monascin as well as thiazolidinediones are PPAR-γ agonists, which have been proven to act as potent and safe pro-survival factors for primary neurons subjected to either excitotoxic insult, oxygen–glucose deprivation (OGD) or H2O2-induced oxidative stress [44, 47, 50] and then attenuate ROS generation. These PPAR-c agonists are proposed to act as endogenous PPAR-γ ligands demonstrate rather limited selectivity towards PPAR-γ with some of its biological activation of Nrf2. Monascin regulated PPAR-γ and Nrf-2 to improve lung oxidative inflammation [51].

Cilostazol, a potent phosphodiesterase type III inhibitor, has been used as a vasodilating antiplatelet drug for the treatment of ischaemic symptoms in chronic peripheral arterial obstruction for preventing recurrence of cerebral infarction [52]. Cilostazol stimulates PPAR-γ transcriptional activity in human endothelial cells and may offer an effective therapeutic window along with complementary effects for individuals at high risk of type 2 diabetes by improving insulin sensitivity with anti-inflammatory effects [53]. Ankaflavin exerted PPAR-γ agonist activity by the up-regulation of the signalling pathway of Nrf2 [54].

The existing evidence showed that dose-dependent neurotoxicity of the

15d–PGJ2 in cerebellar granule cells, primary cortical neurons and spinal cord motor neurons which were believed to be associated with induction of apoptosis and not likely associated with the activation of PPAR-γ [55]. On the other hand, the clinically relevant, more selective PPAR-γ agonist, such as rosiglitazone, was linked to peripheral oedema, increase in body weight, and cardiomyopathies and heart failure [56]. It is likely that PPAR-γ agonist treatment for ICH will be short term, potentially avoiding these side-effects, although this needs further testing.

Nrf2 agonists

Nrf2 as a second important transcription factor involved in the induction of the scavenger receptor CD36 and antioxidant stress genes in atherosclerosis [57]. Nrf2 transcription factor could be an alternative target to PPAR-γ in the control of severe malaria through parasite clearance [58]. Nrf2 plays an essential role in the effective clean-up process after ICH, perhaps via co-ordinated efforts to enhance phagocytosis while concomitantly limiting oxidative stress[1]. Sulforaphane was capable of enhancing RBC phagocytosis and improving haematoma resolution via activating Nrf2 and inducing CD36 expression in microglias[1]. Monascin acts as a novel natural Nrf2 activator with PPAR-γ agonist activity was confirmed by Nrf2 and PPAR-γ reporter assays [59]. Protective effects of ankaflavin against diabetes are mediated by the upregulation of the signalling pathway of Nrf2, which enhances antioxidant activity and serves as a PPAR-c agonist to enhance insulin sensitivity [54]. Monascin and ankaflavin, the yellow pigments produced by Monascus species, have been proven to possess hypolipidaemic functions and less side-effects [60]. Dimethyl fumarate is an orally administered fumarate ester recently FDA approved for first-line monotherapy of multiple sclerosis, which stimulates Nrf2 activity to attenuate hyperphosphataemia in vitro or vitamin D3-induced in vivo vascular calcification [61]. Carnosol increased the nuclear levels of Nrf2 and involved in the cytoprotective effects [62].

The agonists for the other scavenger receptors

CD163 agonists

To date, the Hb–haptoglobin (Hp) complex is the only known ligand of CD163, and neither Hp alone nor free Hb has been found to display high-affinity binding to the receptor. Because the Hb–Hp complex binds to CD163 with high affinity and the receptor system has a high endocytotic capacity, CD163 is thought to mediate the clearance of Hb–Hp complexes from the blood [27]. Glucocorticoid can induce CD163 expression in MMΦ which enhances their capacity to bind and internalize Hb–Hp complexes [63].

Haptoglobin (Hp) and haemopexin (Hx) agonists

Hp expression is induced by inflammatory cytokines, dexamethasone and adrenoceptor agonists. In contrast, Hp was inhibited by nicotinic acid and the PPARc agonist, rosiglitazone [64]. The transcription rate of Hx increased by the calcium ionophore A23187, ionomycin and phorbol 12-myristate 13-acetate (PMA) in serum-starved H4IIE rat hepatoma cells [65]. Activated Nrf2 binds to antioxidant response elements (ARE), which promotes the transcription of haptoglobin and haemopexin [66].

LRP1 agonists

LRP1/CD91 contributed to haem clearance and blood–brain barrier protection after ICH in mice. Our research showed that recombinant LRP1 as supplement provides a novel approach to ameliorate intracerebral haemorrhage brain injury via its pleiotropic neuroprotective effects [33]. Intrathecal infusions of LRP1 agonists—RBD (the Receptor Binding Domain of alpha-2-macroglobulin) or PEX (the haemopexin domain of MMP-9) result in axonal sprouting and regeneration after spinal cord injury via activating ERK and Akt pathways [67]. Imatinib promotes LRP1-dependent ERK activation and helps to the pro-survival effects on b-cells [68].

SRA agonists

Fucoidan, a SRA agonist, could promote macrophage apoptosis by repressing ER stressor triggered autophagy [69]. Heptapeptide XD4 activates SRA on the glia by increasing the binding of Ab to SRA, thereby promoting glial phagocytosis of Ab oligomer in microglia and astrocytes [70].

CD47 agonists

CD47 stimulated by its ligands, thrombospondins (TSPs), the agonist sequences occur in all five isoforms of TSP, it is possible that any TSP isoform could be pro-apoptotic [71]. PKHB1, the serum-stable CD47 agonist peptide, might overcome drug refractoriness of chronic lymphocytic leukaemia by the pro-apoptotic potential of targeting cell [72].

Iron chelators

Our study showed that ferric iron chelators such as deferoxamine and deferiprone lowered iron deposition in brain following ICH [73]. However, ferric iron chelation does not improve the outcome after ICH [33, 74]. Clioquinol, a ferrous iron chelator, improved the neurological outcome and attenuated brain oedema and ROS production besides reducing iron levels [73]. Another ferrous chelator, 2,20-bipyridine, is a potential means of ameliorating iron-induced injury after ICH [75]; unfortunately, another results failed to support the use of bipyridine against ICH [76], and the function of bipyridine on ICH is uncertain so far.

Conclusion

Hp–Hb–CD163 as well as Hx–haem–LRP1 is believed to be the most important endogenous garbage scavenging pathway which participates in haematoma/ blood components resolution following ICH.

PPARγ–Nrf2 activates the aforementioned clearance pathway and then accelerates haematoma removal. So the above-mentioned haematoma scavenger pathway as a novel targets for therapeutic interventions to treat

ICH is prospective and valuable.

Acknowledgements

Funding source: This work was supported by a project from National Natural Science Foundation of China (Project number: 81771294).

Conflict of interest

The authors confirm that there is no conflict of interests.

References

1. Zhao X, Sun G, Ting SM, et al. Cleaning up after ICH: the role of Nrf2 in modulating microglia function and hematoma clearance. J Neurochem. 2015; 133: 144–52.

2. Zhao X, Sun G, Zhang J, et al. Hematoma resolution as a target for intracerebral hemorrhage treatment: role for peroxisome proliferator-activated receptor gamma in microglia/macrophages. Ann Neurol. 2007;61: 352–62.

3. Zhao X, Grotta J, Gonzales N, et al. Hematoma resolution as a therapeutic target: the role of microglia/macrophages. Stroke. 2009; 40: S92–4.

4. Fang H, Wang PF, Zhou Y, et al. Toll-like receptor 4 signaling in intracerebral hemorrhage-induced inflammation and injury. J Neuroinflammation. 2013; 10: 27.

5. Husemann J, Loike JD, Anankov R, et al. Scavenger receptors in neurobiology and neuropathology: their role on microglia and other cells of the nervous system. Glia.2002; 40: 195–205.

6. Keep RF, Hua Y, Xi G. Intracerebral haemorrhage: mechanisms of injury and therapeutic targets. Lancet Neurol. 2012; 11: 720–31.

7. Xi G, Wagner KR, Keep RF, et al. Role of blood clot formation on early edema development after experimental intracerebral hemorrhage. Stroke. 1998; 29: 2580–6.

8. Wu J, Hua Y, Keep RF, et al. Oxidative brain injury from extravasated erythrocytes after intracerebral hemorrhage. Brain Res. 2002; 953: 45–52.

9. Schilling M, Besselmann M, Muller M, et al. Predominant phagocytic activity of resident microglia over hematogenous macrophages following transient focal cerebral ischemia: an investigation using green fluorescent protein transgenic bone marrow chimeric mice. Exp Neurol. 2005; 196: 290–7.

10. Hu X, Li P, Guo Y, et al. Microglia/macrophage polarization dynamics reveal novel mechanism of injury expansion after focal cerebral ischemia. Stroke. 2012; 43: 3063–70.

11. Yu X, Guo C, Fisher PB, et al. Scavenger receptors: emerging roles in cancer

biology
and immunology. Adv Cancer Res. 2015; 128: 309–64.

12. Cao D, Luo J, Chen D, et al. CD36 regulates lipopolysaccharide-induced signaling pathways and mediates the internalization of Escherichia coli in cooperation with TLR4 in goat mammary gland epithelial cells. Sci Rep. 2016; 6: 23132.

13. van Schravendijk MR, Handunnetti SM, Barnwell JW, et al. Normal human erythrocytes express CD36, an adhesion molecule of monocytes, platelets, and endothelial cells. Blood. 1992; 80: 2105–14.

14. Burger P, de Korte D, van den Berg TK, et al. CD47 in Erythrocyte Ageing and Clearance – the Dutch Point of View. Transfus Med Hemother. 2012; 39: 348–52.

15. Olsson M, Nilsson A, Oldenborg PA. Target cell CD47 regulates macrophage activation and erythrophagocytosis. Transfus Clin Biol. 2006; 13: 39–43.

16. Zhou X, Xie Q, Xi G, et al. Brain CD47 expression in a swine model of intracerebral hemorrhage. Brain Res. 2014; 1574: 70–6.

17. Ni W, Mao S, Xi G, et al. Role of erythrocyte CD47 in intracerebral hematoma clearance. Stroke. 2016; 47: 505–11.

18. Platt N, Gordon S. Is the class A macrophage scavenger receptor (SR-A) multifunctional? - The mouse's tale. J Clin Invest. 2001; 108: 649–54.

19. Kelley JL, Ozment TR, Li C, et al. Scavenger receptor-A (CD204): a two-edged sword in health and disease. Crit Rev Immunol. 2014; 34: 241–61.

20. Wilkinson K, El Khoury J. Microglial scavenger receptors and their roles in the pathogenesis of Alzheimer's disease. Int J Alzheimers Dis. 2012; 2012: 489456.

21. Yang Z, Zhong S, Liu Y, et al. Scavenger receptor SRA attenuates microglia activation and protects neuroinflammatory injury in intracerebral hemorrhage. J Neuroimmunol. 2015; 278: 232–8.

22. Yuan B, Shen H, Lin L, et al. Scavenger receptor SRA attenuates TLR4-induced microglia activation in intracerebral hemorrhage. J Neuroimmunol. 2015; 289: 87–92.

23. Schaer DJ, Alayash AI, Buehler PW. Gating the radical hemoglobin to macrophages: the anti-inflammatory role of CD163, a scavenger receptor. Antioxid Redox Signal. 2007; 9: 991–9.

24. Wang X, Mori T, Sumii T, et al. Hemoglobin-induced cytotoxicity in rat cerebral cortical neurons: caspase activation and oxidative stress. Stroke. 2002; 33: 1882–8.

25. Qu Y, Chen J, Benvenisti-Zarom L, et al. Effect of targeted deletion of the heme oxygenase-2 gene on hemoglobin toxicity in the striatum. J Cereb Blood Flow Metab. 2005; 25: 1466–75.

26. Garton TP, He Y, Garton HJ, et al. Hemoglobin-induced neuronal degeneration in the hippocampus after neonatal intraventricular hemorrhage. Brain Res. 2016; 1635:

86–94.

27. Moestrup SK, Moller HJ. CD163: a regulated hemoglobin scavenger receptor with a role in the anti-inflammatory response. Ann Med. 2004; 36: 347–54.

28. Ma B, Day JP, Phillips H, et al. Deletion of the hemopexin or heme oxygenase-2 gene aggravates brain injury following stroma free hemoglobin-induced intracerebral hemorrhage.J Neuroinflammation. 2016; 13: 26.

29. Aronowski J, Zhao X. Molecular pathophysiology of cerebral hemorrhage: secondary brain injury. Stroke. 2011; 42: 1781–6.

30. Schaer DJ, Vinchi F, Ingoglia G, et al. Haptoglobin, hemopexin, and related defense pathways-basic science, clinical perspectives, and drug development. Front Physiol.2014; 5: 415.

31. Deuel JW, Vallelian F, Schaer CA, et al. Different target specificities of haptoglobin and hemopexin define a sequential protection system against vascular hemoglobin toxicity. Free Radic Biol Med. 2015; 89:931–43.

32. Hvidberg V, Maniecki MB, Jacobsen C, et al. Identification of the receptor scavenging hemopexin-heme complexes. Blood.2005; 106: 2572–9.

33. Wang G, Manaenko A, Shao A, et al. Low-density lipoprotein receptor-related protein-1 facilitates heme scavenging after intracerebral hemorrhage in mice. J Cereb Blood Flow Metab. 2016; 37: 1299–310.

34. Storck SE, Meister S, Nahrath J, et al. Endothelial LRP1 transports amyloid-beta1-42 across the blood-brain barrier. J Clin Invest. 2016; 126: 123–36.

35. Garland P, Durnford AJ, Okemefuna AI, et al. Heme-hemopexin scavenging is activein the brain and associates with outcome after subarachnoid hemorrhage. Stroke. 2016; 47: 872–6.

36. Zhao H, Hao S, Xu H, et al. Protective role of nuclear factor erythroid 2-related factor 2 in the hemorrhagic shock-induced inflammatory response. Int J Mol Med. 2016; 37: 1014–22.

37. Ma Q. Role of nrf2 in oxidative stress and toxicity. Annu Rev Pharmacol Toxicol. 2013;53: 401–26.

38. Jo C, Gundemir S, Pritchard S, et al. Nrf2 reduces levels of phosphorylated tau protein by inducing autophagy adaptor protein NDP52. Nat Commun. 2014; 5: 3496.

39. Kim S, Choi KJ, Cho SJ, et al. Fisetin stimulates autophagic degradation of phosphorylated tau via the activation of TFEB and Nrf2 transcription factors. Sci Rep. 2016; 6:24933.

40. Boyle JJ, Johns M, Lo J, et al. Heme induces heme oxygenase 1 via Nrf2: role in the homeostatic macrophage response to intraplaque hemorrhage. Arterioscler Thromb Vasc Biol. 2011; 31: 2685–91.

41. Ikeda Y, Sugawara A, Taniyama Y, et al. Suppression of rat thromboxane synthase gene transcription by peroxisome proliferator-activated receptor gamma in

macrophages via an interaction with NRF2. J Biol Chem. 2000; 275: 33142–50.

42. Wu JS, Cheung WM, Tsai YS, et al. Ligand activated peroxisome proliferator-activated receptor-gamma protects against ischemic cerebral infarction and neuronal apoptosis by 14-3-3 epsilon upregulation. Circulation. 2009; 119: 1124–34.

43. Reddy RC. Immunomodulatory role of PPAR-gamma in alveolar macrophages. J Investig Med. 2008; 56: 522–7.

44. Zhao XR, Gonzales N, Aronowski J. Pleiotropic role of PPARgamma in intracerebral hemorrhage: an intricate system involving Nrf2, RXR, and NF-kappaB. CNS Neurosci Ther. 2015; 21: 357–66.

45. Cho HY, Gladwell W, Wang X, et al. Nrf2-regulated PPAR{gamma} expression is critical to protection against acute lung injury in mice. Am J Respir Crit Care Med. 2010; 182:170–82.

46. Luo Z, Aslam S, Welch WJ, et al. Activation of nuclear factor erythroid 2-related factor 2 coordinates dimethylarginine dimethylaminohydrolase/PPAR-gamma/ endothelial nitric oxide synthase pathways that enhance nitric oxide generation in human glomerular endothelial cells. Hypertension. 2015; 65: 896–902.

47. Lehmann JM, Moore LB, Smith-Oliver TA,et al. An antidiabetic thiazolidinedione is a high affinity ligand for peroxisome proliferator-activated receptor gamma (PPAR gamma). J Biol Chem. 1995; 270: 12953–6.

48. Liu J, Wang LN, Jia JP. Peroxisome proliferator- activated receptor-gamma agonists for Alzheimer's disease and amnestic mild cognitive impairment: a systematic review and meta-analysis. Drugs Aging. 2015; 32: 57–65.

49. Gonzales NR, Shah J, Sangha N, et al. Design of a prospective, dose-escalation study evaluating the Safety of Pioglitazone for Hematoma Resolution in Intracerebral Hemorrhage (SHRINC). Int J Stroke. 2013;8: 388–96.

50. Zhao X, Zhang Y, Strong R, et al. 15d-Prostaglandin J2 activates peroxisome proliferator- activated receptor-gamma, promotes expression of catalase, and reduces inflammation, behavioral dysfunction, and neuronal loss after intracerebral hemorrhage in rats. J Cereb Blood Flow Metab. 2006; 26: 811–20.

51. Hsu WH, Lee BH, Pan TM. Monascin attenuates oxidative stress-mediated lung inflammation via peroxisome proliferator-activated receptor-gamma (PPAR-gamma) and nuclear factor-erythroid 2 related factor 2 (Nrf-2) modulation. J Agric Food Chem. 2014; 62: 5337–44.

52. Kambayashi J, Liu Y, Sun B, et al. Cilostazol as a unique antithrombotic agent. Curr Pharm Des. 2003; 9: 2289–302.

53. Park SY, Shin HK, Lee JH, et al. Cilostazol ameliorates metabolic abnormalities with suppression of proinflammatory markers in a db/db mouse model of type 2 diabetes via activation of peroxisome proliferator-activated receptor gamma transcription. J Pharmacol Exp Ther. 2009; 329: 571–9.

54. Lee BH, Hsu WH, Chang YY, et al. Ankaflavin: a natural novel PPARgamma agonist upregulates Nrf2 to attenuate methylglyoxal induced diabetes in vivo. Free Radic Biol Med. 2012; 53: 2008–16.

55. Yagami T, Ueda K, Asakura K, et al. Novel binding sites of 15-deoxy-Delta 12,14-prostaglandin J2 in plasma membranes from primary rat cortical neurons. Exp Cell Res. 2003; 291: 212–27.

56. Nissen SE, Wolski K. Effect of rosiglitazone on the risk of myocardial infarction and death from cardiovascular causes. N Engl J Med. 2007; 356: 2457–71.

57. Ishii T, Itoh K, Ruiz E, et al. Role of Nrf2 in the regulation of CD36 and stress protein expression in murine macrophages: activation by oxidatively modified LDL and 4-hydroxynonenal. Circ Res. 2004; 94: 609–16.

58. Olagnier D, Lavergne RA, Meunier E, et al. Nrf2, a PPARgamma alternative pathway to promote CD36 expression on inflammatory macrophages: implication for malaria. PLoS Pathog. 2011; 7: e1002254.

59. Hsu WH, Lee BH, Chang YY, et al. A novel natural Nrf2 activator with PPARgamma agonist (monascin) attenuates the toxicity of methylglyoxal and hyperglycemia. Toxicol Appl Pharmacol. 2013; 272: 842–51.

60. Lee CL, Hung YP, Hsu YW, et al. Monascin and ankaflavin have more anti-atherosclerosis effect and less side effect involving increasing creatinine phosphokinase activity than monacolin K under the same dosages. J Agric Food Chem. 2013; 61: 143–50.

61. Ha CM, Park S, Choi YK, et al. Activation of Nrf2 by dimethyl fumarate improves vascular calcification. Vascul Pharmacol. 2014;63: 29–36.

62. Chen CC, Chen HL, Hsieh CW, et al. Upregulation of NF-E2-related factor-2-dependent glutathione by carnosol provokes a cytoprotective esponse and enhances cell survival. Acta Pharmacol Sin. 2011; 32: 62–9.

63. Schaer DJ, Boretti FS, Schoedon G, et al. Induction of the CD163-dependent haemoglobin uptake by macrophages as a novel anti-inflammatory action of glucocorticoids. Br J Haematol. 2002; 119: 239–43.

64. do Nascimento CO, Hunter L, Trayhurn P. Regulation of haptoglobin gene expression in 3T3-L1 adipocytes by cytokines, catecholamines, and PPARgamma. Biochem Biophys Res Commun. 2004; 313: 702–8.

65. Stred SE, Cote D, Weinstock RS, et al. Regulation of hemopexin transcription by calcium ionophores and phorbol ester in hepatoma cells. Mol Cell Endocrinol. 2003; 204: 111–6.

66. Belcher JD, Nath KA, Vercellotti GM. Vasculotoxic and Proinflammatory Effects of Plasma Heme: cell Signaling and Cytoprotective Responses. ISRN Oxidative Med. 2013; 2013: pii. 831596.

67. Yoon C, Van Niekerk EA, Henry K, et al. Low-density lipoprotein receptor-related

protein 1 (LRP1)-dependent cell signaling promotes axonal regeneration. J Biol Chem. 2013; 288: 26557–68.

68. Fred RG, Boddeti SK, Lundberg M, et al. Imatinib mesylate stimulates low-density lipoprotein receptor-related protein 1-mediated ERK phosphorylation in insulin-producing cells. Clin Sci (Lond). 2015; 128: 17–28.

69. Huang H, Li X, Zhuang Y, et al. Class A scavenger receptor activation inhibits endoplasmic reticulum stress-induced autophagy in macrophage. J Biomed Res. 2014; 28:213–21.

70. Zhang H, Su YJ, Zhou WW, et al. Activated scavenger receptor A promotes glial internalization of abeta. PLoS ONE. 2014; 9: e94197.

71. Manna PP, Frazier WA. The mechanism of CD47-dependent killing of T cells: heterotrimeric Gi-dependent inhibition of protein kinase A. J Immunol. 2003; 170:3544–53.

72. Martinez-Torres AC, Quiney C, Attout T, et al. CD47 agonist peptides induce programmed cell death in refractory chronic lymphocytic leukemia B cells via PLCgamma1 activation: evidence from mice and humans. PLoS Med. 2015; 12: e1001796.

73. Wang G, Hu W, Tang Q, et al. Effect comparison of both iron chelators on outcomes, iron deposit, and iron transporters after intracerebral hemorrhage in rats. Mol Neurobiol. 2016; 53: 3576–85.

74. Auriat AM, Silasi G, Wei Z, et al. Ferric iron chelation lowers brain iron levels after intracerebral hemorrhage in rats but does not improve outcome. Exp Neurol. 2012; 234: 136–43.

75. Wu H, Wu T, Li M, et al. Efficacy of the lipid-soluble iron chelator 2,2'-dipyridyl against hemorrhagic brain injury. Neurobiol Dis. 2012; 45: 388–94.

76. Caliaperumal J, Wowk S, Jones S, et al. Bipyridine, an iron chelator, does not lessen intracerebral iron-induced damage or improve outcome after intracerebral hemorrhagic stroke in rats. Transl Stroke Res. 2013; 4: 719–28.

DECLARATION: This chapter was authored by Gaiqing Wang, Li Wang, Xin-gang Sun and Jiping Tang published as "Hematoma scavenging in intracerebral hemorrhage: From mechanisms to the clinic" in "Journal of Cellular and Molecular Medicine",2018;22(2):768-777

CHAPTER 14:

Aquaporin-4 in glymphatic system, and its implication for central nervous system disorders

ABSTRACT:

The clearance function is essential for maintaining brain tissue homeostasis, and the glymphatic system is the main pathway for removing brain interstitial solutes. Aquaporin-4 (AQP4) is the most abundantly expressed aquaporin in the central nervous system (CNS) and is an integral component of the glymphatic system. In recent years, many studies have shown that AQP4 affects the morbidity and recovery process of CNS disorders through the glymphatic system, and AQP4 shows notable variability in CNS disorders and is part of the pathogenesis of these diseases. Therefore, there has been considerable interest in AQP4 as a potential and promising target for regulating and improving neurological impairment. This review aims to summarize the pathophysiological role that AQP4 plays in several CNS disorders by affecting the clearance function of the glymphatic system. The findings can contribute to a better understanding of the self-regulatory functions in CNS disorders that AQP4 were involved in and provide new therapeutic alternatives for incurable debilitating neurodegenerative disorders of CNS in the future.

KEY WORDS: Aquaporin 4; Glymphatic system; Central nervous system; Intracerebral hemorrhage; Alzheimer's disease; Traumatic brain injury;

Status epilepticus; Migraine; Neuromyelitis optical; Idiopathic normal pressure hydrocephalus

【Introduction】

CNS diseases are prevalent in middle-aged and older adults. Several common CNS diseases have become a heavy social burden. Most of the pathogenesis has yet to be elucidated, leading to treatment difficulties. The brain tissue has a high metabolite level, which produces many potential neurotoxic proteins, cell fragments, and other metabolites in metabolism. Iliff et al. (Jeffrey J. Iliff 2012) found that there is a rapid exchange flow system between cerebrospinal fluid and brain tissue fluid widely in the brain, which can promote the clearance of soluble proteins in the brain. This system, one of the ways for the brain to remove metabolites and foreign bodies, has the function of flushing and cleaning brain tissues. In the CNS, AQP4 is the most critical part of the glymphatic system, the most abundant aquaporin in the brain, spinal cord, and optic nerve, controls cerebral water balance and is highly expressed in astrocyte foot processes around blood vessels(J E Rash 1998;S Nielsen 1997).

Characterization of the glymphatic system clarified the critical role of AQP4 in this clearance network, with AQP4-deficient animals showing astrocytes exhibiting slowed CSF influx through this system and an approximately 70% reduction in interstitial solute clearance, suggesting that the glymphatic system is AQP4-dependent (Jeffrey J. Iliff 2012). The localization of AQP4 also around blood vessels promotes the flow of CSF (Humberto Mestre 2018). Studies have shown that AQP4 activation can enhance interstitial fluid transport from the glial border to the capillaries of the peripapillary membrane (Vincent J Huber 2018). Recent studies have shown that altered AQP4 localization in the brain of aged rodents results in significantly increased retention of adeno-associated viral (AAV) vectors in the brain parenchyma, supporting the importance of AQP4 as an effective promoter of lymphatic transport and clearance (Giridhar Murlidharan 2016). Research has recently focused on AQP4 in the glymphatic system as a hotspot for CNS diseases. Many diseases of the CNS are associated with AQP4 expression and glymphatic system dysfunction. In this article, we will briefly describe AQP4 and glymphatic function. Then, the relationship between AQP4 and common CNS diseases and their possible mechanism is reviewed.

1. The structure and function of the glymphatic system

The pathway of the glymphatic system is a highly organized fluid transport system and has been well described in animal models(Martin Kaag Rasmussen 2018). The glymphatic fluid exchange and drainage system dependent on astrocytes include the entire perivascular space (PVS) network surrounding the arteries, arterioles, capillaries, venules, and veins in the brain parenchyma. PVS is a network of low-resistance tubes formed by astrocyte foot processes surrounding blood vessels. Specifically, PVS is constructed as a coaxial system in which the inner cylinder is the cerebral vascular wall, and the outer cylinder is the glial boundary that wraps around blood vessels or the ends of astrocytes that penetrate arterioles (Thomas Misje Mathiisen 2010). The flow of cerebrospinal fluid into and out of the glymphatic system has been described in detail. At the beginning of the pericapillary pathway, cerebrospinal fluid from the subarachnoid space flows into the brain through the perivascular space of the grand pia meningeal artery. As the vascular tree branches, cerebrospinal fluid enters the brain parenchyma through the perivascular space in the artery (Jeffrey J Iliff 2013; Jeffrey J. Iliff 2012; Qiaoli Ma 2017). Then from the perivascular space, CSF passes through the glial basement membrane and astrocyte terminal processes, wrapping the cerebrovascular system(Jeffrey J. Iliff 2012;Melanie-Jane Hannocks 2018). Furthermore, in brain interstitial fluid, fluid is dispersed by the movement of polarized net fluid toward veins and the space around nerves (Benjamin T Kress 2014;Jeffrey J. Iliff 2012). Eventually, CSF is expelled along the schwannomas, meningeal lymphatics, and arachnoid granulations of cranial and spinal nerves (Jeffrey J. Iliff 2012) (Fig.1). Thus, it can be inferred that under certain conditions, waste products produced by brain tissue can be removed along with cerebrospinal fluid through these pathways.

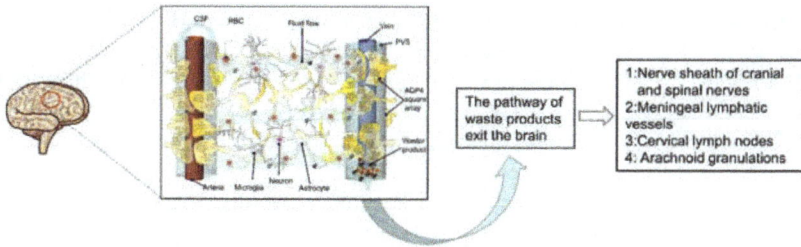

Figure 1. The pathways of the glymphatic system.
The glymphatic system is one of the most important metabolic pathways in the brain, and its normal function depends on the polarization distribution of AQP4 on the astrocyte extremities. This polarized distribution of AQP4 can promote the rapid movement of cerebrospinal fluid from the periarterial space to the perivenous space. This process promotes the metabolism of damaged red blood cells and metabolic waste from the body, which is beneficial for the recovery of nerve function. Finally, these metabolites are excreted outside the brain from four pathways, including the nerve sheath of cranial and spinal nerves, meningeal lymphatic vessels, cervical lymph node and arachnoid granulations.

The specific mechanisms of solute transport and waste excretion in the glymphatic system remain unclear. There are two ways for solute transport through the brain, including diffusion and convection. Furthermore, the importance of convection in the subarachnoid and perivascular has long been recognized. Iliff et al.(Jeffrey J. Iliff 2012) proposed that the glymphatic system clearance mechanism showed that AQP4 promotes the convective transport of brain parenchyma. Besides, Nedergaard et al.(Nadia Aalling Jessen 2015) proposed that cerebrospinal fluid is spatially transferred from pararenal to paracentral through the extracellular space (ECS), and solute transport in ECS depends on the glymphatic flow. Moreover, ECS consists of the ventricular system and subarachnoid space containing cerebrospinal fluid, parenchyma in grey and white matter, and perivascular space surrounding blood vessels(Stephen B Hladky 2014). Moreover, the glymphatic system is a highly polarized cerebrospinal fluid (CSF) transport system that facilitates the clearance of neurotoxic molecules through a network of perivascular pathways (Anne Sofie Munk 2019). Furthermore, the transport of solutes through brain ECS is essential for transporting nutrients and drugs to brain cells and removing metabolites, neurotransmitters, and toxic macromolecules (Stephen B Hladky 2014).

2. The structure, function and regulation of AQP4

In the brain, it has been found that there are three types of AQPs, including AQP4(K Oshio 2004), AQP1(Daniela Boassa 2005;Kotaro Oshio 2005), and AQP9(Zelenina 2010). Furthermore, AQP4 was almost expressed in astrocytes and ependymal cells (Zelenina 2010). It has been reported that AQP4 is a homologous tetramer assembled by AQP4 monomer with independent water molecular channels on the cell membrane. There are two subtypes, AQP4-M1 and AQP4-M23, which mainly exist in brain tissues (Thomas Walz 2009). The monomer is about 30 KD, and each monomer crosses the membrane six times to form three extracellular rings (A, C, E) and two intracellular rings (B, D). The free N-terminal and C-terminal are distributed in the cytoplasm, and the B and E ring containing the NPA conserved sequence return to the lipid bilayer of the membrane (Fig.2). In addition, the whole AQP4 monomer is composed of the widely open ends on both sides of the membrane and the constriction part of the NPA conserved sequence in the central of the membrane, forming a three-dimensional "funnel model"(Erlend A Nagelhus 2013). Studies have shown that AQP4 tetramers form orthogonal arrays of particles (OAPs) on astrocyte membranes (Hartwig Wolburg 2011;Manuela de Bellis 2021), mainly composed of AQP4-M1 and AQP4-M23. And the size of OAPs is determined by the proportion of AQP4-M1 and AQP4-M23. Moreover, there is a conclusion that the more AQP4-M23 is, the more stable the OAPs structure will be (Jérôme Badaut 2014) (Jesse A Stokum 2015) (G P Nicchia 2010). In addition, as reported, the M23 isoform exhibits a much stronger water transport capacity than the M1 isoform (Claudia Silberstein 2004). In the case of astrocytes, tetrameric AQP4 is not inserted into the membrane as a supramolecular assembly of water channel molecules independently, and AQP4 molecules form functional complexes with other membrane proteins such as the dystrophin glycoprotein complex (DGC)(T Haenggi 2006). It was found that AQP4 was enriched at three critical locations in astrocytes. Furthermore, it is vital for blood-brain barrier function at the end of perivascular astrocytes. In addition, AQP4 is involved in neurotransmitter clearance in peri-synaptic astrocytes and K+ clearance during contact with Ranvier nodes and unmyelinated axons (Zelenina 2010). It has also been reported that AQP4 is mainly expressed in the cell membrane at the junction of the brain parenchyma and brain fluid components, such as, on the podocytes of astrocytes adjacent to microvascular endothelial cells, on the side of the basement membrane of ependymal cells in the ventricles, and on the cell membrane of astrocytes composing the glial boundary membrane. This polar distribution of AQP4 suggests that AQP4 may be involved in regulating the flow of brain water into and out of the CNS (Hubbard, et al. 2015).

There are mainly two ways of regulating AQP4 expression: short-term and long-term. Conformational alterations or channel gating can affect short-term regulation (E S McCoy 2010;H B Moeller 2009;Monica Carmosino 2007). Besides, because of dynamic regulation, the permeability of AQP channels or the subcellular localization of AQP channels (their abundance in the membrane) may change within seconds or minutes, resulting in an immediate change in membrane permeability (Zelenina 2010).

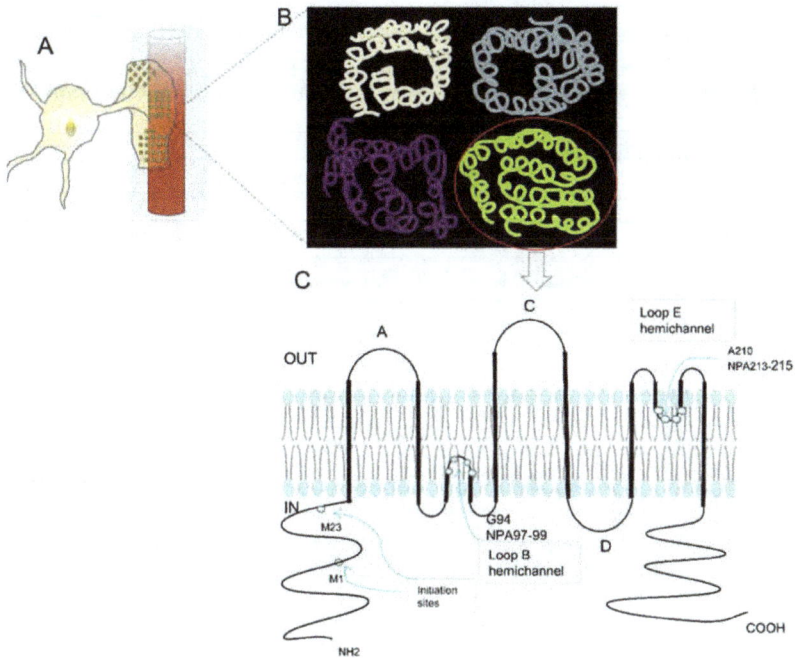

Figure 2. Structure of AQP4 molecule.

(A) AQP4 was distributed in orthogonal arrays of particles on the astrocyte's end foot. (B) Aquaporins, in general, form tetrameric protein complexes within the membrane plane. (C) The proposed membrane topology of AQP4 comprises six presumed bilayer-spanning domains and five connecting loops. Furthermore, the initiation sites at methionines1 and 23 are shown at the N-terminus.

Unlike short-term adjustment, long-term regulation is mediated by changes in AQP mRNA and protein synthesis or degradation rates. These changes alter the abundance of AQP4 over hours or days, thereby altering the permeability of the AQP4 membrane. As more and more studies have been conducted on AQP4's involvement in nervous system diseases, pharmacological interventions have become more prevalent. Activators and inhibitors of AQP4 are summarized in table 1. Therefore, it is reasonable to assume that the regulation of AQP4 is a highly complex process. For an investigator, it would be beneficial to study the function of the glymphatic system by using pharmacological methods to regulate the expression of AQP4.

The type of drug	Drug' name	The pattern of drugs to regulate the expression of AQP4
Activators of AQP4	Dexamethasone	by inducing small ubiquitin-like modifiers (SUMO) (Xiaoling Zhang 2020).
	Testosterone	Being attenuated by the protein kinase C activator 12-O-tetradecanoylphorbol 13-acetate (Feng Gu 2003).
	Genistein	through the cAMP/PKA/CREB signaling pathway(Haohai Huang 2015).
Inhibitors of AQP4	TGN-020	Direct binding inhibition likely mediated by binding to D69, M70, I73, F77, V145 (rat)/L145 (human), I205, and R216.(Arno Vandebroek 2020;Ionica Pirici 2017)
	Minocycline	by reversing the translocation of AQP4 from astrocyte processes to cell bodies.(Qi Lu 2022)
	Methylene blue	through the ERK1/2 pathway(Zhong-Fang Shi 2021).

Table 1. The regulation of AQP4 through drugs.
AQP4: aquaporin4; TGN-020: N-(1,3,4-thiadiazol-2-yl) pyridine-3-carboxamide

3. The effects of AQP4 in glymphatic system on CNS disorders

3.1 Intracerebral hemorrhage (ICH)

ICH is a subtype of stroke caused by intracerebral vascular rupture, with high mortality and disability rates (Adnan I Qureshi 2009;He Wu 2011). Intracerebral hemorrhage accounts for 10-15% of strokes worldwide and is often associated with inadequate blood pressure control and excessive use of anticoagulants, thrombolytic agents, and antiplatelet drugs (Adnan I Qureshi 2009; C L Sudlow 1997). Several hours after intracerebral hemorrhage, the primary brain injury is mainly caused by the compression and destruction of nearby tissues caused by hematoma. Inflammation, thrombin activation and erythrocyte lysis caused by primary brain injury can promote the formation of brain edema, which has a poor prognosis and can cause more severe and lasting damage (Richard F Keep 2012). Jeon et al. (Hanwool Jeon 2021) found that AQP4 enhancer attenuated peri-hematoma edema by improving the integrity of the blood-brain barrier by up-regulating AQP4 expression on astrocytes with the AQP4 enhancer BQ-788. Besides, Liu et al. (Xichang Liu 2021) used a collagenase-induced rat model of ICH. Ligation and resection of cervical lymph nodes could lead to cerebral lymphatic vessel obstruction. They found that cerebral lymphatic obstruction down-regulated the expression of AQP4, up-regulated the expression of inflammatory TNF-α and inhibited the expression of IL-10, and aggravated brain edema, neuroinflammation and neuronal apoptosis in rats with cerebral hemorrhage, resulting in neurological deficits. Thus, it is concluded that AQP4 is involved in ICH-induced brain edema, BBB destruction and neuronal apoptosis.

Subarachnoid hemorrhage (SAH) is a highly prevalent ICH disorder (Aizawa 1971; Gijn 1992; Jolobe 2007; R Bonita 1985). SAH refers to blood flow into the subarachnoid space due to intracranial vascular rupture, often accompanied by permanent brain damage. Moreover, after SAH, blood components would enter the perivascular space, resulting in varying degrees of coagulation and macrophage chemotaxis, which could impede fluid exchange between cerebrospinal and interstitial fluid (A Jackowski 1990). A report showed that after SAH, for AQP4 knockout rats, CSF flow would significantly reduce through interstitial and parenchyma. The glymphatic system function was also impaired, and there was no improvement in neurological function and neuroinflammation compared with WT rats at seven days. The report indicated that the glymphatic system significantly removes harmful metabolites and excess fluid produced after SAH and plays a positive role in the recovery of neurological function (E Liu 2020). In addition, studies have shown persistent lymphatic and meningeal lymphatic drainage dysfunction and associated neuropathological damage after SAH (Pu, et al. 2019). Therefore, improving the clearance function of the glymphatic system in injured brain tissue after SAH may become a new strategy for treating SAH.

3.2 Ischemic stroke

Ischemic stroke is a disorder of cerebral blood flow caused by vascular obstruction (Wang, et al. 2023). The pathophysiology includes excitotoxicity, free radical release, protein misfolding, mitochondrial response, and inflammatory changes, leading to neuronal death and neurological deficits (George and Steinberg 2015; Jiang, et al. 2022; Li, et al. 2022). In rodent models of acute ischaemic stroke, MRI and histological examination showed impaired CSF inflow in the ipsilateral cortex at 3 h after middle cerebral artery occlusion, and glymphatic influx had recovered 24 h after spontaneous arterial recanalization (Gaberel, et al. 2014). Notably, a murine study evaluating clearance of fluorescent tracers from the necrotic infarct core at 7 weeks after a hypoxic middle cerebral artery occlusion showed that solutes trapped in the core leaked through the glial scar and were transported from the brain along perivascular spaces. Otherwise, they also found that the ISF within the core contained elevated levels of proinflammatory cytokines and was toxic to cultured cortical and hippocampal neurons, even at 7 weeks after the middle cerebral artery occlusion, suggesting a beneficial role of glymphatic clearance in disease resolution (Zbesko, et al. 2018). Toh and Siow found that the autoimmune lymphoproliferative syndrome (ALPS) index showed lower values in ischemic stroke suggesting impaired glymphatic function. Following initial impairment, the ALPS index increased with the time since stroke onset, which is suggestive of glymphatic function recovery (Toh and Siow 2021). Cortical spreading depression (mass depolarization of neurons, initiating in the ischaemic core, potentially leading to neuronal death in surrounding hypoxic tissue after stroke) has also been implicated in impaired glymphatic flow (Schain, et al. 2017). In mice, cortical spreading depression-induced in the non-hypoxic brain led to a complete transient closure of the perivascular spaces around both arteries and veins lasting up to 10 min, followed by a gradual reopening that did not recover to the baseline calibre within the first 30 min, and resulted in a reduction of interstitial flow (Schain et al. 2017). A mass of studies on astrocytes' roles in ischemic stroke has been conducted. Astrocyte-related structures/

proteins play different roles in the activation of astrocytes at different developmental stages of ischemic stroke. In the acute phase of ischemic stroke, the proliferation and hypertrophy of astrocytes in the peri-infarct area are conducive to sealing the site of injury, remodeling the tissue, and controlling the local immune response both spatially and temporally (Wang, et al. 2012). However, in the chronic phase, the formation of glial scarring by excessive astrocyte proliferation may limit the recovery of central nervous function (Daneman and Prat 2015). In addition, many studies have shown the effect of AQP4 on ischemic stroke. For example, a study showed that deletion of AQP4 or TRPV4 channels alone leads to a significant worsening of ischemic brain injury at both time points, whereas their simultaneous deletion results in a smaller brain lesion at day 1 but equal tissue damage at day 2 when compared with controls. The data indicate that the interplay between AQP4 and TRPV4 channels is critical during neuronal and non-neuronal swelling in the acute phase of ischemic injury (Sucha, et al. 2022). Sun and collaborators have found that acutely inhibiting AQP4 using TGN-020 promoted neurological recovery by diminishing brain edema at the early stage and attenuating peri-infarct astrogliosis and AQP4 depolarization at the subacute stage after stroke (Sun, et al. 2022). In addition, oxytocin (OXT) significantly suppresses neuronal damage in the early stage of stroke by inhibiting apoptotic and NF-κB signaling pathways, increasing the expression of VEGF, AQP4 and

BDNF proteins and reducing the BBB leakage (Wang et al. 2012). Furthermore, experts concluded that miR-29b could potentially predict stroke outcomes as a novel circulating biomarker, and miR-29b overexpression reduced BBB disruption after ischemic stroke via downregulating AQP-4(Wang, et al. 2015). Now, evidence of the involvement of the glymphatic pathway in stroke, at present, comes from findings in animal research, and the pathway must be investigated in human trials.

3.3 Traumatic brain injury (TBI)

TBI refers to the organic brain tissue lesions caused by trauma, resulting in brain dysfunction (Ann C Mckee 2015; Benjamin L Brett 2022; Hardman 1979; Kara N Corps 2015). TBI patients often perform neurodegenerative features of neurofibrillary tangles composed of Tau aggregates and Aβ amyloid aggregation. By injecting human Tau protein into the brain tissue of a moderate TBI animal model and tracking its clearance path, it was found that human Tau protein was mainly concentrated around the large veins(Jessen, et al. 2015). Studies have shown that TBI significantly inhibited the entry of cerebrospinal fluid tracer (OA-45) in mice, resulting in a glymphatic system function decline of about 60%. Researchers also found that impairing cerebrospinal fluid entry and Aβ clearance could be observed in the ipsilateral hippocampus one day after the onset of TBI, and the functional inhibition of the glial lymphatic system caused by TBI was still significant 28 days later(Iliff, et al. 2014). Those results suggest that the AQP4-mediated removal of Tau from the glymphatic system is essential for limiting secondary neuronal damage after trauma.

3.4 Alzheimer's disease (AD)

AD is common dementia in the elderly, accounting for about 50-70% of dementia in the elderly (Dhamidhu Eratne 2018; Jose A Soria Lopez 2019; Morgan Robinson 2017). Genetic variants in AQP4 are associated with Aβ accumulation, disease stage progression, and cognitive decline, which may correspond to changes in glymphatic system function and brain Aβ clearance and may be useful biomarkers for predicting the burden of disease in patients with dementia (Chandra, et al. 2021). It has also been shown that loss of perivascular AQP4 localization in neurodegenerative diseases such as AD may be a factor that makes the ageing brain vulnerable to protein mis-aggregation (Zeppenfeld, et al. 2017). Andrea et al. (Arighi, et al. 2019) measured the levels of AQP4 in cerebrospinal fluid (CSF) in 11 AD patients, ten normal pressure hydrocephalus (NPH) patients and nine controls, finding that AQP4 was significantly decreased in AD patients and tended to decrease in NPH patients. Besides, there was also a correlation between AQP4 and the levels of amyloid beta and CSF. This study suggests a potential role of AQP4 and the glymphatic system's pathophysiology of neurodegenerative diseases. The relationship between the glymphatic system and AD is being further studied, and the strategy for treating AD by regulating the glymphatic system is also gradually developing. For example, an experiment found that the β- lactam antibiotics such as ceftriaxone can be efficiently activated by the N F − κ B pathway activation of astrocyte glutamate transfer eggs (glutamate transporter, GLT1) express. It alleviated the problems of memory loss and cognitive impairment caused by excessive accumulation of glutamate and glutamatergic N-methyl-d-aspartate (NMDA) receptors, such as Ca2+isorder, massive production of NO, increase of free radicals, activation of proteasome and proliferation of cytotoxic transcription factors (Brhane Teklebrhan Assefa 2018). Now, the most promising drug is the target of AQP4, and its therapeutic effect has been proved by comparison. For example, AQP4 can help regulate the Ca2+ signaling pathway, K+ balance, glutamate transport, astrocyte proliferation and activation, and neuroinflammatory response of astrocytes (Yu-Long Lan 2017).

3.5 Parkinson's disease (PD)

Parkinson's disease (PD) is a multisystem alpha-synucleinopathic neurodegenerative disease and the most prevalent neurodegenerative disorder after Alzheimer's disease, with a high incidence rate in the elderly population (Scott-Massey, et al. 2022). Moreover, its characteristic motor symptoms are tremor, rigidity, bradykinesia/akinesia, and postural stability, but the clinical picture includes other motor and non-motor symptoms (NMSs) (Taylor, et al. 2002). Several studies indicated that extracellular alpha-synuclein might lead to neurotoxic responses by microglia and astrocytes, and deposition and spreading of misfolded proteins (α-synuclein and tau) have been linked to Parkinson's disease cognitive dysfunction. (Han, et al. 2021; Henderson, et al. 2019). Alpha-synucleinopathy is postulated to be central to idiopathic rapid eye movement sleep behaviour disorder (iRBD) and Parkinson's disease (PD). And there is an association between the diminished clearance of α-synuclein and glymphatic system dysfunction (Si, et al. 2022). In PD, the impact of dopaminergic deterioration may be crucial in the disruption of sleep and CSF-ISF flow in the glymphatic system, given the significant involvement of dopaminergic contributions to the disease and waste clearance system (Gratwicke, et al. 2015). Recent studies have indicated that aquaporin 4 (AQP4), as a predominant water channel protein in the brain, is involved in the progression of Parkinson's disease (PD) as well. Dopamine has been shown to reduce the proliferation of striatal glial cells and the expression of AQP4 within these cells (Küppers, et al. 2008). Additionally, AQP4 deficiency has been associated with aggravated dopaminergic degeneration and, in particular, enhanced susceptibility to the insult of the dopaminergic neurons between the substantia nigra and ventral tegmental area (Zhang, et al. 2016). Cui and colleagues established a progressive PD model by subjecting AQP4 null (AQP4(+/-)) mice to bilateral intrastriatal injection of α-syn preformed fibrils (PFFs) and investigated the effect of decreased AQP4 expression on the development of PD. Meanwhile, they found that decreased expression of AQP4 accelerated pathologic deposition of α-syn and facilitated the loss of dopamine neurons and behavioral disorders. Draining of macromolecules from the brain via the glymphatic pathway was slowed due to decreased AQP4 expression (Cui, et al. 2021). Additionally, Chi et al. found that AQP4-deficient mice were hypersensitive to stimulations such as 1-methyl-4-phenyl-1,2,3,6-tetrahydropyridine (MPTP) or lipopolysaccharide compared to wild-type (WT) littermates. In a mouse model of MPTP-induced Parkinson's disease (PD), AQP4-deficient animals show more robust microglial inflammatory responses and more severe loss of dopaminergic neurons (DNS) compared with WT mice (Chi, et al. 2011). A study of three-hundred and eighty-two patients with PD and 180 healthy controls with a mean follow-up time of 66.1 months from the Parkinson's Progression Marker Initiative study were analyzed. The result showed that genetic variations of AQP4 and subsequent alterations of glymphatic efficacy might contribute to an altered rate of cognitive decline in PD. AQP4 rs162009 is likely a novel genetic prognostic marker of glymphatic function and cognitive decline in PD (Fang, et al. 2021).

3.6 Vascular dementia (VaD)

Vascular dementia (VaD) is one of the most common causes of dementia after Alzheimer's disease, causing around 15% of cases (O'Brien and

Thomas 2015). Furthermore, Vascular and neurodegenerative dementia has emerged as the leading cause of age-related cognitive impairment (Iadecola 2013). Among these cerebrovascular disorders, major stroke, and cerebral small vessel disease (cSVD) constitute the major risk factors for VaD. These conditions alter neurovascular functions leading to blood-brain barrier (BBB) deregulation, neurovascular coupling dysfunction, and inflammation (Lecordier, et al. 2021). The entry of blood-borne macromolecular substances into the brain parenchyma from cerebral vessels is blocked by the blood-brain barrier (BBB) function. Accordingly, increased permeability of the vessels induced by insult noted in patients suffering from vascular dementia likely contributes to cognitive impairment (Ueno, et al. 2019). The glymphatic system plays an essential role in the pathophysiological processes of many cognitive disorders. AQP4 shows noteworthy changes in various cognitive disorders and is part of the pathogenesis of these diseases (Wang, et al. 2022b). Yu and colleagues employed a multiple microinfarction (MMI) model to induce VaD in mice, and investigate VaD-induced cognitive dysfunction, white matter (WM) damage, glymphatic dysfunction and the role of miR-126 in mediating these effects. Results showed that MMI in WT mice decreases synaptic plasticity and dendritic spine density, instigates water channel and glymphatic dysfunction, and decreases serum miR-126 expression. Furthermore, the reduction of endothelial miR-126 expression may mediate cognitive impairment in MMI-induced VaD. (Yu, et al. 2019).

Moreover, Venkat's team have investigated the therapeutic effects of human umbilical cord blood cells (HUCBC) treatment on the cognitive outcome, white matter (WM) integrity, and glymphatic system function in rats subject to a multiple microinfarction (MMI) model of VaD. Data indicated that HUCBC treatment of an MMI rat model of VaD promotes WM remodeling and improves glymphatic function, which may aid in improving cognitive function and memory (Venkat, et al. 2020). Therefore, we may infer from the above that a therapeutic strategy to clear brain metabolic waste through the glymphatic pathway may be a promising approach to prevent neurodegenerative diseases.

3.7 Idiopathic normal pressure hydrocephalus (iNPH)

iNPH, one of NPH and with no apparent cause, often occurs in the elderly, and imaging analysis shows normal cerebrospinal fluid (CSF) pressure and ventricular enlargement (Changwu Tan 2021) (Michael A Williams 2016). Moreover, this disease is characterized by progressive ventricular enlargement and the clinical tread of gait ataxia, urinary incontinence, and dementia (Basant R. Nassar and Carol F. Lippa 2016). iNPH presents with similar symptoms to AD, with pathological findings: cortical biopsies of brains with iNPH have shown Aβ deposition, reactive astrocyte proliferation, and AQP4 depolarization (G V Gavrilov 2019). Studies have shown that the inflow and outflow functions of the glymphatic system are impaired in iNPH patients, especially in the entorhinal cortex (ERC)(Per K Eide 2019). ERC is one of the essential bases of hippocampal function, directly affecting memory function. Hasan-Olive et al. (Md Mahdi Hasan-Olive 2019) found that immunohistochemical analysis of AQP4 in cortical brain biopsies from 30 iNPH patients and 12 normal subjects showed decreased AQP4 density at the end arterial end peri-cerebrovascular astrocytes in iNPH compared with control brains. Using intrathecal injection of gadolinium-diethylenetriaminepentacetate (Gd-DTPA), a magnetic resonance imaging (MRI) paramagnetic contrast agent, Ringstad et al. (Per K Eide 2019), and Eide et al. (Geir Ringstad 2018) found that Gd-DTPA extends anteriorly along the great arachnoid artery into the subarachnoid space and then enters the brain parenchyma along the extravascular space. Moreover, compared with ordinary people, the clearance of Gd-DTPA is delayed in patients with idiopathic hydrocephalus, suggesting that the glial lymphatic system is related to the pathogenesis of idiopathic normal pressure hydrocephalus. According to clinical guidelines, patients with iNPH are still advised to undergo early shunt surgery to improve intracranial lymphatic dysfunction (Basant R. Nassar and Carol F. Lippa 2016; Etsuro Mori 2012) and help regulate the rate of cerebrospinal fluid drainage (Albert M Isaacs 2019). In one study, changes in cerebrospinal fluid biomarkers after shunt surgery were found, which suggested that shunt surgery improves the glymphatic system function

(Madoka Nakajima 2018). In the end, an in-depth study of the relationship between the glymphatic system and the pathogenesis of iNPH can optimize the current clinical diagnostic methods and prevent the early deterioration of the disease.

3.8 Status epilepticus (SE)

SE is a neurologic emergency characterized by persistent epileptic activity or frequent seizures without return to baseline, with high mortality and morbidity (Bhavpreet S Dham 2014). Moreover, many patients have persistent neurocognitive impairment after completion of SE(Khalil S Husari 2020;Kjersti N Power 2018). In addition to the direct neuronal damage caused by SE, the deposition of hyperphosphorylated tau (p-tau) is thought to contribute to post-SE neurodegeneration (Ali, et al. 2019). In addition, cerebral edema after SE is considered almost inevitable and is associated with a poor prognosis in SE(Amélia Mendes 2016). Liu et al. (Kewei Liu 2021) found that Glymphatic system function was temporarily impaired after SE, and the time course of lymphatic system dysfunction was well matched with the progression of brain edema after SE. In addition, when cerebral edema was relieved by Glibenclamide treatment or Trpm4 gene deletion, the function of the glymphatic system recovered earlier. At the same time, p-tau deposition and neuronal degeneration were reduced, and cognitive function was improved. Furthermore, the results suggest that SE-induced brain edema may lead to lymphatic dysfunction and make the post-SE brain vulnerable to p-tau aggregation and neurocognitive impairment. The cerebellar AQP4 levels in SE were evaluated by constructing pilocarpine-induced SE mouse models. The results showed that the expression of aquaporin decreased from day three after SE and recovered on day 7. In addition, mice showed impaired motor coordination and learning in the acute post-SE phase. Thus, SE is implicated in changes in AQP4 expression and cerebellar injury (Hui Tang 2017). Another study investigated the role of 67-kDa laminin receptor (LR) in SE-induced vasogenic edema formation in rat piriform cortex (PC). SE reduced the expression of 67-kDa LR and SMI-71(a rat BBB barrier marker) in endothelial cells and astrocytes. An additional 67-kDa LR neutralization also reduced dystrophin and aquaporin 4 (AQP4) expression. Therefore, the findings indicate that 67-kDa LR dysfunction may disrupt the dystrophin-AQP4 complex, which would evoke vasogenic edema formation and subsequent laminin over-expression via activating p38 MAPK/VEGF axis (Hana Park 2019). It is concluded that AQP4 is involved in the occurrence and development of SE.

3.9 Migraine and other pathologic pain

Migraine is a common primary headache in clinical practice (Diamond 1991; Elithorn 1969; Michel D Ferrari 2022; Tfelt-Hansen 1994; Walter 2022; William Qubty 2020). It is characterized by paroxysmal, primarily unilateral, moderate to severe, pulsatile headache, generally lasting 4-72 hours, and can be accompanied by nausea, vomiting, sound stimulation, light stimulation or daily activities, which can aggravate the headache. Furthermore, cortical spreading inhibition (CSD), a cell depolarization autogenous wave, is associated with progressive neuronal damage after migraine (Takano, et al. 2007). Because CSD can be regarded as a neurophysiological precursor of migraine, animal models of migraine are often induced by CSD (Zhang, et al. 2010). Schain et al.(Schain et al. 2017) injected dextran labelled with different fluorescent dyes into the frontal cortex of the cerebral cortex of induced CSD mice and control mice. Through using two-photon imaging technology, the VRS around the arteries and veins on the cerebral cortex of CSD mice were rapidly closed. The ependyma of VRS is mainly surrounded by astrocyte terminus, and Takano et al. (Schain et al. 2017) previously reported that CSD would cause swelling of neurons and astrocyte terminus. Schain et al. (Nadia Aalling Jessen 2015) suggested that VRS closure was related to this swelling. Moreover, VRS closure was accompanied by a decrease in dye clearance at the injection site, indicating that CSD impeded ISF outflow from brain tissue through the glymphatic system, which would also slow fluid flow in the VRS. This phenomenon is consistent with previous studies on the role of the glymphatic system in the clearance of ISF solutes(Erik N T P Bakker 2016). However, ROSIC et al.(Brana Rosic 2019) used AQP4-/ - and wild-type mice as models to induce CSD and found that the time and volume of astrocyte terminal foot swelling in the two mice were consistent, suggesting that CSD caused astrocyte terminal foot swelling in an AQP4-independent manner. Combined with their previous studies, they hypothesized that astrocyte end foot swelling might be related to abnormal Ca2+ signaling of functional molecules assembled in the end foot and that astrocyte end foot swelling may be mediated by membrane proteins such as chloride cotransporters rather than aquaporins. Although the abnormal mechanics of the glymphatic system in migraine is still controversial, the fact that VRS is closed suggests that if the homeostasis of astrocyte terminal foot function is disrupted, this entry point may provide a new therapeutic direction for migraine treatment.

Pain is a common symptom in patients with all types of demyelinating-ON (Ayzenberg, et al. 2021; Kang, et al. 2022) and MOG-IgG-pos(Asseyer, et al. 2018) . Moreover, intractable neuropathic pain is a common symptom of neuromyelitis optica spectrum disorder (NMOSD)(Ishikura, et al. 2021). The immune system has long been recognised as important in pain regulation through inflammatory cytokine modulation of peripheral nociceptive fibres (Xu, et al. 2020). However, emerging clinical and experimental evidence demonstrates that neuroinflammation is essential in cognitive impairment associated with neuropathic pain (Mai, et al. 2021). Notably, Lu and collaborators found that Complete Freund's adjuvant-induced chronic inflammatory pain and spared nerve injury-induced neuropathic pain models, AQP4(-/-) mice attenuated pain-related behavioral responses compared with AQP4(+/+) mice, demonstrating that AQP4 deficiency relieved chronic inflammatory pain and neuropathic pain. In the formalin and capsaicin tests, two models of chemical stimuli-induced acute pain, no differences in the durations of licking the injected hind-paw were found between AQP4(+/+) and AQP4(-/-) mice (Lu, et al. 2020). In AQP4-ON, loss of AQP4, impairment of astrocytes and parallel injury in AQP4-coexpressed molecules (such as excitatory amino acid transporter 2, EAAT2), may lead to an excessive accumulation of glutamate in the extracellular space, interrupting the glutamine-glutamate-GABA axis (Kang et al. 2022). In addition, recent studies have found that astrocytes can regulate nociceptive synaptic transmission via neuronal-glial and glial-glial cell interactions and are involved in the modulation of pain signaling and the maintenance of neuropathic pain (Ji, et al. 2019). Many recent studies have shown that the glymphatic system is also associated with other pathologic pain in addition to migraine. The study of Wang and collaborators verified that alterations in glymphatic function are closely related to cancer pain, and the quantification of functional changes reflects pain severity (Wang, et al. 2022a). Goldman and his partners' study showed that the glymphatic system is regulated by sleep and norepinephrine, with increased levels of norepinephrine during wakefulness inhibiting fluid movement. Norepinephrine is also essential for transitioning from acute to chronic pain, and sufferers of chronic neuropathic pain frequently present with sleep disruption (Goldman, et al. 2020). However, it remains unclear how AQP4 mediates the glymphatic system specifically to affect the pathophysiology of pathologic pain

3.10 Neuromyelitis optical (NMO)

NMO is a chronic inflammatory autoimmune disease of the CNS associated with a characteristic pattern of astrocyte dysfunction and loss, leading to secondary demyelination and neurodegeneration (Izumi Kawachi and Lassmann 2017). In most patients, NMO is caused by pathogenic serum IgG antibodies against AQP4(Carnero Contentti and Correale 2021). In most patients, NMO is caused by pathogenic serum IgG antibodies against AQP4[87]. The binding of AQP4-antibody (AQP4-ab) to AQP4 expressed by astrocytes triggers activation of a classical complement cascade, followed by granulocyte, eosinophil, and lymphocyte infiltration. Eventually, astrocytes are injured first, followed by oligodendrocytes, demyelination, neuronal loss, and neurodegeneration (Carnero Contentti and Correale 2021). However, how AQP4-IgG enters the brain from the periphery must be clarified. It has been suggested that the blood-brain barrier may not be fully developed in the anterior lamina part of the optic nerve and the root entrance area of the spinal cord, making IgG more likely to enter the circulation than elsewhere in the CNS (Hofman, et al. 2001;Iorio, et al. 2011). Here somebody also hypothesized that infection temporarily preferentially destroys the blood-brain barrier in the optic nerve or spinal cord, allowing AQP4-IgG entry (Koga, et al. 2011). There are many methods to treat NMO, currently available methylprednisolone and maintenance plasmapheresis in resistant cases, including corticosteroids, azathioprine, rituximab, mitoxantrone, cyclophosphamide, and mycophenolate salts (Collongues and Seze 2011). Besides, an emerging approach to targeted therapy that prevents AQP4-IgG from binding to AQP4 has recently been proposed (Verkman, et al. 2012). In brain tissue, AQP4 is mainly expressed in the astrocyte terminus, and both AQP4 and astrocytes are related to the pathogenesis of NMO. Therefore, we might hypothesize that the glymphatic system influences NMO, but further research is required.

Disease	The effects of AQP4 in CNS disorders
ICH	• AQP4 might improve the integrity of the blood-brain barrier • AQP4 up-regulated the expression of inflammatory cytokines, such as TNF-α and IL-10
Ischemic stroke	•AQP4 expression is altered in a stage-specific manner •AQP4 expression may be regulated by oxytocin and miR-29b
TBI	•AQP4 mediated removal of Tau from the glymphatic system
AD	•The loss of perivascular AQP4 localization may be a factor to make protein mis-aggregation •AQP4 could help regulate the Ca2+ signaling pathway, K+ balance, glutamate transport, astrocyte proliferation and activation, and neuroinflammatory response of astrocytes
PD	• AQP4 deficiency was associated with aggravated dopaminergic degeneration • Decreased expression of AQP4 accelerated pathologic deposition of α-syn and facilitated the loss of dopamine neurons and behavioral disorders. •The genetic variations of AQP4 might contribute to an altered rate of cognitive decline in PD
VaD	•AQP4 showed noteworthy changes in various cognitive disorders and is part of the pathogenesis of these diseases
iNPH	•AQP4 depolarization may help regulate the rate of cerebrospinal fluid drainage
SE	•The changes in AQP4 expression

	•67-kDa laminin receptor (LR) dysfunction may disrupt the dystrophin-AQP4 complex
Migraine	•AQP4 may be not participate in the process of astrocyte end foot swelling
pathologic pain	•AQP4 deficiency relieved chronic inflammatory pain and neuropathic pain
	•The AQP4-coexpressed molecules may lead to an excessive accumulation of glutamate in the extracellular space, interrupting the glutamine-glutamate-GABA axis
NMO	•Often defined by the presence of anti-AQP IgGs
	•The binding of AQP4-antibody (AQP4-ab) to AQP4 expressed by astrocytes triggers activation of a classical complement cascade

Table.2 Summary of AQP4 regulation in various neurological disorders.

Summary

As the most abundantly expressed aquaporin in the CNS, AQP4 has always been the focus of research on related CNS disorders. The glymphatic system has emerged as a major clearance pathway for brain metabolic waste, with AQP4 being an essential component. As a result, AQP4 provides a new avenue for research in various disorders of the CNS.

There is a brief review of the mechanisms and effects of AQP4 in several common disorders of the central nervous system (Table.2). In ICH diseases, AQP4 and the glymphatic system play a critical role in maintaining the integrity of the blood-brain barrier, removing hematoma and reducing edema. In the case of AD is to clear away the deposits of Aβ and tau, and in PD, AQP4 is a significant effect on the accumulation of α-Synuclein and dopamine secretion. But as for the VaD, it is not clear about the role of AQP4. In iNPH may be caused by insufficient drainage of the glymphatic system and AQP4 depolarization. In SE, it is likely that the integrity of the BBB and the dystrophin-AQP4 complex are disrupted. In migraine, AQP4 may affect the homeostasis of astrocyte foot processes. In other pathologic pain, AQP4 is associated with interrupting the glutamine-glutamate-GABA axis and synaptic transmission. Moreover, triggering the closure of the VRS. And the pathogenesis of NMO is correlated with pathogenic serum IgG antibodies to AQP4.

In summary, the pathogenesis of the central nervous system is challenging to elucidate. Usually, it results from multiple factors, which undoubtedly increases the difficulty and complexity of patient treatment. This review indicates that AQP4 plays a non-negligible role in neurological disorders due to its location in the glymphatic system, which means that AQP4 is a promising therapeutic target. It has been shown that regulating the expression of AQP4 in the glymphatic system can delay or improve the occurrence and development of disorders related to the central nervous system. Although research on AQP4 and the glymphatic system has increased in recent years, the field is still in its infancy. As a result of the pathway's distribution throughout the brain, it is difficult to pinpoint the exact routes of glymphatic system in brain. More researches should be conducted to strengthen the function of the waste clearance system in brain by regulating phagocytosis and AQP4 in order to treat CNS diseases precisely, which provides new possibilities for incurable debilitating neurodegenerative disorders of CNS in the future.

Author Contributions Statement

All authors listed have made a substantial, direct and intellectual contribution to the work, and approved it for publication.

Conflict of Interest Statement

The authors declare that the research was conducted in the absence of any commercial or financial relationships that could be construed as a potential conflict of interest.

Acknowledgments:

This work was supported by Hainan Province Clinical Medical Center, National Natural Science Foundation of China (No.81771294; 82160237) and Shenzhen Municipal Science, Technology and Innovation Commission (No. JCYJ 20190808161013492).

REFERENCE:

A Jackowski AC, G Burnstock,R R Russell,F Kristek. 1990.The Time Course of Intracranial Pathophysiological Changes Following Experimental Subarachnoid Haemorrhage in the Rat. J Cereb Blood Flow Metab.10(6),835-849 https://doi.org /10.1038/jcbfm.1990.140

Adnan I Qureshi ADM, Daniel F Hanley. 2009.Intracerebral Haemorrhage. Lancet.373(9675),1632-1644 https://doi.org/10.1016/S0140-6736(09)60371-8

Aizawa T. 1971.Subarachnoid Hemorrhage. Nihon Ishikai Zasshi.66(12),1423-1428

Albert M Isaacs MAW, Mark G Hamilton. 2019.Current Update on Treatment Strategies for Idiopathic Normal Pressure Hydrocephalus. Curr Treat Options Neurol.21(12),65 https://doi.org/10.1007/s11940-019-0604-z

Ali I, Silva JC, Liu S, Shultz SR, Kwan P, Jones NC, O'Brien TJ. 2019.Targeting Neurodegeneration to Prevent Post-Traumatic Epilepsy. Neurobiology of Disease. 123, 100-109 https://doi.org/10.1016/j.nbd.2018.08.006

Amélia Mendes LS. 2016.Brain Magnetic Resonance in Status Epilepticus: A Focused Review. Seizure.38,63-67 https://doi.org/10.1016/j.seizure.2016.04.007

Ann C Mckee DHD. 2015.The Neuropathology of Traumatic Brain Injury. Handb Clin Neurol.127,45-66 https://doi.org/10.1016/B978-0-444-52892-6.00004-0

Anne Sofie Munk WW, Nicholas Burdon Bèchet,Ahmed M Eltanahy,Anne Xiaoan Cheng,Björn Sigurdsson,Abdellatif Benraiss,Maarja A Mäe,Benjamin Travis Kress,Douglas H Kelley,Christer Betsholtz,Kjeld Møllgård,Anja Meissner,Maiken Nedergaard,Iben Lundgaard. 2019.Pdgf-B Is Required for Development of the Glymphatic System. Cell Rep.26(11),2955-2969.e2953 https://doi.org/10.1016/j.celrep. 2019.02.050

Arighi A, Di Cristofori A, Fenoglio C, Borsa S, D'Anca M, Fumagalli GG, Locatelli M, Carrabba G, Pietroboni AM, Ghezzi L, Carandini T, Colombi A, Scarioni M, De Riz MA, Serpente M, Rampini PM, Scarpini E, Galimberti D, Bozzali M. 2019.Cerebrospinal Fluid Level of Aquaporin4: A New Window on Glymphatic System Involvement in Neurodegenerative Disease? Journal of Alzheimer's Disease. 69(No.3), 663-669 https://doi.org/10.3233/JAD-190119

Arno Vandebroek MY. 2020.Regulation of Aqp4 in the Central Nervous System. Int J Mol Sci.21(5),1603 https://doi.org/10.3390/ijms21051603

Asseyer S, Schmidt F, Chien C, Scheel M, Ruprecht K, Bellmann-Strobl J, Brandt AU, Paul F. 2018.Pain in Aqp4-Igg-Positive and Mog-Igg-Positive Neuromyelitis Optica Spectrum Disorders. Mult Scler J Exp Transl Clin.4(3),2055217318796684 https:// doi. org/10.1177/2055217318796684

Ayzenberg I, Richter D, Henke E, Asseyer S, Paul F, Trebst C, Hümmert MW, Havla J, Kümpfel T, Ringelstein M, Aktas O, Wildemann B, Jarius S, Häußler V, Stellmann JP, Senel M, Klotz L, Pellkofer HL, Weber MS, Pawlitzki M, Rommer PS, Berthele A, Wernecke KD, Hellwig K, Gold R, Kleiter I. 2021.Pain, Depression, and Quality of Life in Neuromyelitis Optica Spectrum Disorder: A Cross-Sectional Study of 166 Aqp4 Antibody-Seropositive Patients. Neurol Neuroimmunol Neuroinflamm.8(3) https: // doi. org/10.1212/nxi.0000000000000985

Basant R. Nassar B, Carol F. Lippa M. 2016. Idiopathic Normal Pressure Hydrocephalus: A Review for General Practitioners. Gerontology and Geriatric Medicine (3) https://doi.org/10.1177/2333721416643702

Benjamin L Brett RCG, Jonathan Godbout, Kristen Dams-O'Connor,C Dirk Keene. 2022.Traumatic Brain Injury and Risk of Neurodegenerative Disorder. Biol Psychiatry.91(5),498-507 https://doi.org/10.1016/j.biopsych.2021.05.025

Benjamin T Kress JJI, Maosheng Xia,Minghuan Wang,Helen S Wei,Douglas Zeppenfeld, Lulu Xie,Hongyi Kang,Qiwu Xu,Jason A Liew,Benjamin A Plog,Fengfei Ding, Rashid Deane,Maiken Nedergaard. 2014.Impairment of Paravascular Clearance Pathways in the Aging Brain. Ann Neurol.76(6),845-861 https://doi.org/10.1002/ana. 24271

Bhavpreet S Dham KH, Fred Rincon. 2014.The Epidemiology of Status

Epilepticus in the United States. Neurocrit Care.20(3),476-483 https://doi.org/10.1007/s12028-013-9935-x

Brana Rosic DBD, Knut Sindre Åbjørsbråten,Wannan Tang,Vidar Jensen,Ole Petter Ottersen, Rune Enger, Erlend A Nagelhus. 2019.Aquaporin-4-Independent Volume Dynamics of Astroglial Endfeet During Cortical Spreading Depression. Glia.67(6),1113-1121 https://doi.org/10.1002/glia.23604

Brhane Teklebrhan Assefa AKG, Birhanetensay Masresha Altaye. 2018.Reactive Astrocytes as Drug Target in Alzheimer's Disease. Biomed Res Int.2018,4160247 https://doi.org/10.1155/2018/4160247

C L Sudlow CPW. 1997.Comparable Studies of the Incidence of Stroke and Its Pathological Types: Results from an International Collaboration. International Stroke Incidence Collaboration. Stroke.28(3),491-499 https://doi.org/10.1161/01.str.28.3.491

Carnero Contentti E, Correale JD. 2021.Neuromyelitis Optica Spectrum Disorders: From Pathophysiology to Therapeutic Strategies. Journal of Neuroinflammation. 18(No.1),208 https://doi.org/10.1186/s12974-021-02249-1

Chandra A, Farrell C, Wilson H, b, Dervenoulas G, c, de Natale ER, b, Politis M, b, Initiative AsDN. 2021.Aquaporin-4 Polymorphisms Predict Amyloid Burden and Clinical Outcome in the Alzheimer's Disease Spectrum. Neurobiology of aging.97,1-9 https://doi.org/10.1016/j.neurobiolaging.2020.06.007

Changwu Tan XW, Yuchang Wang, Chuansen Wang,Zhi Tang,Zhiping Zhang, Jingping Liu,Gelei Xiao. 2021.The Pathogenesis Based on the Glymphatic System, Diagnosis, and Treatment of Idiopathic Normal Pressure Hydrocephalus. Clin Interv Aging.16,139-153 https://doi.org/10.2147/CIA.S290709

Chi Y, Fan Y, He L, Liu W, Wen X, Zhou S, Wang X, Zhang C, Kong H, Sonoda L, Tripathi P, Li CJ, Yu MS, Su C, Hu G. 2011.Novel Role of Aquaporin-4 in Cd4+ Cd25+ T Regulatory Cell Development and Severity of Parkinson's Disease. Aging Cell.10(3),368-382 https://doi.org/10.1111/j.1474-9726.2011.00677.x

Claudia Silberstein RB, Yan Huang,Pingke Fang,Nuria Pastor-Soler,Dennis Brown,Alfred N Van Hoek. 2004.Membrane Organization and Function of M1 and M23 Isoforms of Aquaporin-4 in Epithelial Cells. Am J Physiol Renal Physiol.287(3),F501-511 https://doi.org/10.1152/ajprenal.00439.2003

Collongues N, Seze Jd. 2011.Current and Future Treatment Approaches for Neuromyelitis Optica. Therapeutic advances in neurological disorders.4(No.2),111-121 https://doi.org/10.1177/1756285611398939

Cui H, Wang W, Zheng X, Xia D, Liu H, Qin C, Tian H, Teng J. 2021.Decreased Aqp4 Expression Aggravates ɑ-Synuclein Pathology in Parkinson's Disease Mice, Possibly Via Impaired Glymphatic Clearance. J Mol Neurosci.71(12),2500-2513 https:// doi.org/10.1007/s12031-021-01836-4

Daneman R, Prat A. 2015.The Blood-Brain Barrier. Cold Spring Harb Perspect

Biol.7(1), a020412 https://doi.org/10.1101/cshperspect.a020412

Daniela Boassa AJY. 2005.Physiological Roles of Aquaporins in the Choroid Plexus. Curr Top Dev Biol.67,181-206 https://doi.org/10.1016/S0070-2153(05)67005-6

Dhamidhu Eratne SML, Sarah Farrand,Wendy Kelso,Dennis Velakoulis,Jeffrey Cl Looi. 2018.Alzheimer's Disease: Clinical Update on Epidemiology, Pathophysiology and Diagnosis. Australas Psychiatry.26(4),347-357 https://doi.org/10.1177/ 103985621 8762308

Diamond S. 1991.Migraine Headaches. Med Clin North Am.75(3),545-566 https://doi.org/10.1016/S0025-7125(16)30432-1

E Liu XP, Haowen Ma,Yan Zhang,Xiaomei Yang,Yixuan Zhang,Linlin Sun,Junhao Yan. 2020.The Involvement of Aquaporin-4 in the Interstitial Fluid Drainage Impairment Following Subarachnoid Hemorrhage. Front Aging Neurosci.12,611494 https://doi.org/ 10.3389/fnagi.2020.611494

E S McCoy BRH, H Sontheimer. 2010.Water Permeability through Aquaporin-4 Is Regulated by Protein Kinase C and Becomes Rate-Limiting for Glioma Invasion. Neuroscience.168(4),971-981 https://doi.org/10.1016/j.neuroscience.2009.09.020

Elithorn A. 1969.Migraine. Br Med J.4(5680),411-413 https://doi.org/ 10.1136/ bmj. 4.5680.411

Erik N T P Bakker BJB, Michal Arbel-Ornath,Roxana Aldea,Beatrice Bedussi,Alan W J Morris,Roy O Weller,Roxana O Carare. 2016.Lymphatic Clearance of the Brain: Perivascular, Paravascular and Significance for Neurodegenerative Diseases. Cell Mol Neurobiol.36(2),181-194 https://doi.org/10.1007/s10571-015-0273-8

Erlend A Nagelhus OPO. 2013.Physiological Roles of Aquaporin-4 in Brain. Physiol Rev.93(4),1543-1562 https://doi.org/10.1152/physrev.00011.2013

Etsuro Mori MI, Takeo Kato,Hiroaki Kazui,Hiroji Miyake,Masakazu Miyajima,Madoka Nakajima,Masaaki Hashimoto,Nagato Kuriyama,Takahiko Tokuda,Kazunari Ishii,Mitsunobu Kaijima,Yoshihumi Hirata,Makoto Saito,Hajime Arai,. 2012.Guidelines for Management of Idiopathic Normal Pressure Hydrocephalus: Second Edition. Neurol Med Chir (Tokyo).52(11),775-809 https://doi.org/10.2176/nmc.52.775

Fang Y, Dai S, Jin C, Si X, Gu L, Song Z, Gao T, Chen Y, Yan Y, Yin X, Pu J, Zhang B. 2021.Aquaporin-4 Polymorphisms Are Associated with Cognitive Performance in Parkinson's Disease. Front Aging Neurosci.13,740491 https://doi.org/10.3389/ fnagi. 2021.740491

Feng Gu RH, Kazuko Toku,Lihua Yang,Yong-Jie Ma,Nobuji Maeda,Masahiro Sakanaka,Junya Tanaka. 2003.Testosterone up-Regulates Aquaporin-4 Expression in Cultured Astrocytes. J Neurosci Res.72(6),709-715 https://doi.org/10.1002/jnr.10603

G P Nicchia AR, M G Mola,F Pisani,C Stigliano,D Basco,M Mastrototaro,M Svelto, A Frigeri. 2010.Higher Order Structure of Aquaporin-4. Neuroscience. 168(4), 903-91 https://doi.org/10.1016/j.neuroscience.2010.02.008

G V Gavrilov AVS, B V Gaydar,N M Paramonova,O N Gaykova,D V Svistov. 2019.Pathological Changes in Human Brain Biopsies from Patients with Idiopathic Normal Pressure Hydrocephalus. Zh Nevrol Psikhiatr Im S S Korsakova.119(3),50-54 https://doi.org/10.17116/jnevro201911903150

Gaberel T, Gakuba C, Goulay R, Martinez De Lizarrondo S, Hanouz JL, Emery E, Touze E, Vivien D, Gauberti M. 2014.Impaired Glymphatic Perfusion after Strokes Revealed by Contrast-Enhanced Mri: A New Target for Fibrinolysis? Stroke.45(10),3092-3096 https://doi.org/10.1161/strokeaha.114.006617

Geir Ringstad LMV, Anders M Dale,Are H Pripp,Svein-Are S Vatnehol, Kyrre E Emblem, Kent-Andre Mardal,Per K Eide. 2018.Brain-Wide Glymphatic Enhancement and Clearance in Humans Assessed with Mri. JCI Insight.3(13),M 29997300 https://doi.org/10.1172/jci.insight.121537

George PM, Steinberg GK. 2015.Novel Stroke Therapeutics: Unraveling Stroke Pathophysiology and Its Impact on Clinical Treatments. Neuron.87(2),297-309 https://doi.org/10.1016/j.neuron.2015.05.041

Gijn Jv. 1992.Subarachnoid Haemorrhage. Lancet.339(8794),653-655 https:// doi. org /10.1016/0140-6736(92)90803-B

Giridhar Murlidharan AC, Rebecca A Reardon,Juan Song,Aravind Asokan. 2016. Glymphatic Fluid Transport Controls Paravascular Clearance of Aav Vectors from the Brain. JCI Insight.1(14),e88034 https://doi.org/10.1172/jci.insight.88034

Goldman N, Hablitz LM, Mori Y, Nedergaard M. 2020.The Glymphatic System and Pain. Med Acupunct.32(6),373-376 https://doi.org/10.1089/acu.2020.1489

Gratwicke J, Jahanshahi M, Foltynie T. 2015.Parkinson's Disease Dementia: A Neural Networks Perspective. Brain.138(Pt 6),1454-1476 https://doi.org/10.1093/ brain/ awv104

H B Moeller RAF, T Zeuthen,N Macaulay. 2009.Vasopressin-Dependent Short-Term Regulation of Aquaporin 4 Expressed in Xenopus Oocytes. Neuroscience.164(4),1674-1684 https://doi.org/10.1016/j.neuroscience.2009.09.072

Han F, Brown GL, Zhu Y, Belkin-Rosen AE, Lewis MM, Du G, Gu Y, Eslinger PJ, Mailman RB, Huang X, Liu X. 2021.Decoupling of Global Brain Activity and Cerebrospinal Fluid Flow in Parkinson's Disease Cognitive Decline. Mov Disord. 36(9), 2066-2076 https://doi.org/10.1002/mds.28643

Hana Park S-HC, Min-Jeong Kong,Tae-Cheon Kang. 2019.Dysfunction of 67-Kda Laminin Receptor Disrupts Bbb Integrity Via Impaired Dystrophin/Aqp4 Complex and P38 Mapk/Vegf Activation Following Status Epilepticus. Front Cell Neurosci.13,236 https://doi.org/10.3389/fncel.2019.00236

Hanwool Jeon MK, Wonhyoung Park,Joon Seo Lim,Eunyeup Lee,Hyeuk Cha,Jae Sung Ahn,Jeong Hoon Kim,Seok Ho Hong,Ji Eun Park, Eun-Jae Lee,Chul-Woong Woo,Seungjoo Lee. 2021.Upregulation of Aqp4 Improves Blood-Brain Barrier Integrity and Perihematomal Edema Following Intracerebral Hemorrhage. Neurotherapeutics. 18(4),2692-2706 https://doi.org/10.1007/s13311-021-01126-2

Haohai Huang DL, Liping Liang,Lijun Song,Wenchang Zhao. 2015.Genistein Inhibits Rotavirus Replication and Upregulates Aqp4 Expression in Rotavirus-Infected Caco-2 Cells. Arch Virol.160(6),1421-1433 https://doi.org/10.1007/s00705-015-2404-4

Hardman JM. 1979.The Pathology of Traumatic Brain Injuries. Adv Neurol.22,15-50

Hartwig Wolburg KW-B, Petra Fallier-Becker,Susan Noell,Andreas F Mack. 2011.Structure and Functions of Aquaporin-4-Based Orthogonal Arrays of Particles. Int Rev Cell Mol Biol.287,1-41 https://doi.org/10.1016/B978-0-12-386043-9.00001-3

He Wu TW, Xueying Xu,Jessica Wang,Jian Wang. 2011.Iron Toxicity in Mice with Collagenase-Induced Intracerebral Hemorrhage. J Cereb Blood Flow Metab.31(5),1243-1250 https://doi.org/10.1038/jcbfm.2010.209

Henderson MX, Trojanowski JQ, Lee VM. 2019.A-Synuclein Pathology in Parkinson's Disease and Related A-Synucleinopathies. Neurosci Lett.709,134316 https://doi.org/10.1016/j.neulet.2019.134316

Hofman P, Hoyng P, vanderWerf F, Vrensen GF, Schlingemann RO. 2001.Lack of Blood-Brain Barrier Properties in Microvessels of the Prelaminar Optic Nerve Head. Investigative ophthalmology & visual science.42(No.5),895-901

Hubbard J, Hsu M, Seldin M, Binder D. 2015.Expression of the Astrocyte Water Channel Aquaporin-4 in the Mouse Brain. ASN Neuro.7(No.5) https://doi.org/10.1177 /1759091415605486

Hui Tang CS, Jiaquan He. 2017.Down-Regulated Expression of Aquaporin-4 in the Cerebellum after Status Epilepticus. Cogn Neurodyn.11(2),183-188 https://doi.org/ 10.1007/s11571-016-9420-2

Humberto Mestre LMH, Anna Lr Xavier,Weixi Feng,Wenyan Zou,Tinglin Pu,Hiromu Monai,Giridhar Murlidharan,Ruth M Castellanos Rivera,Matthew J Simon,Martin M Pike,Virginia Plá,Ting Du,Benjamin T Kress,Xiaowen Wang,Benjamin A Plog,Alexander S Thrane,Iben Lundgaard,Yoichiro Abe,Masato Yasui,John H Thomas, Ming Xiao, Hajime Hirase,Aravind Asokan,Jeffrey J Iliff,Maiken Nedergaard. 2018.Aquaporin-4-Dependent Glymphatic Solute Transport in the Rodent Brain. Elife.7,M 30561329 https://doi.org/10.7554/eLife.40070

Iadecola C. 2013.The Pathobiology of Vascular Dementia. Neuron.80(4),844-866 https://doi.org/10.1016/j.neuron.2013.10.008

Iliff JJDoGD, Therapeutics CfTN, Department of Neurosurgery, University of

Rochester Medical Center, Rochester, NY, US, iliffj@ohsu.edu, Chen MJDoGD, Therapeutics CfTN, Department of Neurosurgery, University of Rochester Medical Center, Rochester, NY, US, Plog BADoGD, Therapeutics CfTN, Department of Neurosurgery, University of Rochester Medical Center, Rochester, NY, US, Zeppenfeld DMDoA, Peri-Operative Medicine OH, Science University P, OR, US, Soltero MDoA, Peri-Operative Medicine OH, Science University P, OR, US, Yang LDoGD, Therapeutics CfTN, Department of Neurosurgery, University of Rochester Medical Center, Rochester, NY, US, Singh IDoGD, Therapeutics CfTN, Department of Neurosurgery, University of Rochester Medical Center, Rochester, NY, US, Deane RDoGD, Therapeutics CfTN, Department of Neurosurgery, University of Rochester Medical Center, Rochester, NY, US, Nedergaard MDoGD, Therapeutics CfTN, Department of Neurosurgery, University of Rochester Medical Center, Rochester, NY, US. 2014.Impairment of Glymphatic Pathway Function Promotes Tau Pathology after Traumatic Brain Injury. The Journal of Neuroscience.Vol.34(No.49),16180-16193 https://doi.org/10.1523/JNEUROSCI.3020-14.2014

Ionica Pirici TAB, Catalin Bogdan,Claudiu Margaritescu,Tamir Divan,Vacaras Vitalie,Laurentiu Mogoanta,Daniel Pirici,Roxana Octavia Carare,Dafin Fior Muresanu. 2017.Inhibition of Aquaporin-4 Improves the Outcome of Ischaemic Stroke and Modulates Brain Paravascular Drainage Pathways. Int J Mol Sci.19(1),M29295526 https: //doi.org/10.3390/ijms19010046

Iorio RDoLM, Mayo Clinic College of Medicine, Rochester, MN, US, Lucchinetti CFDoN, Mayo Clinic College of Medicine, Rochester, MN, US, Lennon VADoN, Mayo Clinic College of Medicine, Rochester, MN, US, Costanzi CDoN, Mayo Clinic College of Medicine, Rochester, MN, US, Hinson SDoLM, Mayo Clinic College of Medicine, Rochester, MN, US, Weinshenker BGDoN, Mayo Clinic College of Medicine, Rochester, MN, US, Pittock SJDoLM, Mayo Clinic College of Medicine, Rochester, MN, US, pittock.sean@mayo.edu. 2011.Syndrome of Inappropriate Antidiuresis May Herald or Accompany Neuromyelitis Optica. Neurology.Vol.77(No.17),1644-1646 https://doi.org/ 10.1212/WNL.0b013e3182343377

Ishikura T, Kinoshita M, Shimizu M, Yasumizu Y, Motooka D, Okuzaki D, Yamashita K, Murata H, Beppu S, Koda T, Tada S, Shiraishi N, Sugiyama Y, Miyamoto K, Kusunoki S, Sugimoto T, Kumanogoh A, Okuno T, Mochizuki H. 2021.Anti-Aqp4 Autoantibodies Promote Atp Release from Astrocytes and Induce Mechanical Pain in Rats. J Neuroinflammation.18(1),181 https://doi.org/10.1186/s12974-021-02232-w

Izumi Kawachi, Lassmann H. 2017.Neurodegeneration in Multiple Sclerosis and Neuromyelitis Optica. Journal of Neurology, Neurosurgery & Psychiatry. Vol.88(No.2), 137-145 https://doi.org/10.1136/jnnp-2016-313300

J E Rash TY, C S Hudson,P Agre,S Nielsen. 1998.Direct Immunogold Labeling of

Aquaporin-4 in Square Arrays of Astrocyte and Ependymocyte Plasma Membranes in Rat Brain and Spinal Cord. Proc Natl Acad Sci U S A.95(20),11981-11986 https://doi.org/10.1073/pnas.95.20.11981

Jeffrey J Iliff HL, Mei Yu,Tian Feng,Jean Logan,Maiken Nedergaard,Helene Benveniste. 2013.Brain-Wide Pathway for Waste Clearance Captured by Contrast-Enhanced Mri. J Clin Invest.123(3),1299-1309 https://doi.org/10.1172/JCI67677

Jeffrey J. Iliff MW, 1,2 Yonghong Liao,1 2012.A Paravascular Pathway Facilitates Csf Flow through the Brain Parenchyma and the Clearance of Interstitial Solutes, Including Amyloid B. CEREBROSPINAL FLUID C I RCULATION. 4(No.147), 147ra111 https://doi.org/10.1126/scitranslmed.3003748

Jérôme Badaut AMF, Amandine Jullienne,Klaus G Petry. 2014.Aquaporin and Brain Diseases. Biochim Biophys Acta.1840(5),1554-1565 https://doi.org/10.1016/j.bbagen. 2013.10.032

Jesse A Stokum DBK, Volodymyr Gerzanich,J Marc Simard. 2015.Mechanisms of Astrocyte-Mediated Cerebral Edema. Neurochem Res.40(2),317-328 https://doi.org/10.1007/s11064-014-1374-3

Jessen NA, Munk ASF, Lundgaard I, Nedergaard M. 2015.The Glymphatic System: A Beginner's Guide(Article). Neurochemical Research (No.12),2583-2599 https://doi.org /10.1007/s11064-015-1581-6

Ji RR, Donnelly CR, Nedergaard M. 2019.Astrocytes in Chronic Pain and Itch. Nat Rev Neurosci.20(11),667-685 https://doi.org/10.1038/s41583-019-0218-1

Jiang C, Wang ZN, Kang YC, Chen Y, Lu WX, Ren HJ, Hou BR. 2022.Ki20227 Aggravates Apoptosis, Inflammatory Response, and Oxidative Stress after Focal Cerebral Ischemia Injury. Neural Regen Res.17(1),137-143 https://doi.org/ 10.4103/1673-5374.314318

Jolobe OM, 2007. Subarachnoid Haemorrhage, Vol 369, 904 p.

Jose A Soria Lopez HMG, Gabriel C Léger. 2019.Alzheimer's Disease. Handb Clin Neurol.167,231-255 https://doi.org/10.1016/B978-0-12-804766-8.00013-3

K Oshio DKB, B Yang,S Schecter,A S Verkman,G T Manley. 2004.Expression of Aquaporin Water Channels in Mouse Spinal Cord. Neuroscience.127(3),685-693 https://doi.org/10.1016/j.neuroscience.2004.03.016

Kang H, Qiu H, Hu X, Wei S, Tao Y. 2022.Differences in Neuropathic Pain and Radiological Features between Aqp4-on, Mog-on, and Idon. Front Pain Res (Lausanne). 3,870211 https://doi.org/10.3389/fpain.2022.870211

Kara N Corps TLR, Dorian B McGavern. 2015.Inflammation and Neuroprotection in Traumatic Brain Injury. JAMA Neurol.72(3),355-362 https://doi.org/10.1001/jamaneurol.2014.3558

Kewei Liu JZ, Yuan Chang,Zhenzhou Lin,Zhu Shi,Xing Li,Xing Chen,Chuman Lin,Suyue Pan,Kaibin Huang. 2021.Attenuation of Cerebral Edema Facilitates

Recovery of Glymphatic System Function after Status Epilepticus. JCI Insight.6(17),M 34494549 https://doi.org/10.1172/jci.insight.151835

Khalil S Husari KL, Rong Huang,Rana R Said. 2020.New-Onset Refractory Status Epilepticus in Children: Etiologies, Treatments, and Outcomes. Pediatr Crit Care Med. 21(1),59-66 https://doi.org/10.1097/PCC.0000000000002108

Kjersti N Power AG, Nils Erik Gilhus,Karl Ove Hufthammer,Bernt A Engelsen. 2018.Cognitive Function after Status Epilepticus Versus after Multiple Generalized Tonic-Clonic Seizures. Epilepsy Res.140,39-45 https://doi.org/10.1016/j.eplepsyres. 2017.11.014

Koga M, Takahashi T, Kawai M, Fujihara K, Kanda T. 2011.A Serological Analysis of Viral and Bacterial Infections Associated with Neuromyelitis Optica. Journal of the neurological sciences.Vol.300(No.1-2),19-22 https://doi.org/10.1016/j.jns.2010.10.013

Kotaro Oshio HW, Yaunlin Song, A S Verkman,Geoffrey T Manley. 2005.Reduced Cerebrospinal Fluid Production and Intracranial Pressure in Mice Lacking Choroid Plexus Water Channel Aquaporin-1. FASEB J.19(1),76-78 https://doi.org/ 10.1096/ fj.04-1711fje

Küppers E, Gleiser C, Brito V, Wachter B, Pauly T, Hirt B, Grissmer S. 2008.Aqp4 Expression in Striatal Primary Cultures Is Regulated by Dopamine--Implications for Proliferation of Astrocytes. Eur J Neurosci.28(11),2173-2182 https://doi.org/10.1111/ j.1460-9568.2008.06531.x

Lecordier S, Manrique-Castano D, El Moghrabi Y, ElAli A. 2021.Neurovascular Alterations in Vascular Dementia: Emphasis on Risk Factors. Front Aging Neurosci.13,727590 https://doi.org/10.3389/fnagi.2021.727590

Li TT, Wan Q, Zhang X, Xiao Y, Sun LY, Zhang YR, Liu XN, Yang WC. 2022.Stellate Ganglion Block Reduces Inflammation and Improves Neurological Function in Diabetic Rats During Ischemic Stroke. Neural Regen Res.17(9),1991-1997 https://doi.org/10.4103/1673-5374.335162

Lu G, Pang C, Chen Y, Wu N, Li J. 2020.Aquaporin 4 Is Involved in Chronic Pain but Not Acute Pain. Behav Brain Res.393,112810 https://doi.org/ 10.1016/j.bbr. 2020. 112810

Madoka Nakajima MM, Ikuko Ogino,Chihiro Akiba,Kaito Kawamura,Chihiro Kamohara,Keiko Fusegi,Yoshinao Harada,Takeshi Hara,Hidenori Sugano,Yuichi Tange,Kostadin Karagiozov,Kensaku Kasuga,Takeshi Ikeuchi,Takahiko Tokuda,Hajime Arai. 2018.Preoperative Phosphorylated Tau Concentration in the Cerebrospinal Fluid Can Predict Cognitive Function Three Years after Shunt Surgery in Patients with Idiopathic Normal Pressure Hydrocephalus. J Alzheimers Dis. 66(1), 319-331 https://doi. org/10.3233/JAD-180557

Mai CL, Tan Z, Xu YN, Zhang JJ, Huang ZH, Wang D, Zhang H, Gui WS, Zhang J, Lin ZJ, Meng YT, Wei X, Jie YT, Grace PM, Wu LJ, Zhou LJ, Liu XG. 2021.Cxcl12-

Mediated Monocyte Transmigration into Brain Perivascular Space Leads to Neuroinflammation and Memory Deficit in Neuropathic Pain. Theranostics. 11(3), 1059-1078 https://doi.org/10.7150/thno.44364

Manuela de Bellis AC, Maria Grazia Mola,Francesco Pisani,Barbara Barile,Maria Mastrodonato,Shervin Banitalebi,Mahmood Amiry-Moghaddam, Pasqua Abbrescia, Antonio Frigeri, Maria Svelto,Grazia Paola Nicchia. 2021.Orthogonal Arrays of Particle Assembly Are Essential for Normal Aquaporin-4 Expression Level in the Brain. Glia. 69(2),473-488 https://doi.org/10.1002/glia.23909

Martin Kaag Rasmussen HM, Maiken Nedergaard. 2018.The Glymphatic Pathway in Neurological Disorders. Lancet Neurol.17(11),1016-1024 https://doi.org/ 10.1016/ S1474-4422(18)30318-1

Md Mahdi Hasan-Olive RE, Hans-Arne Hansson, Erlend A Nagelhus, Per Kristian Eide. 2019.Loss of Perivascular Aquaporin-4 in Idiopathic Normal Pressure Hydrocephalus. Glia.67(1),91-100 https://doi.org/10.1002/glia.23528

Melanie-Jane Hannocks MEP, Jula Huppert,Tushar Deshpande,N Joan Abbott, Robert G Thorne, Lydia Sorokin. 2018. Molecular Characterization of Perivascular Drainage Pathways in the Murine Brain. J Cereb Blood Flow Metab. 38(4), 669-686 https://doi.org/10.1177/0271678X17749689

Michael A Williams JM. 2016.Diagnosis and Treatment of Idiopathic Normal Pressure Hydrocephalus. Continuum (Minneap Minn).Vol.22(No.2),579-599 https:// doi. org/10.1212/CON.0000000000000305

Michel D Ferrari PJG, Rami Burstein,Tobias Kurth,Cenk Ayata,Andrew Charles,Messoud Ashina,Arn M J M van den Maagdenberg,David W Dodick. 2022. Migraine.Nat Rev Dis Primers.8(1),2 https://doi.org/10.1038/s41572-022-00335-z

Monica Carmosino GP, Grazia Tamma,Roberta Mannucci,Maria Svelto,Giovanna Valenti. 2007.Trafficking and Phosphorylation Dynamics of Aqp4 in Histamine-Treated Human Gastric Cells. Biol Cell.99(1),25-36 https://doi.org/10.1042/BC2006 0068

Morgan Robinson BYL, Francis T Hane. 2017.Recent Progress in Alzheimer's Disease Research, Part 2: Genetics and Epidemiology. J Alzheimers Dis.57(2),317-330 https://doi.org/10.3233/JAD-161149

Nadia Aalling Jessen ASFM, Iben Lundgaard,Maiken Nedergaard. 2015.The Glymphatic System: A Beginner's Guide. Neurochem Res.40(12),2583-2599 https:// doi. org/10.1007/s11064-015-1581-6

O'Brien JT, Thomas A. 2015.Vascular Dementia. Lancet.386(10004),1698-1706 https://doi.org/10.1016/s0140-6736(15)00463-8

Per K Eide GR. 2019.Delayed Clearance of Cerebrospinal Fluid Tracer from Entorhinal Cortex in Idiopathic Normal Pressure Hydrocephalus: A Glymphatic Magnetic Resonance Imaging Study. J Cereb Blood Flow Metab.39(7),1355-1368 https://doi.org/10.1177/0271678X18760974

Pu T, Zou W, Feng W, Zhang Y, Wang L, Wang H, Xiao M. 2019.Persistent Malfunction of Glymphatic and Meningeal Lymphatic Drainage in a Mouse Model of Subarachnoid Hemorrhage. Experimental Neurobiology.Vol.28(No.1),104-118 https://doi.org/ 10.5607/en.2019.28.1.104

Qi Lu JX, Yuan Yuan,Zhanwei Ruan,Yu Zhang,Bo Chai,Lei Li,Shufang Cai,Jian Xiao,Yanqing Wu,Peng Huang,Hongyu Zhang. 2022.Minocycline Improves the Functional Recovery after Traumatic Brain Injury Via Inhibition of Aquaporin-4. Int J Biol Sci.18(1),441-458 https://doi.org/10.7150/ijbs.64187

Qiaoli Ma BVI, Michael Detmar,Steven T Proulx. 2017.Outflow of Cerebrospinal Fluid Is Predominantly through Lymphatic Vessels and Is Reduced in Aged Mice. Nat Commun.8(1),1434 https://doi.org/10.1038/s41467-017-01484-6

R Bonita ST. 1985.Subarachnoid Hemorrhage: Epidemiology, Diagnosis, Management, and Outcome. Stroke.16(4),591-594 https://doi.org/10.1161/01.STR. 16.4. 591

Richard F Keep YH, Guohua Xi. 2012.Intracerebral Haemorrhage: Mechanisms of Injury and Therapeutic Targets. Lancet Neurol.11(8),720-731 https://doi.org/10.1016/ S1474- 4422 (12)70104-7

S Nielsen EAN, M Amiry-Moghaddam,C Bourque,P Agre,O P Ottersen. 1997.Specialized Membrane Domains for Water Transport in Glial Cells: High-Resolution Immunogold Cytochemistry of Aquaporin-4 in Rat Brain. J Neurosci.17(1),171-180 https://doi.org/10.1523/jneurosci.17-01-00171.1997

Schain AJ, Melo-Carrillo A, Strassman AM, Burstein R. 2017.Cortical Spreading Depression Closes Paravascular Space and Impairs Glymphatic Flow: Implications for Migraine Headache. J Neurosci.37(11),2904-2915 https://doi.org/10.1523/ jneurosci. 3390-16.2017

Scott-Massey A, Boag MK, Magnier A, Bispo D, Khoo TK, Pountney DL. 2022.Glymphatic System Dysfunction and Sleep Disturbance May Contribute to the Pathogenesis and Progression of Parkinson's Disease. Int J Mol Sci.23(21) https://doi.org/10.3390/ijms232112928

Si X, Guo T, Wang Z, Fang Y, Gu L, Cao L, Yang W, Gao T, Song Z, Tian J, Yin X, Guan X, Zhou C, Wu J, Bai X, Liu X, Zhao G, Zhang M, Pu J, Zhang B. 2022.Neuroimaging Evidence of Glymphatic System Dysfunction in Possible Rem Sleep Behavior Disorder and Parkinson's Disease. NPJ Parkinsons Dis.8(1),54 https://doi.org/ 10.1038/s41531-022-00316-9

Stephen B Hladky MAB. 2014.Mechanisms of Fluid Movement into, through and out of the Brain: Evaluation of the Evidence. Fluids Barriers CNS.11(1),26 https:// doi.org/10.1186/2045-8118-11-26

Sucha P, Hermanova Z, Chmelova M, Kirdajova D, Camacho Garcia S, Marchetti

V, Vorisek I, Tureckova J, Shany E, Jirak D, Anderova M, Vargova L. 2022.The Absence of Aqp4/Trpv4 Complex Substantially Reduces Acute Cytotoxic Edema Following Ischemic Injury. Front Cell Neurosci.16,1054919 https://doi.org/10.3389/ fncel.2022. 1054919

Sun C, Lin L, Yin L, Hao X, Tian J, Zhang X, Ren Y, Li C, Yang Y. 2022.Acutely Inhibiting Aqp4 with Tgn-020 Improves Functional Outcome by Attenuating Edema and Peri-Infarct Astrogliosis after Cerebral Ischemia. Front Immunol.13,870029 https:// doi.org/10.3389/fimmu.2022.870029

T Haenggi J-MF. 2006.Role of Dystrophin and Utrophin for Assembly and Function of the Dystrophin Glycoprotein Complex in Non-Muscle Tissue. Cell Mol Life Sci. 63 (14),1614-1631 https://doi.org/10.1007/s00018-005-5461-0

Takano T, Tian GF, Peng W, Lou N, Lovatt D, Hansen AJ, Kasischke KA, Nedergaard M. 2007.Cortical Spreading Depression Causes and Coincides with Tissue Hypoxia. Nat Neurosci.10(6),754-762 https://doi.org/10.1038/nn1902

Taylor JP, Hardy J, Fischbeck KH. 2002.Toxic Proteins in Neurodegenerative Disease. Science.296(5575),1991-1995 https://doi.org/10.1126/science.1067122

Tfelt-Hansen P. 1994.Migraine--Diagnosis and Pathophysiology. Pharmacol Toxicol.75 Suppl 2,72-75 https://doi.org/10.1111/j.1600-0773.1994.tb02003.x

Thomas Misje Mathiisen KPL, Niels Christian Danbolt,Ole Petter Ottersen. 2010.The Perivascular Astroglial Sheath Provides a Complete Covering of the Brain Microvessels: An Electron Microscopic 3d Reconstruction. Glia.58(9),1094-1103

Thomas Walz YF, Andreas Engel. 2009.The Aqp Structure and Functional Implications. Handb Exp Pharmacol (190),31-56

Toh CH, Siow TY. 2021.Glymphatic Dysfunction in Patients with Ischemic Stroke. Front Aging Neurosci.13,756249 https://doi.org/10.3389/fnagi.2021.756249

Ueno M, Chiba Y, Murakami R, Matsumoto K, Fujihara R, Uemura N, Yanase K, Kamada M. 2019.Disturbance of Intracerebral Fluid Clearance and Blood-Brain Barrier in Vascular Cognitive Impairment. Int J Mol Sci.20(10) https://doi.org/ 10.3390/ ijms 20102600

Venkat P, Culmone L, Chopp M, Landschoot-Ward J, Wang F, Zacharek A, Chen J. 2020.Hucbc Treatment Improves Cognitive Outcome in Rats with Vascular Dementia. Front Aging Neurosci.12,258 https://doi.org/10.3389/fnagi.2020.00258

Verkman AS, Phuan P-W, Zhang H, Papadopoulos MC, Lam C, Bennett JL, Saadoun S, Tradtrantip L. 2012.Anti–Aquaporin-4 Monoclonal Antibody Blocker Therapy for Neuromyelitis Optica. Annals of Neurology.Vol.71(No.3),314-322 https://doi.org/10. 1002/ana.22657

Vincent J Huber HI, Satoshi Ueki,Ingrid L Kwee,Tsutomu Nakada. 2018.Aquaporin-4 Facilitator Tgn-073 Promotes Interstitial Fluid Circulation within the Blood-Brain Barrier: [17o]H2o Jjvcpe Mri Study. Neuroreport.29(9),697-703 https://doi.org/ 10.1097/WNR.0000000000000990

Walter K, 2022. What Is Migraine?, Vol 327, 93 p.

Wang A, Chen L, Tian C, Yin X, Wang X, Zhao Y, Zhang M, Yang L, Ye Z. 2022a.Evaluation of the Glymphatic System with Diffusion Tensor Imaging-Along the Perivascular Space in Cancer Pain. Front Neurosci.16,823701 https://doi.org/ 10.3389 /fnins.2022.823701

Wang R, Zhang X, Zhang J, Fan Y, Shen Y, Hu W, Chen Z. 2012.Oxygen-Glucose Deprivation Induced Glial Scar-Like Change in Astrocytes. PLoS One.7(5),e37574 https://doi.org/10.1371/journal.pone.0037574

Wang Y, Huang C, Guo Q, Chu H. 2022b.Aquaporin-4 and Cognitive Disorders. Aging Dis.13(1),61-72 https://doi.org/10.14336/ad.2021.0731

Wang Y, Huang J, Ma Y, Tang G, Liu Y, Chen X, Zhang Z, Zeng L, Wang Y, Ouyang YB, Yang GY. 2015.Microrna-29b Is a Therapeutic Target in Cerebral Ischemia Associated with Aquaporin 4. J Cereb Blood Flow Metab.35(12),1977-1984 https:// doi.org/10.1038/jcbfm.2015.156

Wang YJ, Sun YR, Pei YH, Ma HW, Mu YK, Qin LH, Yan JH. 2023.The Lymphatic Drainage Systems in the Brain: A Novel Target for Ischemic Stroke? Neural Regen Res.18(3),485-491 https://doi.org/10.4103/1673-5374.346484

William Qubty IP. 2020.Migraine Pathophysiology. Pediatr Neurol.107,1-6 https:// doi.org/10.1016/j.pediatrneurol.2019.12.014

Xiaoling Zhang XM, Yanxia Li,Weiheng Yan,Quan Zheng,Lili Li,Yulan Yan,Xiaozhi Liu,Jun Zheng. 2020.Dexamethasone Upregulates the Expression of Aquaporin4 by Increasing Sumoylation in A549 Cells. Inflammation.43(5),1925-1935 https://doi.org/ 10. 1007/s10753-020-01267-0

Xichang Liu GW, Na Tang,Li Li,Cuimin Liu,Feng Wang,Shaofa Ke. 2021.Glymphatic Drainage Blocking Aggravates Brain Edema, Neuroinflammation Via Modulating Tnf-A, Il-10, and Aqp4 after Intracerebral Hemorrhage in Rats. Front Cell Neurosci.15,784154 https://doi.org/10.3389/fncel.2021.784154

Xu M, Bennett DLH, Querol LA, Wu LJ, Irani SR, Watson JC, Pittock SJ, Klein CJ. 2020.Pain and the Immune System: Emerging Concepts of Igg-Mediated Autoimmune Pain and Immunotherapies. J Neurol Neurosurg Psychiatry.91(2),177-188 https:// doi. org/10.1136/jnnp-2018-318556

Yu-Long Lan J-JC, Gang Hu,Jun Xu,Ming Xiao,Shao Li. 2017.Aquaporin 4 in Astrocytes Is a Target for Therapy in Alzheimer's Disease. Curr Pharm Des.23(33),4948-4957 https://doi.org/10.2174/1381612823666170714144844

Yu P, Venkat P, Chopp M, Zacharek A, Shen Y, Ning R, Liang L, Li W, Zhang L, Landschoot-Ward J, Jiang R, Chen J. 2019.Role of Microrna-126 in Vascular Cognitive Impairment in Mice. J Cereb Blood Flow Metab.39(12),2497-2511 https://doi.org /10. 1177/0271678x18800593

Zbesko JC, Nguyen TV, Yang T, Frye JB, Hussain O, Hayes M, Chung A, Day WA, Stepanovic K, Krumberger M, Mona J, Longo FM, Doyle KP. 2018.Glial Scars Are Permeable to the Neurotoxic Environment of Chronic Stroke Infarcts. Neurobiol Dis. 112, 63-78 https://doi.org/10.1016/j.nbd.2018.01.007

Zelenina M. 2010.Regulation of Brain Aquaporins. Neurochem Int.57(4),468-488 https://doi.org/10.1016/j.neuint.2010.03.022

Zeppenfeld DMB, Simon MB, Haswell JDB, DAbreo D, Murchison CM, Quinn JFM, Grafe MRM, PhD, Woltjer RLM, PhD, Kaye JM, Iliff JJP. 2017.Association of Perivascular Localization of Aquaporin-4 with Cognition and Alzheimer Disease in Aging Brains. JAMA Neurology.Vol.74(No.1),91-99 https://doi.org/10.1001/ jamaneurol. 2016.4370

Zhang J, Yang B, Sun H, Zhou Y, Liu M, Ding J, Fang F, Fan Y, Hu G. 2016.Aquaporin-4 Deficiency Diminishes the Differential Degeneration of Midbrain Dopaminergic Neurons in Experimental Parkinson's Disease. Neurosci Lett.614,7-15 https://doi.org/10.1016/j.neulet.2015.12.057

Zhang X, Levy D, Noseda R, Kainz V, Jakubowski M, Burstein R. 2010.Activation of Meningeal Nociceptors by Cortical Spreading Depression: Implications for Migraine with Aura. J Neurosci.30(26),8807-8814 https://doi.org/10.1523/JNEUROSCI.0511-10.2010

Zhong-Fang Shi QF, Ye Chen,Li-Xin Xu,Min Wu,Mei Jia,Yi Lu,Xiao-Xuan Wang,Yu-Jiao Wang,Xu Yan,Li-Ping Dong,Fang Yuan. 2021.Methylene Blue Ameliorates Brain Edema in Rats with Experimental Ischemic Stroke Via Inhibiting Aquaporin 4 Expression. Acta Pharmacol Sin.42(3),382-392 https://doi.org/ 10.1038/ s41401-020-0468-5

DECLARATION: This chapter was authored by Shasha Peng, Jiachen Liu, Chuntian Liang, Lijun Yang and Gaiqing Wang published as "Aquaporin-4 in glymphatic system, and its implication for central nervous system disorders" in "Neurobiology of Disease", 2023; 179:106035

CHAPTER 15:

Research Progress on Endogenous Hematoma Clearance Mechanisms after Intracerebral Hemorrhage

ABSTRACT:

Intracerebral hemorrhage (ICH) is one of the most common refractory diseases of the nervous system, characterized by high incidence, high disability rate, and high mortality rate, imposing a heavy burden on families and society. Studies have shown that the components and degradation products of hematomas after cerebral hemorrhage are the main causes of secondary brain damage. Recent research has shown that the brain tissue itself has the ability to spontaneously absorb and clear hematomas after cerebral hemorrhage. Therefore, timely and effective promotion of the endogenous absorption of hematomas is of great significance for preventing and alleviating brain tissue damage after cerebral hemorrhage. This article reviews the research progress in recent years, aiming to provide new treatment strategies for cerebral hemorrhage.

KEY WORDS: Hematoma; Scavenger receptors; Intracerebral hemorrhage

Intracerebral hemorrhage (ICH) is one of the most common refractory diseases of the nervous system, characterized by high incidence, high disability rate, and high mortality rate, imposing a heavy burden on families and society. Studies have shown that the components and degradation products of hematomas after cerebral hemorrhage are the main causes of secondary brain damage. Recent research has shown that the brain tissue itself has the ability to spontaneously absorb and clear hematomas after cerebral hemorrhage. Therefore, timely and effective promotion of the endogenous absorption of hematomas is of great significance for preventing and alleviating brain tissue damage after cerebral hemorrhage. This article reviews the research progress in recent years, aiming to provide new treatment strategies for cerebral hemorrhage.

1. Main components of intracerebral hematomas after ICH

Red blood cells and their degradation products are the main components of hematomas. After ICH, extravasation and destruction of red blood cells occur, with a large amount of hemoglobin (Hb) exposed extracellularly. Methemoglobin can spontaneously oxidize to form high iron hemoglobin peroxide, continuing reactions lead to the formation of free hemoglobin (heme). Heme, under the action of Heme Oxygenase (HO), oxidizes to generate free iron, carbon monoxide (CO), and biliverdin. Biliverdin is quickly reduced to bilirubin. These metabolic products all have damaging effects on brain tissue. Therefore, finding effective methods to control the degradation of red blood cells, avoid or reduce the toxic effects of hematoma degradation products, and effectively promote the absorption of these metabolic products are key to hematoma clearance and preventing further neurological damage.

2. Internal Clearance Mechanisms Targeting Red Blood Cells After Intracerebral Hemorrhage

2.1 CD36-Mediated Phagocytosis of Red Blood Cells

CD36 is recognized as one of the scavenger receptors in brain tissue, mediating the phagocytosis and clearance of apoptotic and damaged cells, including red blood cells. Studies have shown that CD36 mediates the absorption of hematomas in animal models of intracerebral hemorrhage (ICH), and upregulating CD36 can promote the clearance of extravasated red blood cells by microglia/macrophages. Moreover, in ICH patients, those with CD36 deficiency exhibit significantly lower hematoma absorption rates compared to those with normal CD36 levels. These findings suggest a positive role for CD36 in promoting hematoma absorption, thus actively enhancing CD36 expression may serve as a novel therapeutic target for treating ICH. In recent years, peroxisome proliferator-activated receptor gamma (PPARγ), nuclear factor-2 (Nrf2), and Toll-like receptor 4 (TLR4) have garnered attention for their roles in regulating CD36-mediated phagocytic clearance processes. Administration of PPARγ agonists such as rosiglitazone, pioglitazone, and 15-deoxy-delta-12,14-prostaglandin J2 in vitro and in vivo models of ICH has been shown to enhance CD36 expression in microglia, thereby augmenting their phagocytic capacity for red blood cells and promoting hematoma clearance. Activation of Nrf2 upregulates CD36-mediated phagocytosis, reinforcing microglial phagocytic activity and consequently enhancing hematoma absorption. Similarly, genetic deletion of TLR4 in vitro and in vivo models of ICH results in increased CD36 expression in microglia/macrophages, enhanced red blood cell phagocytic capability, and accelerated hematoma absorption. Additionally, the TLR4 inhibitor TAK242 has been shown to enhance CD36 expression, further promoting hematoma clearance. These findings suggest that stimulating PPARγ and Nrf2 expression or blocking the TLR4 pathway may facilitate hematoma absorption and could potentially serve as a therapeutic strategy for ICH.

2.2 CD47-Mediated Phagocytosis of Red Blood Cells

CD47, a crucial member of the immunoglobulin superfamily, is primarily expressed on the surface of macrophages, dendritic cells, and neuronal cells, regulating cell migration, phagocytosis, and immune homeostasis. Following ICH, CD47 interacts with the inhibitory receptor signal regulatory protein alpha (SIRPα) on the surface of macrophages, forming a negative regulatory signal that inhibits the phagocytosis of red blood cells by macrophages. In murine models of ICH, hematoma clearance is significantly faster in CD47-deficient mice compared to normal controls, resulting in less severe damage to brain tissue. Recent studies have demonstrated that deferoxamine reduces CD47 expression after ICH by chelating iron, thereby accelerating hematoma absorption. However, further research is needed to elucidate the regulatory mechanisms of CD47 expression and the signaling pathways involved in CD47-SIRPα interactions following ICH.

3. Endogenous Clearance Mechanisms Targeting Hemoglobin and Its Degradation Products After Intracerebral Hemorrhage

3.1 Mechanisms for Hemoglobin Clearance

Following intracerebral hemorrhage, ruptured red blood cells release large amounts of free hemoglobin (Hb) into the brain parenchyma, which binds to haptoglobin (Hp) to form hemoglobin-haptoglobin complexes (Hb-Hp). CD163, as a scavenger receptor on monocyte-derived macrophages, specifically recognizes Hb-Hp complexes and clears free Hb through phagocytic internalization, thereby accelerating the clearance of Hb after ICH and reducing associated toxic effects. Importantly, multiple studies have shown that Nrf2 upregulates CD163 expression on phagocytic cell membranes, facilitating the clearance of free Hb and accelerating hematoma absorption after ICH. Furthermore, Nrf2 agonists such as lefutrozole can increase Hp expression in blood and brain tissues, promoting the upregulation of CD163 expression and mitigating the toxic effects of hemolysis after ICH.

3.2 Endogenous Clearance Mechanisms for Heme

Heme released from hemoglobin after ICH binds to hemopexin (Hx) to form hemopexin-heme complexes (Hx-heme), which are engulfed by scavenger receptor CD91/LRP1. CD91 is a cell surface immunoreceptor that, upon binding to Hx-heme complexes, facilitates the reduction of heme and its degradation products in tissues, promoting their uptake by phagocytic cells. Additionally, studies have shown that Hx enhances the phagocytic capacity of microglial cells, and knockout of Hx and HO2 genes in mice reduces their phagocytic function, exacerbating brain tissue damage and neurological deficits after ICH. Currently, there is limited research on the expression mechanisms of CD91 after ICH, highlighting the need for further investigation into its role in hematoma clearance after ICH.

3.3 Endogenous Clearance Mechanisms for Iron

After intracerebral hemorrhage, red blood cell lysis releases iron ions. Iron chelators exhibit high specificity and affinity for iron ions, effectively binding to intracellular and extracellular ferrous or ferric ions or transferrin, forming iron ion complexes and promoting their excretion, thereby alleviating pathological iron deposition and iron overload in tissues. Numerous studies have shown that exogenous iron chelators, including deferoxamine, deferiprone, and minocycline, can alleviate post-ICH brain edema and improve neurological function in rats. Additionally, deferoxamine can reduce CD47 expression after ICH, regulating CD47-mediated phagocytosis of red blood cells and accelerating endogenous hematoma absorption. In humans, there are also many endogenous iron chelators, such as ascorbic acid, ferritin, transferrin, ATP, and sugars, but there is currently a lack of relevant reports on endogenous iron clearance mechanisms. Therefore, active research on endogenous iron chelators for the clearance of iron overload after intracerebral hemorrhage is essential.

4. Exploration of the Role of SRA (CD204) in Hematoma Clearance After ICH

Scavenger receptor A (SRA), also known as CD204, is a pattern recognition receptor primarily expressed on microglia/macrophages, playing a crucial role in lipid metabolism, atherosclerosis, ischemic injury, and some metabolic processes. Recent studies have shown that SRA can inhibit the activation of microglia/macrophages induced by Toll-like receptor 4 (TLR4) after ICH, exerting a protective effect against neuroinflammation-induced damage. However, there is currently no literature reporting on the role of SRA in hematoma clearance after ICH, necessitating further research to explore its involvement.

5. Conclusion

In summary, the internal hematoma clearance systems described in current research mainly include CD36-red blood cells, CD47-red blood cells, CD163-Hp-Hb, CD91-Hx-heme, SRA, and endogenous iron clearance mechanisms. However, there is scarce literature on the coordinated actions of scavenger receptors, and the specific expression mechanisms and influencing factors are not yet fully understood, necessitating further research by clinicians to provide new and effective strategies for the clinical treatment of intracerebral hemorrhage.

REFERENCE:

1. ZHOU Y, WANG Y, WANG J, et al. Inflammation in intracerebral hemorrhage: from mechanisms to clinical translation [J]. Prog Neurobiol, 2013, 115(2):25-44.
2. HUANG F, JING CH, SEN L, et al. CD36-mediated hematoma absorption following intracerebral hemorrhage: Negative regulation by TLR4 signaling [J]. The Journal of Immunology, 2014,192(12):5984–5992.
3. VAN ASCH CJ, LUITSE MJ, RINKEL GJ, et al. Incidence case fatality, and functional outcome of intracerebral haemorrhage over time, according to age, sex, and ethnic origin: A systematic review and meta-analysis [J]. Lancet Neurology, 2010, 9(2): 167-176.
4. GASSCH JA, LOCKMAN PR, GELDENHUYS WJ, et al. Brain iron toxicity: Differential responses of astrocytes, neurons, and endothelial cell [J]. Neurochemical Res, 2007, 32(7): 1196-1208.
5. ZHAO X, AUN G, ZHANG J, et al. Hematoma resolution as a target for intracerebral hemorrhage treatment: Role for peroxisome proliferator-activated receptor γ in microglia/macrophages[J]. Annalsof neurology, 2007, 61(4): 352-362.
6. LI X, MELIEF E, POSTUPNA N, et al. Prostaglandin E2 receptor subtype 2 regulation of scavenger receptor CD36 modulates microglial Aβ42 phagocytosis [J]. Am J Pathol, 2015, 185(1):230-239.
7. FLORES JJ, KLEBE D, ROLLAND WB, et al. PPARγ-induced upregulation of CD36 enhances hematoma resolution and attenuates long-term neurological deficits after germinal matrix hemorrhage in neonatal rats [J]. Neurobiology of Disease, 2015, 87:124-133.
8. ZHAO XR, GONZALES N, ARONOWSKI J. Pleiotropic role of PPARγ in intracerebral hemorrhage: an intricate system involving Nrf2, RXR, and NF-κB [J]. CNS Neurosci Ther, 2015, 21(4):357-366.
9. ZHAO X, SUN G, TING SM, et al. Cleaning up after ICH: the role of Nrf2 in modulating microglia function and hematoma clearance [J]. J Neurochem, 2015, 133(1): 144-152.
10. WANG YC, WANG PF, FANG H, et al. Toll-like receptor 4 antagonist attenuates intracerebral hemorrhage induced brain injury [J]. Stroke, 2013, 44(9):2545-2552.
11. ZHOU X, XIE Q, XI G, et al. Brain CD47 expression in a swine model of intracerebral hemorrhage [J]. Brain Res, 2014, 1574(1):70-76.
12. BROWN GC, NEHER JJ. Eaten alive Cell death by primary phagocytosis: 'phagoptosis'[J]. Trends in Biochemical Sciences,2012, 37(8): 325–332.
13. WEI NI, GUOHUA XI, JIAWEI SONG, et al. Role of erythrocyte CD47 in

intracerebral hematoma clearance [J]. Stroke, 2016, 47(2): 505-511.

14. CAO S, ZHENG M, HUA Y, et al. Hematoma changes during clot resolution after experimental intracerebral hemorrhage [J]. Stroke, 2016 ,47(6): 1626-1631.

15. MOESTRUP SK, MOLLER HJ. CD163: A regulated hemoglobin scavenger receptor with a role in the anti – inflammatory response [J]. AnnMed, 2004, 36(5): 347 -354.

16. MARTIN-VENTURA, MADRIQAL-MATUTE J, MARTI-NEZ-PINNA R, et al. Erythrocytes, leukocytes and platelets as a source of oxidative stress in chronic vascular diseases: detoxifying mechanisms and potential therapeutic options [J]. Thromb Haemost, 2012, 108(3): 435-442.

17. ZHAO X, SUN G, ZHANG J, et al. Transcription factor Nrf2 protects the brain from damage produced by intracerebral hemorrhage [J]. Stroke, 2007, 38(12):3280–3286.

18. ZHAO X, SUN G, TING SM, et al. Cleaning up after ICH: the role of Nrf2 in modulating microglia function and hematoma clearance [J]. J Neurochem, 2015, 133(1): 144-152.

19. ZHAO X, SONG S, SUN G, et al. Neuroprotective role of haptoglobin after intracerebral hemorrhage [J]. J Neurosci, 2009. 29(50): 15819-15827.

20. SCHAER DJ, VINCHI F, INQOQLIA G, et al. Haptoglobin, hemopexin, and related defense pathways-basic science, clinical perspectives, and drug development[J]. Front Physiol, 2014, 5: 415.

21. NIELSEN MJ, MOLLER HJ, MOESTRUP SK. Moestrup, Hemoglobin and heme scavenger receptors [J]. Antioxid Redox Signal, 2010, 12(2): 261-273.

22. VIBEKE H, MACIEJ B, MANIECKI, et all. Identification of the receptor scavenging hemopexin-heme complexes [J]. Blood,2005, 106(7): 2572-2579.

23. MA B, DAY JP, PHILLIPS H, et al. Deletion of the hemopexin or heme oxygenase-2 gene aggravates brain injury following stroma-free hemoglobin-induced intracerebral hemorrhage[J]. J Neuroinflammation, 2016, 13(1): 26.

24. HUANG FP, XI G, KEEP RF, et al. Brain edema after experimental intracerebral hemorrhage: role of hemoglobin degradation products[J]. J Neurosurg, 2002, 96(2):287-293.

25. SELIM M, YEATTS S, GOLDSTEIN JN, et al. Safety and tolerability of deferoxamine mesylate in patients with acuteintracerebral hemorrhage[J]. Stroke, 2011, 42(11): 3067-3074.

26. KELLEY JL, OZMENT TR, LI C, et al. Scavenger receptor-A (CD204): a two-edged sword in health and disease[J]. Crit Rev Immunol, 2014, 34(3): 241-261.

27. YANG Z, ZHONG S, LIU Y, et al. Scavenger receptor SRA attenuates microglia activation and protects neuroinflammatory injury in intracerebral hemorrhage[J]. J Neuroimmunol, 2015, 278:232-238.

28. YUAN B, SHEN H, LIN L, et al. Scavenger receptor SRA attenuates TLR4-induced microglia activation in intracerebral hemorrhage[J]. J Neuroimmunol, 2015, 289: 87-92.

DECLARATION: This chapter was authored by Juan Wang and Gaiqing Wang published as "Research Progress on Endogenous Hematoma Clearance Mechanisms After Intracerebral Hemorrhage" in "Chinese Journal of Neurology and Psychiatry", 2016;42(7):438-440

CHAPTER 16:

Clearance Systems in the Brain, From Structure to Function

ABSTRACT:

As the most metabolically active organ in the body, there is a recognized need for pathways that remove waste proteins and neurotoxins from the brain. Previous research has indicated potential associations between the clearance system in the brain and the pathological conditions of the central nervous system (CNS), due to its importance, which has attracted considerable attention recently. In the last decade, studies of the clearance system have been restricted to the glymphatic system. However, removal of toxic and catabolic waste by-products cannot be completed independently by the glymphatic system, while no known research or article has focused on a comprehensive overview of the structure and function of the clearance system. This thesis addresses a neglected aspect of linkage between the structural composition and main components as well as the role of neural cells throughout the clearance system, which found evidence that the components of CNS including the glymphatic system and the meningeal lymphatic system interact with a neural cell, such as astrocytes and microglia, to carry out vital clearance functions. As a result of this evidence that can contribute to a better understanding of the clearance system, suggestions were identified for further clinical intervention development of severe conditions caused by the accumulation of metabolic waste products and neurotoxins in the brain, such as Alzheimer's disease (AD) and Parkinson's disease (PD).

KEY WORDS: Brain waste clearance; Glymphatic system; Meningeal lymphatic vessels; Blood-brain barrier; Neuroglia

Introduction

It has previously been observed that despite a high metabolic rate, the brain lacks an actual lymphatic system that aids in removing metabolic waste and toxic agents from the brain (1). Therefore, the clearance system in the brain has long been a subject of great interest in a wide range of neuroscience fields since it was discovered in the 1960s (2). In recent years, there has been growing recognition of the vital links between the clearance system and disease of the central nervous system (CNS). Therefore there is an urgent need to have a comprehensive understanding of the clearance system (3). So far, however, the whole clearance system, including structural characterization and a possible connection between them, has received scant attention in the research literature. Most of these previous studies have generally been restricted to analyzing the glymphatic system, which has suffered from a lack of a comprehensive theoretical framework (4). Because of this, the research to date has not been able to provide robust evidence for promising clinical intervention based on clearance system in brain disorders due to the accumulation of waste products (5). This paper seeks to remedy these problems and propose a conceptual, theoretical framework based on the clearance system in the brain by systematically review the literature of main structural components, including nerve cells and extracellular vesicles (EVs) on date. (Fig. 1) The viewpoint presented in this review is one of the first overviews to explore the overall structure and function of the clearance system, which will shed new light on future research that will lead to the further potential development of preventive and therapeutic interventions of brain disorders mentioned above.

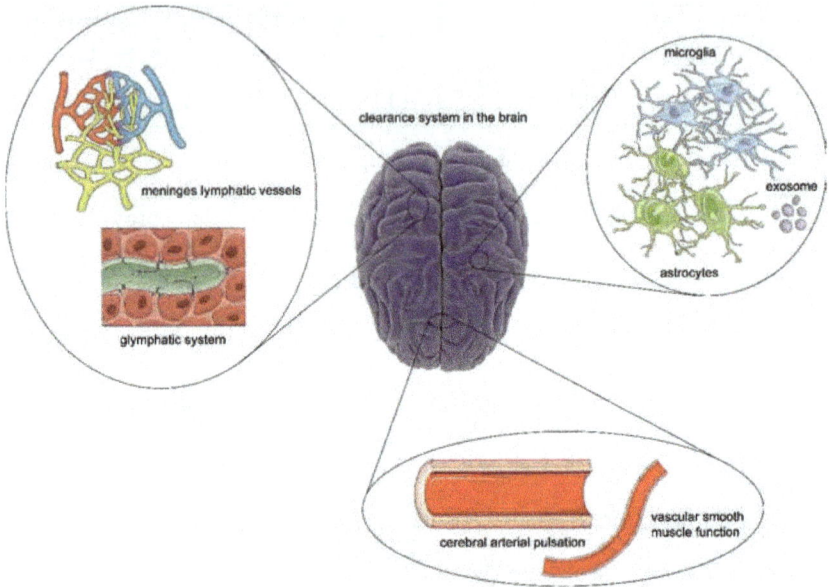

Figure1. A comprehensive overview of clearance system in the brain.

As paucity of lymphoid tissue, brain has unique clearance system to eliminate metabolic waste. Construction of framework based on glymphatic system and meninges lymphatic vessels to provide a platform for CSF flow, which is essential for exchange and transport of metabolic waste. Besides, the driving force for CSF flow is provided by cerebral arterial pulsation and smooth muscle function. While the steady-states of the process are guaranteed by astrocytes and microglia coupled with EVs like exosome.

Structural basis of clearance system in the brain

The proper functioning of the clearance system in the brain requires a stable structure. And it has been reported that the glymphatic and meningeal lymphatic have brain lymphoid function. So the following section will establishe the framework of the structure, function, and interactions of two systems, which contributes to a better understanding of physiological and pathological conditions of the clearance system in the brain.

The glymphatic system

The first pioneering study in 2012 identified a brain-wide pathway in mice with small fluorescent tracers and termed it as a "glymphatic" system for its dependence on astrocytic aquaporin-4 (AQP4) water channels and its subservience of a lymphatic function in the waste clearance (6). With the development of the diffusion MR technique and diffusion tensor imaging, subsequent researches indicated the presence of the glymphatic system in the human brain (7,8).

The glymphatic system maintains the delicate balance in CNS by delivering soluble waste and metabolic products from the brain parenchyma to the major cerebrospinal fluid (CSF) egress routes. And there are several critical components in this system, including CSF, interstitial fluid (ISF), perivascular space (PVS), cerebral vascular, glial cells, and the astrocyte aquaporin4(AQP4)-controlled water channels. Produced by the choroid plexus, CSF flows through the lateral ventricles, the third ventricles, and the fourth ventricles into the subarachnoid compartment connected to the glymphatics' perivascular tunnels (6,9). CSF is then driven into the PVS under the pulsatility of the penetrating arteries. PVS is an open, low-resistance space formed by the vascular endfeet of the astrocyte, which serves as a wall strengthening the entire cerebral vascular bed. Therefore, CSF can be thought of as river-carrying sediment, which is metabolic waste, and PVS is the conduit where CSF flows. AQP4 is one of the subtypes of AQP that are highly expressed in the endfeet of the astrocyte. Working like sluice gates, AQP4 allows CSF to enter the brain parenchyma to exchanges metabolites(10). ISF takes up 12-20% of the fluid compartments in the brain and it mixes with the CSF influx within the tissue toward the perivenous spaces. Eventually, the CSF-ISF fluid and small-size and hydrophilic waste drain to meningeal lymphatic vessels and the blood circulation. (Fig. 2)

Having discussed how to construct the glymphatic system, it's essential to probe into the significant roles in neurophysiology (11). The function of the glymphatic system in waste clearance includes three aspects. 1) Since the PVS serves as a conduit sink for CSF/ISF movement, the glymphatic system constructs a trans-arteriovenous network in transmitting hydrophilic waste like lactate (12). 2) The perivascular influx of CSF also involves in the clearance of macromolecules which are then absorbed by the downstream lymphatic network, forming a "front end" of the Glymphatic-lymphatic connection (13,14). 3) It serves complementary roles with the blood-brain barrier (BBB) in providing a well-conditioned neuronal environment in the prevention of mechanical disruption and waste accumulation (15).

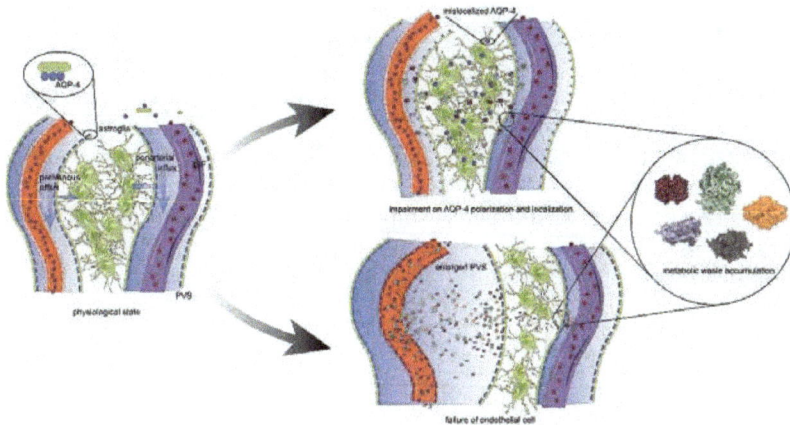

Figure2. The glymphatic pathway and pathological changes.

In the healthy brain, CSF is driven into the PVS in the brain parenchyma and flows across the glial basement membrane and astroglial endfeet to enter the interstitial space. The AQP4 is highly expressed on the endfeet of astrocytes, forming the outer wall of the PVS and facilitating the CSF influx into the interstitium. To mix with ISF and waste metabolites, CSF is transported towards to peri-venous space in a polarized net fluid movement. Ultimately, CSF exits along the lymphatic vessels and arachnoid granulations for removal of solutes from the brain parenchyma accumulated during neural activity. Under pathologic conditions, the brain may have a impairment on AQP4 polarization and localization, result in the reduced influx of CSF as well as a decrease of CSF clearance rate. And with that came the aggregation of Aβ and tau protein, which is relevant for AD. Vascular pathology causes the failure of endothelial cell, producing the cell debris and protein deposition that give rise to the obstruction and inflammation of PVS. Increased PVS fluid along with the factors mentioned above causes enlarged PVS, which then leads to a further accumulation of toxic metabolic byproducts like Aβ and tau.

With multiple critical roles in CNS physiology, it's not difficult to comprehend that the lesions of the major structures of the glymphatic system can weaken its capabilities to remove waste and have a devastating impact on brain health. For example, the depolarization, mislocalization and deletion of AQP4 in the aging brain associated with the impairment of perivascular CSF recirculation, which may contribute to the accumulation of amyloid β-protein (Aβ) and Tau proteins in the brain (16,17) (Fig. 2). The mechanism can be further explained as follows: due to a loss of AQP4 localization, the extracellular fluid containing amyloid-ß, which should have proceeded on to the perivenous spaces, now flows back into the periarterial space. And it results in the elevated extracellular concentration of the protein of interest (9). Given the combination of other factors such as shear stress, ionic strength, and local pH, waste accumulation comes into existence (18). A recent study that used pharmacological blockade to perturb AQP4 polarization in rTg4510 mice has observed an ~85% reduction in MRI quantified CSF-ISF exchange and a similar decrease in tau clearance from the brain (19), which is consistent with what mentioned above. It suggests that AQP4 may serve as a significant predictor for the status of certain diseases, including chronic sleep disruption (20), Alzheimer's disease (AD) (16), and traumatic brain injury (TBI) (21), whose pathogenesis are all related to the inefficient waste removal process. To further discuss the imaging progress of AQP4 detection, it is known that the diffusion methods can evaluate the molecular dynamics of water in brain tissue by the signal changes of motion-probing gradients (22). Diffusion tensor image analysis along the perivascular space (DTI-ALPS) has the advantage of being non-invasive. It is applied to measure the motion of water molecules along the PVS direction in recent studies, indicating that diffusion MRI can evaluate the CSF-ISF exchange (23,24).

The expression of AQP4 plays an essential role in CSF-ISF exchange, and the apparent diffusion coefficient (ADC) can be regarded as a biomarker of AQP gene expression (25), suggesting that diffusion MRI can monitor the changes of AQP4 molecules while evaluating the glymphatic system. What's more, a study of Sindex and sADC, two biomarkers that are more sensitive to tissue microstructure than ADC, further makes it possible to monitor the expression of AQP4 in vivo(26).

PVS are spaces filled with CSF-like fluid, which follow penetrating vessels (6,27). The pulsatility of the penetrating arteries drives CSF into the neuropil along with the periarterial spaces. Typically, vascular cell debris, particulate, and protein deposition can cause the enlargement of PVS. However, the driving forces within the glymphatic system do not change synchronously, resulting in the slowdown of the flow and further accumulation of toxins and tissue damage, which are risk factors for PVS inflammation and perivascular edema. (Fig. 2). Therefore, it's reasonable to work on the principle that ePVS are pathological changes that occurs early in minor vessel diseases (28,29), in which secondary neuroinflammation is often observed. In addition to the associations between ePVS burden and minor vessel diseases, mounting evidence also suggests that ePVS may be modulated by sleep and TBI (30), revealing ePVS as a potential state marker impaired clearance. While researchers have recently started to assess the role of astroglial biology in ePVS (31), more studies are needed to confirm the relationship between the pathological states of AQP-4 and ePVS. Previous studies have been carried out on single structural dysfunction and its role in waste accumulation and disease, which may neglect their interrelation and interaction with one another in the glymphatic system. Further work is necessary to uncover their close connection to the waste clearance process. Thus, new insights can be given to discovering drugs and therapeutics for neurodegenerative diseases that involve multiple pathological changes.

Meningeal lymphatic vessels

The first serious discussions and analyses of meningeal lymphatic vessels emerged during the 1800s with Paolo Mascagni (32). By far, evidence of meningeal lymphatic vessels was obtained at autopsy (33) that at the level of the superior sagittal sinus, there were lymphatic vessels in the human dura mater. In 2017, Absinta et al. visualized the lymphatic vessels in the dura mater by brain magnetic resonance imaging (MRI) (34) which innovatively and concretely demonstrates the existence of meningeal lymphatic vessels.

The meningeal lymphatic vessels were initially considered mainly residing in the base of the skull (35). The development of MRI has enabled a more delicate and precise structure of meningeal lymphatic vessels. Through 3D-rendering of subtraction MRI images, dural lymphatics are discerned running parallel to the dural venous sinuses and along with branches of the middle meningeal artery (34). Besides, arteries, veins, and cranial nerves draining the contents into the deep cervical lymph nodes (dCLN) were also detected by MRI (35,36), which includes immune cells, CSF, and ISF from the subarachnoid space. Accordingly, meningeal lymphatic vessels are the main drainage of soluble and cellular components in CSF (37).

Like the initial lymphatic vessels in anatomy and molecular characteristics, the meningeal lymphatic vessels express all the traditional markers of endothelial cells (EC) of the lymphatic vessels, without smooth muscle cells and valves (38). While, a potential lymphatic valve has been detected at the bottom of the skull(37), suggesting that these lymphatic vessels transition from the initial vessel to the collection vessel. Moreover, the diameter of meningeal lymphatic vessels is smaller than peripheral lymphatic vessels (38).

One way to remove cellular debris and toxic molecules such as Aβ peptides in the brain is that CSF influx and ISF efflux through the paravascular (lymphatic) pathway (6,39), as previously demonstrated. As far as pathologic changes are concerned, meningeal lymphatic vessel disorders can impair the efflux of substantial / ISF macromolecules and their drainage to dCLNs, which functionally links the meningeal lymphatics with the CSF influx / ISF efflux mechanism (13).

As the functions of CSF and ISF in the glymphatic system mentioned earlier, it is speculated that the glymphatic system and the meningeal lymphatic system are inextricably linked in exerting immune and clean functions. CSF, ISF, and meningeal lymphatic flows can be regarded as a holistic model when exploring the mechanism of brain immune surveillance and waste removal. Meningeal lymphatic vessels were proved to be located downstream of glymphatic system using MRI (40), and rather than dorsal MLVs, basal MLVs are the main pathways to uptake and clear macromolecule and could be hotspots for drainage of CSF and ISF (37). Researches show that injected brain-derived antigens efflux by CSF through meningeal lymphatic vessels can trigger T cell immune response after passing through dCLNs (41). In comparison, impairment of CSF-ISF exchange leads to reduced clearance of tracers in the brain and damage of drainage to dCLN(6).

The regular operation of the CNS of the brain has strict requirements for the brain environment. Therefore, when the meningeal lymphatic vessels are damaged or CNS changes, it will affect the function. Recent evidence from animal studies demonstrates that impaired meningeal lymphatic drainage function caused spatial learning and memory impairment (42). Additionally, mice with long-term ablation of meningeal lymphatic vessels show abnormal gene expression in the hippocampus related to neurodegenerative diseases (13), which all suggest that neurodegenerative diseases might be related to meningeal lymphatic disorders. As mentioned above, the meningeal lymphatic vessel is an immune tissue structure closely related to CSF. Impaired function of the meningeal lymphatic vessel may affect the removal of metabolic waste in CSF, providing new possibilities for the preventive treatment of certain elder brain diseases manifested as cognitive impairment.

Take AD, one of the common neurodegenerative diseases as an example. We infer above that the obstruction of Aβ precipitation removal may lead to AD. Previously mentioned, drainage of meningeal lymphatic vessels is one of the pathways for Aβ clearance, so it is inferred that the damage of meningeal lymphatics is related to AD. Recent observations suggest that the decline in meningeal lymphatic function during aging may aggravate the pathological state of the brain and meningeal amyloid (43). It is hypothesized that impaired meningeal lymphatic drainage of CSF will affect Aβ clearance, thus increasing the amyloid load of the brain (44). Since VEGF-C can regulate the development of meningeal lymphatic vessels, promoting the clearance of amyloid (45) makes hope for a novel therapy for elderly AD.

Previous studies have confirmed CSF efflux movement from the brain parenchyma to downstream lymphatic circulation (6). With new studies on the function of the glymphatic system and meningeal lymphatic vessels emerging (46), it's significant to understand their interaction in detail.

Based on former research, the connection between glymphatic system and meningeal lymphatic vessels was demonstrated with fluorescent tracer and dye in 2015 (38). It's found that the meningeal lymphatic vessels could absorb the fluid from CSF through the glymphatic system and transported it into dCLN (47). Anatomically, Aspelund et al indicated that the waste products might gain access to the lymphatic vessels through the adjacent subarachnoid space and drainage veins merging into dura sinubrain (47). The meningeal lymphangiogenesis was found coupled with the enhanced glymphatic influx under chronically implanted electroencephalography electrodes, which confirmed a close association between glymphatic activity and the meningeal lymphatic vasculature (48). When devastating cerebrovascular events like Subarachnoid hemorrhage occurred, a decrease of meningeal lymphatic drainage and depolarization of AQP4 were observed at the same time (49), suggesting a pathological link under the glymphatic-lymphatic connection. Conclusively, the function and dysfunction of meningeal lymphatic vessels and their relationship to the glymphatic system shed light on a hypothesis that the two systems work as a whole clearance system in the brain. Still, the hypothesis needs to be validated and strengthened by future works.

Components and barrier protection of clearance system in the brain

Based on the complete structure, maintaining the normal biological function of the clearance system in the brain still requires that waste capture and directional movement and barrier protective effects of the process ensure metabolic homeostasis in the brain. A more detailed account of components and barrier protection, including drivers and impact factors, is given in the following section.

Cerebrospinal fluid

Produced by the choroid plexus, CSF fills the brain ventricles and the subarachnoid space and surrounds the spinal cord in the adult human brain (50,51). CSF flows are a prerequisite for a clearance system to maintain normal biological function. Therefore, exploring the effect of the driving force is required to construct a framework for a complete system (50). The flow direction of CSF along the intracranial artery was confirmed according to the studies mentioned above, which implies the importance of cerebral arterial pulsation to the driving force (52). Further observations relating to the flow velocity in CSF confirmed the pulsatile flow of CSF that matches the cerebral arterial pulse (53). Subsequently, more and more evidence has indicated the pulsatile flow in the arterial wall is a significant driver of the CSF (54). However, as research in the fields of clearance system surges forward, cerebral arterial pulsation driven by the cardiac pump is strong enough to support efficient CSF flows is questionable (55). Arguments have been put forward that vascular smooth muscle function is also considered important for CSF pressure and dynamics based on increased vascular smooth muscle reactivity modulate clearance of intracranial metabolic waste (56).

In addition, the activity of CSF circulation is also one of the factors affecting brain clearance system function. According to the "glymphatic system" hypothesis, CSF enters the brain via periarterial spaces, passes into the interstitium via perivascular astrocytic AQP4, and then drives the perivenous drainage of ISF and its solute (11). Previous researches pointed out that this cerebral CSF circulation is only active during sleep or general anesthesia (57). More and more evidence suggest that regular sleep time ensures the efficiency of the brain clearance system (58). Given the latest discoveries, the brain clearance system is closely related to neurodegenerative diseases like AD, improving sleep is an essential means of preventing neurodegenerative diseases (59). However, the effect of anesthesia on CSF circulation is still controversial (60). By far, the most influential account of anesthesia on CSF circulation is found in the work of Gakuba et al., which used MRI and near-infrared fluorescence imaging to investigate the impact of general anesthesia on the intracranial CSF circulation in mice. Contrary to what was initially expected, they found that CSF circulation was more active when awake while significantly impaired during general anesthesia, suggesting that the effects of anesthesia on the brain clearance system are related to the dose (61). Clinical studies on whether anesthesia can be used to regulate the function of the clearance system are still lacking.

Blood-Brain Barrier

BBB cooperates with the glymphatic system in waste clearance, plays a dominant role in separating blood cells, exogenous pathogens, and circulatory wastes from the brain to maintain brain homeostasis (62-64) (Fig. 3). With carrier-mediated transport on epithelium performing waste efflux and the clearance of its cellular components, the BBB prevents CNS from accumulating metabolites and xenobiotics (64). (Table1) It is acknowledged that the BBB can be divided into many a basic functional unit called neurovascular unit (NVU), which consists of neurons, vascular cells such as EC, pericytes, and gliacytes, including astrocytes and microglia. Mounting evidence suggests that NVU regulates BBB permeability, cerebrovascular net function, and neurogenesis (65,66). Under pathological conditions, the dysfunction and breakdown of constituent cells and relevant structures like tight junction (TJ) and cells will lead to neurological disorders and deficits. This section will attempt to describe how the cellular components with their junctions realize barrier function in BBB and elimination of wastes in clearance system, while the role of exosomes in this process.

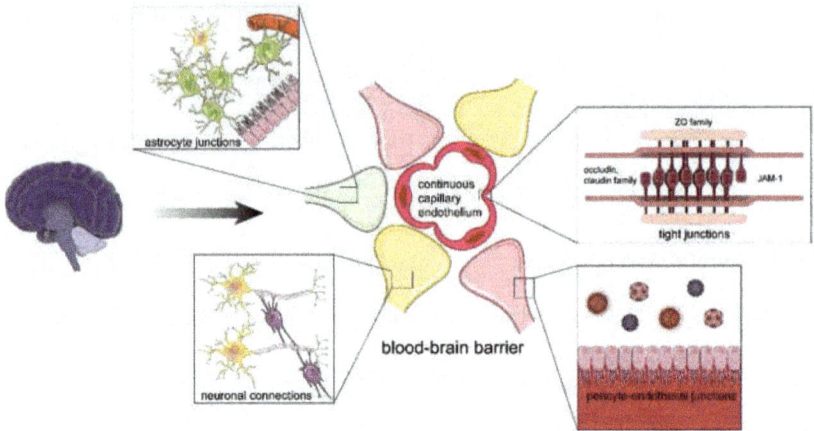

Figure3. The functional structure of blood-brain barrier (BBB).

The BBB is composed of including continuous capillary endothelium with tight junctions (TJ), adherens junctions and gap junctions, pericyte-endothelial junctions, astrocyte junctions, neural connections, intact basement membrane and glial membrane. The TJ is abundant in TJ proteins, for instance, claudin and scaffolding protein like zonnula occludens (ZO) family form the backbone of TJ, occludin helps maintain the intergrity and stability of TJ, junctional adhesion molecule A (JAM-1) mediates cell adhesion to restrict epithelial permeability. In terms of astroytes, they can not only strengthen the BBB by junctions with endothelial cells, but communicate with myelinated nerve fiber and synapses and support them. For neurons, their connections are enhanced by glia cells like oligoderIdrocyte, which can assist efficient jump transmission of bioelectrical signals and the maintain of normal function of neurons.

Tight Junction

TJ is the most substantial supporting structure in the BBB formed on continuous capillary endothelium (67,68). TJ has plenty of specifically marked transmembrane proteins, including the occludin and claudin family, which communicate with other intracellular scaffolding proteins such as the zonnula occludens family (62,68,69)(Fig. 3). However, the TJ can also be passive and changeable for nutrients and metabolites. It has been demonstrated that TJ synergizing with adherens junctions acts as an adjuster to the diffusion of solutes in plasma (68). Recently researchers have identified that appropriate opening of the TJ could promote the values of clearance of CSF and ISF through perivascular gaps. For example, Zn+ highly accumulated in synapses can help open the TJ reversibly via the GSK3β/snail-mediated signal transduction, which facilitates expelling macromolecular metabolites and toxins out of the brain cleaned (70).

Under pathological conditions, the structure of TJ can be damaged, causing the BBB to degrade even break down. The increased Aβ outside the brain, for instance, can lead to the decrease in TJ structure proteins occludin and claudin-5, and the crosstalk between them, during which Aβ can slip into the brain and then deposit without the clearance of gliacytes and ISF, causing a vicious cycle Aβ sedimentation in the brain parenchyma (71). Besides, the TJ leakage can also result in the solute heaped up in vessels and tissues, hindering the drainage of ISF and CSF and causing ischemic lesions like ischemic stroke (69). From the above, opening the TJ can be helpful to deliver drugs targeted at brain parenchyma. Drugs targeting TJ-associated proteins like borneol, bradykinin, and hyperosmotic mannitol and approaches like focused ultrasound have been proven effective in opening TJ currently (72,73).

Cellular components and extracellular vesicles of clearance system in the brain

The glial cell is the executor of the function of the clearance system in the brain. As more adequately correlate with functional status, the following section involves physiological fluctuations and pathological shifts, which can provide perspective guidance and meaningful solutions of diseases caused by the accumulation of metabolic waste products and neurotoxins in the brain in the future.

Vascular endothelial cell

Forming blood vessels by chimerism and connection with each other, vascular endothelial cells build a core barrier between brain parenchyma and external environment, with the assistance of their junctions like TJ. Besides the physical function in BBB mentioned above, vascular endothelial cells also provide a selective passage for the import of macromolecular nutrients and circulating proteins and the efflux of toxins and metabolites (62). Carrier-mediated transporters like nucleotide, hormone, and amino acid transporters, receptor-mediated transporters like insulin and lipoprotein receptors, ATP-binding cassette (ABC), and ion transport channels are all endothelium-dependent, regulating the homeostasis of the material delivery (63) (74). For example, ABC family such as ABCB1 and P-glycoprotein on the endothelium has been proved effective in the removal of Aβ out of the brain (74,75). Factors like gene mutation that can alter the phenotype of vascular endothelial cells may result in the diminishment or disappearance of waste's clearance function (76). In further research, the specific relationship between endothelial cell function-related gene mutation and disease still needs to be clarified, benefiting the symptomatic treatment of specific neurological disorders (76). What's more, the up-regulated expression of translocators on endothelial cells and induced release of endothelial relaxation factor-like NO may also offer a possibility to accelerate the flow of CSF and ISF in PVS, enhancing the function of the clearance system in the brain consequently (77).

Astrocyte

Astrocytes, the coadjutant to build BBB with their endfeet attached to the vascular interface, also function as a doorman to control and clear CSF flow from paravascular spaces (59). In the last few years, more researchers shift their sights to the clearance of metabolic wastes and exogenous toxins that astrocytes perform, during which AQP-4 takes a critical part. The AQP-4 helps to remold to promote synaptic and vascular plasticity and assist astrocytes in eliminating dendritic spines. In the clearance system, the AQP-4 functions as a circulator participating in regulating the diameter of brain capillaries to guarantee interstitial flow and accelerate ISF circulation. It has been demonstrated that the polarized localization of AQP-4 to perivascular endfeet can accelerate the CSF from subarachnoid to flow to brain interstitium in a convective bulk way, helping the glymphatic system clear the ISF and CSF simultaneously (20,78,79). Suppose the AQP-4 localization has been altered or lost. In that case, astrocytes tend to release vascular endothelial growth factors (VEGFs) and matrix metalloproteinases (MMPs) to increase BBB permeability, which will result in the accelerating process of BBB disruption and the deposition of insoluble Aβ along with subsequent reactive gliosis (79,80).

Interestingly, researchers also find a positive correlation between age and the expression of AQP-4, especially in neurodegenerative disorders (such as AD). Therefore, the downregulation and the fine control of the AQP-4 shows potential in the healing and prognosis of these diseases. Shreds of evidence have shown that drugs like zonisamide and topiramate can inhibit the function of AQP-4. At the same time, the synthetic antibody to AQP-4 also benefits a lot in diseases caused by the autoantibody to AQP-4 like neuromyelitis optica (81).

From the perspective of regulating BBB barrier structure, astrocytes are also the hinge cable between BBB and the glymphatic system. As far as can be determined, consciousness and body posture affects the clearance rate of the brain's waste, in which sleep is a stimulating factor (82). While asleep, astrocytes may increase the interstitial volume by shrinking themselves, promoting interstitial fluid flow and the transformation between CSF and ISF. And through this process, glymphatic clearance is straightly facilitated, and the scavenging efficiency of BBB is also indirectly improved by increasing the flow of interstitial solute (15,83,84). Accordingly, the BBB will also up-regulate the activity of efflux transporters like ABCB1 under the control of the circadian clock (83). Consequently, the BBB and the glymphatic system can cooperate and influence each other.

Microglia

Microglia are resident cells in the innate immune system performing as CNS parenchymal macrophages, taking charge of digesting and degrading endogenous wastes in the brain like cellular debris to accomplish neuronal and synaptic surveillance, developmental neuronal apoptosis clearance, and dendritic spine pruning(62,85) (86). Once microglia are exposed to declining and apoptotic cells in the very first stage of apoptosis, the expression of clearance-related genes like PRC2 is promoted, launching a series of clearance reactions in the very first stage of apoptosis (87). Besides, microglia tend to share mutual support and promote phagocytosis, especially the one young microglia give to the older (88). Furthermore, microglia can be divided into pro-inflammatory (M1-like) phenotypes to immunosuppressive (M2-like) phenotypes according to the degree of activation at present (89). Suppose microglia are aberrantly activated, which is common in acute CNS injury and neurodegenerative diseases. In that case, they can shift to M1-like phenotype, which results in theM1/M2-like polarization, and release relative cytokines to speed up the disruption of BBB, consequently exacerbating the destruction of vessels and neurons (89-91).

Moreover, their increased intrinsic function of phagocytosis and elimination can also damage neuron morphology and interconnection with others. Hence, it has been suggested that the detection of regions where the M1-like phenotype of microglia proliferate becomes increasingly significant in diagnosing neurodevelopmental disorders like autistic spectrum disorders, most of which are characterized by microglioma (90). However, microglial activation also has several serious drawbacks, such as transferring microtubule-associated protein tau via exosomes in the brain and failing to clear the toxic metabolite (92,93). Altogether, the mechanism of microglia causing aberrance and dysfunction of neurons in over-clearance circumstances remains to be elucidated, and the moderate regulation of microglia activation also needs to be explored (85). In the next step of research, discovering biomarkers of the M1-like phenotype microglia can be a target, which is beneficial in prompt diagnoses and treatment of neurodevelopmental disorders by more advanced pathological examinations like neuroimaging method.

Pericyte

Pericytes are a group of cells embedded in the basement membrane of capillary ECs in the vasculature, act as ancillary cells to strengthen the BBB and assist functional members in the clearance system. As a member of NVU collaborates with astrocytes, microglia, and other neurons, pericytes participate in vascular development, permeability and remodeling. Currently, pericytes have been proved to have the ability to differentiate into the neural lineage, contributing to the neurogenesis and inflammatory factor clearance after the brain injury or the chronic neuroinflammation like glioblastomas (94-96). In addition, pericytes reach to regulate the blood flow and interstitial flow of capillaries, modulating the clearance values of ISF and CSF. Under pathological conditions, degenerated pericytes can directly decrease the pericyte–glia interface at BBB and then disrupt BBB. Consequently, it allows blood-derived toxins like auto-antibodies mIgG to invade and then deposit in the brain parenchyma, leading to the diminishing clearance of gliocytes (96,97). Although the specific functions and behaviors of various subtypes of pericytes displayed in different life stages in human are not clear currently, the possibility and potential pericytes show in TJ opening and blood flow control is undoubted, which provides us with a novel idea in the therapeutic measures of relative neurodegenerative diseases like AD (98).

The BBB and glymphatic system have in common that they all aim to remove waste from CSF and ISF in the brain and reach mutual promotion and cooperation. Nevertheless, they also differ in the specific way of performing the function on account of structure. For the BBB, barriers formed by cells and tight connections and selection of channels for substances such as proteins are the primary way to execute clearance. For the glymphatic system, however, it mainly separates waste from circulating

CSF by promoting the convective movement of CSF between PVS and interstitial space to achieve the purpose of clearance. On the one hand, when the clearance of more metabolites or toxic substances of BBB transporters reaches operational saturation, it seems that the glymphatic system can undertake the scavenging effect. On the other hand, the activity of convection in the glymphatic system can also stimulate the enhanced responsiveness of the AQP4 water channel and promote the function of BBB, especially astrocytes (17). In the present context, the BBB barrier is more susceptible to aggressive barrier destruction factors like trauma, the collapse of cell junctions like pericyte loss, and internal lesion-like up-regulation of lipoprotein receptors. At the same time, glymphatic system is more susceptible to interference with CSF convection factors like altered pulsations and changed vasomotor tone (10,28,99). In this process, inflammation and sleep disturbances may be the common factors that destroy both and cause the malignant cycle."

Exosome

The exosome is a class of extracellular vesicles of 40-100 mm in size generated from the endosomal membrane and secreted by many cell types in a physiological and pathological state, widely distributed in various body fluids (100). Initially thought to have a function merely in waste disposal, the involvement of exosomes in neuronal development, maintenance, and regeneration through its paracrine and endocrine signaling functions has drawn particular attention in recent years (101). As one of the earlier discovered waste removal organelles, exosome secretion has confirmed emerged as a mode to selectively clear the neurotoxic proteins, such as α-synuclein (102). Furthermore, exosomes seem to possess the ability to reduce brain amyloid beta through microglial uptake (103). However, studies undertaken so far provide conflicting evidence that the exosome is also responsible for the occurrence and development of neurodegenerative diseases (104). Exosomes have been shown to spread toxic amyloid-beta and hyperphosphorylated tau between cells, which appear to act as a seed to spread toxic proteins within the central nervous system, leading to a disorder of clearance system function. For example, some studies have shown that exosomes in patients with Dementia with Lewy Bodies are sufficient for seeding and propagating alpha-syn aggregation in vivo (105). Another concern of exosomes is that by penetrating the BBB, they may be served as accessible biomarkers of neurological dysfunction from the non-invasive separation of body fluids (106) (Fig. 4).

4 Potential therapeutic strategies targeting defects of clearance system in the brain

Exploring the regulatory mechanism of deficiencies in the clearance system may help identify the precise therapeutic target for ICH. Notably, multi-omics technologies have made significant achievements in the research of neurodegenerative diseases (107,108).

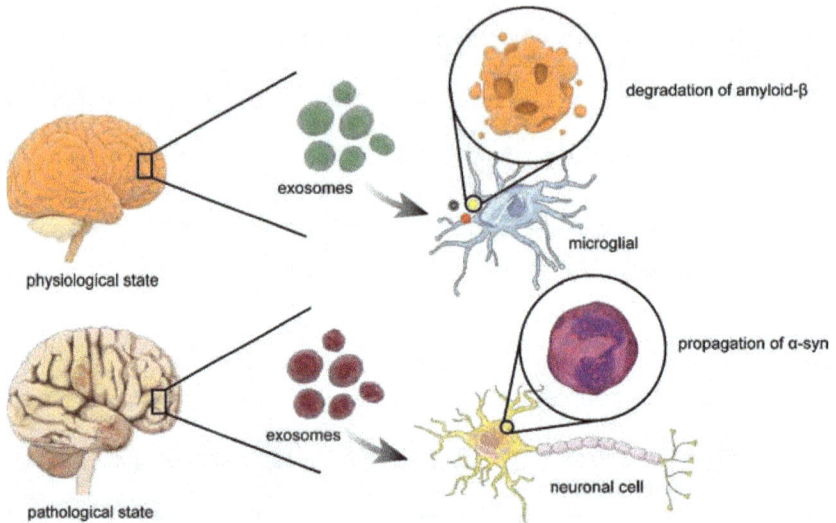

Figure4. Exosomes in brain clearance system. Under physiological conditions, exosomes reduce brain amyloid-β through microglial uptake. Pathologically, for example, in the brain of a patient with DLB, the exosomes propagate α-syn within the central nervous system, leading to a disorder of clearance system function.

A comparative analysis of driving gene expression in the physiological and pathological states of the clearance system will establish preliminary evidence for a link between them (Supplementary Table1). The application of systematic multi-omics approaches to precision medicine and systems biology has great potential to improve the care of patients with dysfunction of clearance system. Besides, the target gene identified by multi-omics studies can potentially be used for drug repositioning in ICH, which is approved to be cheaper, quicker, and effective (109) (Supplementary Table2). For example, Caffeine targeting the PDE1C that is related to brain metabolites has been approved by the FDA for the short-term treatment of apnea of prematurity. Given the same putative drivers of the clearance system, which may maintain clearance system stability via relaxing the vascular smooth muscle, alleviate some pathological conditions caused by the disturbed clearance system. Despite the association among various intracranial diseases, direct evidence linking disease-driven analyses and molecular network dynamics in pathological contexts is lacking. Further research in neurological disorders is an essential next step in confirming diseases-driven networks associated with clearance system, thus developing novel therapeutic strategies that are more pertinent and specific.

Conclusion

This review set out to provide the first systematic account of the clearance system in the brain. The findings indicate that the flow of CSF through the glymphatic system and meninges lymphatic vessels driven by smooth muscle and cerebral arterial pulsation, thus clearing toxic and metabolic waste, including small molecules and biomacromolecules. Notably, BBB that consist of microglia associated with astrocytes and outer-membrane vesicles secreted by them, such as exosome, seems to play a significant role in maintaining the process. These findings have substantial implications for understanding the clearance of metabolic waste from the brain. When the balance of the process is disturbed, how it contributed to pathological changes in the brain lays the groundwork for future research into physiological homeostasis pathophysiologic responses within the brain.

Author Contributions Statement

All authors listed have made a substantial, direct and intellectual contribution to the work, and approved it for publication.

Conflict of Interest Statement

The authors declare that the research was conducted in the absence of any commercial or financial relationships that could be construed as a potential conflict of interest.

Acknowledgments:

This work was supported by a grant from National Natural Science Foundation of China (81771294).

REFERENCE:

1. Kumar A, Ghosh SK, Faiq MA, Deshmukh VR, Kumari C, Pareek V. A brief review of recent discoveries in human anatomy. Qjm. 2019;112(8):567-573.
2. Bedussi B, van Lier MG, Bartstra JW, de Vos J, Siebes M, VanBavel E, Bakker EN. Clearance from the mouse brain by convection of interstitial fluid towards the ventricular system. Fluids Barriers CNS. 2015;12:23.
3. Zhang L, Chopp M, Jiang Q, Zhang Z. Role of the glymphatic system in ageing and diabetes mellitus impaired cognitive function. Stroke Vasc Neurol. 2019;4(2):90-92.
4. Jessen NA, Munk AS, Lundgaard I, Nedergaard M. The Glymphatic System: A Beginner's Guide. Neurochem Res. 2015;40(12):2583-2599.
5. Sun BL, Wang LH, Yang T, Sun JY, Mao LL, Yang MF, Yuan H, Colvin RA, Yang XY. Lymphatic drainage system of the brain: A novel target for intervention of neurological diseases. Prog Neurobiol. 2018;163-164:118-143.
6. Iliff JJ, Wang M, Liao Y, Plogg BA, Peng W, Gundersen GA, Benveniste H, Vates GE, Deane R, Goldman SA, Nagelhus EA, Nedergaard M. A paravascular pathway facilitates CSF flow through the brain parenchyma and the clearance of interstitial solutes, including amyloid beta. Sci Transl Med. 2012;4(147):147ra111.
7. Taoka T, Masutani Y, Kawai H, Nakane T, Matsuoka K, Yasuno F, Kishimoto T, Naganawa S. Evaluation of glymphatic system activity with the diffusion MR technique:

diffusion tensor image analysis along the perivascular space (DTI-ALPS) in Alzheimer's disease cases. Jpn J Radiol. 2017;35(4):172-178.

8. Yokota H, Vijayasarathi A, Cekic M, Hirata Y, Linetsky M, Ho M, Kim W, Salamon N. Diagnostic Performance of Glymphatic System Evaluation Using Diffusion Tensor Imaging in Idiopathic Normal Pressure Hydrocephalus and Mimickers. Curr Gerontol Geriatr Res. 2019; 2019:5675014.

9. Nedergaard M, Goldman SA. Glymphatic failure as a final common pathway to dementia. Science. 2020;370(6512):50-56.

10. Rasmussen MK, Mestre H, Nedergaard M. The glymphatic pathway in neurological disorders. Lancet Neurol. 2018;17(11):1016-1024.

11. Plog BA, Nedergaard M. The Glymphatic System in Central Nervous System Health and Disease: Past, Present, and Future. Annu Rev Pathol. 2018;13:379-394.

12. Lundgaard I, Lu ML, Yang E, Peng W, Mestre H, Hitomi E, Deane R, Nedergaard M. Glymphatic clearance controls state-dependent changes in brain lactate concentration. J Cereb Blood Flow Metab. 2017;37(6):2112-2124.

13. Da Mesquita S, Louveau A, Vaccari A, Smirnov I, Cornelison RC, Kingsmore KM, Contarino C, Onengut-Gumuscu S, Farber E, Raper D, Viar KE, Powell RD, Baker W, Dabhi N, Bai R, Cao R, Hu S, Rich SS, Munson JM, Lopes MB, Overall CC, Acton ST, Kipnis J. Functional aspects of meningeal lymphatics in ageing and Alzheimer's disease. Nature. 2018;560(7717):185-191.

14. Benveniste H, Liu X, Koundal S, Sanggaard S, Lee H, Wardlaw J. The Glymphatic System and Waste Clearance with Brain Aging: A Review. Gerontology. 2019;65(2):106-119.

15. Verheggen ICM, Van Boxtel MPJ, Verhey FRJ, Jansen JFA, Backes WH. Interaction between blood-brain barrier and glymphatic system in solute clearance. Neurosci Biobehav Rev. 2018;90:26-33.

16. Zeppenfeld DM, Simon M, Haswell JD, D'Abreo D, Murchison C, Quinn JF, Grafe MR, Woltjer RL, Kaye J, Iliff JJ. Association of Perivascular Localization of Aquaporin-4 With Cognition and Alzheimer Disease in Aging Brains. JAMA Neurol. 2017;74(1):91-99.

17. Kress BT, Iliff JJ, Xia M, Wang M, Wei HS, Zeppenfeld D, Xie L, Kang H, Xu Q, Liew JA, Plog BA, Ding F, Deane R, Nedergaard M. Impairment of paravascular clearance pathways in the aging brain. Ann Neurol. 2014;76(6):845-861.

18. Burke KA, Yates EA, Legleiter J. Biophysical insights into how surfaces, including lipid membranes, modulate protein aggregation related to neurodegeneration. Front Neurol. 2013;4:17.

19. Harrison IF, Ismail O, Machhada A, Colgan N, Ohene Y, Nahavandi P, Ahmed Z, Fisher A, Meftah S, Murray TK, Ottersen OP, Nagelhus EA, O'Neill MJ, Wells JA, Lythgoe MF. Impaired glymphatic function and clearance of tau in an Alzheimer's

disease model. Brain. 2020;143(8):2576-2593.

20. Zhang R, Liu Y, Chen Y, Li Q, Marshall C, Wu T, Hu G, Xiao M. Aquaporin 4 deletion exacerbates brain impairments in a mouse model of chronic sleep disruption. CNS Neurosci Ther. 2020;26(2):228-239.

21. Piantino J, Lim MM, Newgard CD, Iliff J. Linking Traumatic Brain Injury, Sleep Disruption and Post-Traumatic Headache: a Potential Role for Glymphatic Pathway Dysfunction. Curr Pain Headache Rep. 2019;23(9):62.

22. Taoka T, Naganawa S. Glymphatic imaging using MRI. J Magn Reson Imaging. 2020;51(1):11-24.

23. Harrison IF, Siow B, Akilo AB, Evans PG, Ismail O, Ohene Y, Nahavandi P, Thomas DL, Lythgoe MF, Wells JA. Non-invasive imaging of CSF-mediated brain clearance pathways via assessment of perivascular fluid movement with diffusion tensor MRI. Elife. 2018;7.

24. Taoka T. Neurofluid as Assessed by Diffusion-Weighted Imaging. Magn Reson Imaging Clin N Am. 2021;29(2):243-251.

25. Ohene Y, Harrison IF, Nahavandi P, Ismail O, Bird EV, Ottersen OP, Nagelhus EA, Thomas DL, Lythgoe MF, Wells JA. Non-invasive MRI of brain clearance pathways using multiple echo time arterial spin labelling: an aquaporin-4 study. Neuroimage. 2019; 188:515-523.

26. Debacker C, Djemai B, Ciobanu L, Tsurugizawa T, Le Bihan D. Diffusion MRI reveals in vivo and non-invasively changes in astrocyte function induced by an aquaporin-4 inhibitor. PLoS One. 2020;15(5):e0229702.

27. Mestre H, Kostrikov S, Mehta RI, Nedergaard M. Perivascular spaces, glymphatic dysfunction, and small vessel disease. Clin Sci (Lond). 2017;131(17):2257-2274.

28. Brown R, Benveniste H, Black SE, Charpak S, Dichgans M, Joutel A, Nedergaard M, Smith KJ, Zlokovic BV, Wardlaw JM. Understanding the role of the perivascular space in cerebral small vessel disease. Cardiovasc Res. 2018;114(11):1462-1473.

29. Wardlaw JM, Benveniste H, Nedergaard M, Zlokovic BV, Mestre H, Lee H, Doubal FN, Brown R, Ramirez J, MacIntosh BJ, Tannenbaum A, Ballerini L, Rungta RL, Boido D, Sweeney M, Montagne A, Charpak S, Joutel A, Smith KJ, Black SE. Perivascular spaces in the brain: anatomy, physiology and pathology. Nature reviews Neurology. 2020;16(3):137-153.

30. Opel RA, Christy A, Boespflug EL, Weymann KB, Case B, Pollock JM, Silbert LC, Lim MM. Effects of traumatic brain injury on sleep and enlarged perivascular spaces. J Cereb Blood Flow Metab. 2019;39(11):2258-2267.

31. Boespflug EL, Simon MJ, Leonard E, Grafe M, Woltjer R, Silbert LC, Kaye JA, Iliff JJ. Targeted Assessment of Enlargement of the Perivascular Space in Alzheimer's Disease and Vascular Dementia Subtypes Implicates Astroglial Involvement Specific to Alzheimer's Disease. J Alzheimers Dis. 2018;66(4):1587-1597.

32. Lecco V. [Probable modification of the lymphatic fissures of the walls of the venous sinuses of the dura mater]. Arch Ital Otol Rinol Laringol. 1953;64(3):287-296.

33. Visanji NP, Lang AE, Munoz DG. Lymphatic vasculature in human dural superior sagittal sinus: Implications for neurodegenerative proteinopathies. Neurosci Lett. 2018; 665:18-21.

34. Absinta M, Ha SK, Nair G, Sati P, Luciano NJ, Palisoc M, Louveau A, Zaghloul KA, Pittaluga S, Kipnis J, Reich DS. Human and nonhuman primate meninges harbor lymphatic vessels that can be visualized noninvasively by MRI. Elife. 2017;6.

35. Bakker EN, Bacskai BJ, Arbel-Ornath M, Aldea R, Bedussi B, Morris AW, Weller RO, Carare RO. Lymphatic Clearance of the Brain: Perivascular, Paravascular and Significance for Neurodegenerative Diseases. Cell Mol Neurobiol. 2016;36(2):181-194.

36. Ha SK, Nair G, Absinta M, Luciano NJ, Reich DS. Magnetic Resonance Imaging and Histopathological Visualization of Human Dural Lymphatic Vessels. Bio Protoc. 2018;8(8).

37. Ahn JH, Cho H, Kim JH, Kim SH, Ham JS, Park I, Suh SH, Hong SP, Song JH, Hong YK, Jeong Y, Park SH, Koh GY. Meningeal lymphatic vessels at the skull base drain cerebrospinal fluid. Nature. 2019;572(7767):62-66.

38. Louveau A, Smirnov I, Keyes TJ, Eccles JD, Rouhani SJ, Peske JD, Derecki NC, Castle D, Mandell JW, Lee KS, Harris TH, Kipnis J. Structural and functional features of central nervous system lymphatic vessels. Nature. 2015;523(7560):337-341.

39. Peng W, Achariyar TM, Li B, Liao Y, Mestre H, Hitomi E, Regan S, Kasper T, Peng S, Ding F, Benveniste H, Nedergaard M, Deane R. Suppression of glymphatic fluid transport in a mouse model of Alzheimer's disease. Neurobiol Dis. 2016; 93:215-225.

40. Zhou Y, Cai J, Zhang W, Gong X, Yan S, Zhang K, Luo Z, Sun J, Jiang Q, Lou M. Impairment of the Glymphatic Pathway and Putative Meningeal Lymphatic Vessels in the Aging Human. Ann Neurol. 2020;87(3):357-369.

41. Noé FM, Marchi N. Central nervous system lymphatic unit, immunity, and epilepsy: Is there a link? Epilepsia Open. 2019;4(1):30-39.

42. Wang L, Zhang Y, Zhao Y, Marshall C, Wu T, Xiao M. Deep cervical lymph node ligation aggravates AD-like pathology of APP/PS1 mice. Brain Pathol. 2019;29(2):176-192.

43. Ma Q, Ineichen BV, Detmar M, Proulx ST. Outflow of cerebrospinal fluid is predominantly through lymphatic vessels and is reduced in aged mice. Nat Commun. 2017;8(1):1434.

44. Da Mesquita S, Fu Z, Kipnis J. The Meningeal Lymphatic System: A New Player in Neurophysiology. Neuron. 2018;100(2):375-388.

45. Antila S, Karaman S, Nurmi H, Airavaara M, Voutilainen MH, Mathivet T, Chilov D, Li Z, Koppinen T, Park JH, Fang S, Aspelund A, Saarma M, Eichmann A, Thomas JL, Alitalo K. Development and plasticity of meningeal lymphatic vessels. J Exp Med.

2017;214(12):3645-3667.

46. Louveau A, Plog BA, Antila S, Alitalo K, Nedergaard M, Kipnis J. Understanding the functions and relationships of the glymphatic system and meningeal lymphatics. J Clin Invest. 2017;127(9):3210-3219.

47. Aspelund A, Antila S, Proulx ST, Karlsen TV, Karaman S, Detmar M, Wiig H, Alitalo K. A dural lymphatic vascular system that drains brain interstitial fluid and macromolecules. J Exp Med. 2015;212(7):991-999.

48. Hauglund NL, Kusk P, Kornum BR, Nedergaard M. Meningeal Lymphangiogenesis and Enhanced Glymphatic Activity in Mice with Chronically Implanted EEG Electrodes. J Neurosci. 2020;40(11):2371-2380.

49. Pu T, Zou W, Feng W, Zhang Y, Wang L, Wang H, Xiao M. Persistent Malfunction of Glymphatic and Meningeal Lymphatic Drainage in a Mouse Model of Subarachnoid Hemorrhage. Exp Neurobiol. 2019;28(1):104-118.

50. Benveniste H, Lee H, Volkow ND. The Glymphatic Pathway: Waste Removal from the CNS via Cerebrospinal Fluid Transport. Neuroscientist. 2017;23(5):454-465.

51. Marques F, Sousa JC, Brito MA, Pahnke J, Santos C, Correia-Neves M, Palha JA. The choroid plexus in health and in disease: dialogues into and out of the brain. Neurobiol Dis. 2017;107:32-40.

52. Ringstad G, Vatnehol SAS, Eide PK. Glymphatic MRI in idiopathic normal pressure hydrocephalus. Brain. 2017;140(10):2691-2705.

53. Mestre H, Tithof J, Du T, Song W, Peng W, Sweeney AM, Olveda G, Thomas JH, Nedergaard M, Kelley DH. Flow of cerebrospinal fluid is driven by arterial pulsations and is reduced in hypertension. Nat Commun. 2018;9(1):4878.

54. Taoka T, Naganawa S. Gadolinium-based Contrast Media, Cerebrospinal Fluid and the Glymphatic System: Possible Mechanisms for the Deposition of Gadolinium in the Brain. Magn Reson Med Sci. 2018;17(2):111-119.

55. Aldea R, Weller RO, Wilcock DM, Carare RO, Richardson G. Cerebrovascular Smooth Muscle Cells as the Drivers of Intramural Periarterial Drainage of the Brain. Front Aging Neurosci. 2019;11:1.

56. Cheng Y, Liu X, Ma X, Garcia R, Belfield K, Haorah J. Alcohol promotes waste clearance in the CNS via brain vascular reactivity. Free Radic Biol Med. 2019;143:115-126.

57. Winsky-Sommerer R, de Oliveira P, Loomis S, Wafford K, Dijk D-J, Gilmour G. Disturbances of sleep quality, timing and structure and their relationship with other neuropsychiatric symptoms in Alzheimer's disease and schizophrenia: Insights from studies in patient populations and animal models. Neuroscience & Biobehavioral Reviews. 2019;97:112-137.

58. Aguirre CC. Sleep deprivation: a mind-body approach. Curr Opin Pulm Med. 2016;22(6):583-588.

59. Albrecht U, Ripperger JA. Circadian Clocks and Sleep: Impact of Rhythmic Metabolism and Waste Clearance on the Brain. Trends Neurosci. 2018;41(10):677-688.

60. Taoka T, Jost G, Frenzel T, Naganawa S, Pietsch H. Impact of the Glymphatic System on the Kinetic and Distribution of Gadodiamide in the Rat Brain: Observations by Dynamic MRI and Effect of Circadian Rhythm on Tissue Gadolinium Concentrations. Invest Radiol. 2018;53(9):529-534.

61. Gakuba C, Gaberel T, Goursaud S, Bourges J, Di Palma C, Quenault A, Martinez de Lizarrondo S, Vivien D, Gauberti M. General Anesthesia Inhibits the Activity of the "Glymphatic System". Theranostics. 2018;8(3):710-722.

62. McConnell HL, Kersch CN, Woltjer RL, Neuwelt EA. The Translational Significance of the Neurovascular Unit. J Biol Chem. 2017;292(3):762-770.

63. Sweeney MD, Zhao Z, Montagne A, Nelson AR, Zlokovic BV. Blood-Brain Barrier: From Physiology to Disease and Back. Physiol Rev. 2019;99(1):21-78.

64. Ueno M, Chiba Y, Murakami R, Matsumoto K, Fujihara R, Uemura N, Yanase K, Kamada M. Disturbance of Intracerebral Fluid Clearance and Blood-Brain Barrier in Vascular Cognitive Impairment. Int J Mol Sci. 2019;20(10).

65. Obermeier B, Verma A, Ransohoff RM. The blood-brain barrier. Handb Clin Neurol. 2016; 133:39-59.

66. Saint-Pol J, Gosselet F, Duban-Deweer S, Pottiez G, Karamanos Y. Targeting and Crossing the Blood-Brain Barrier with Extracellular Vesicles. Cells. 2020;9(4).

67. Van Itallie CM, Anderson JM. Architecture of tight junctions and principles of molecular composition. Semin Cell Dev Biol. 2014;36:157-165.

68. Tietz S, Engelhardt B. Brain barriers: Crosstalk between complex tight junctions and adherens junctions. J Cell Biol. 2015;209(4):493-506.

69. Abdullahi W, Tripathi D, Ronaldson PT. Blood-brain barrier dysfunction in ischemic stroke: targeting tight junctions and transporters for vascular protection. Am J Physiol Cell Physiol. 2018;315(3):C343-C356.

70. Xiao R, Yuan L, He W, Yang X. Zinc ions regulate opening of tight junction favouring efflux of macromolecules via the GSK3beta/snail-mediated pathway. Metallomics. 2018;10(1):169-179.

71. Keaney J, Walsh DM, O'Malley T, Hudson N, Crosbie DE, Loftus T, Sheehan F, McDaid J, Humphries MM, Callanan JJ, Brett FM, Farrell MA, Humphries P, Campbell M. Autoregulated paracellular clearance of amyloid-beta across the blood-brain barrier. Sci Adv. 2015;1(8):e1500472.

72. Duan M, Xing Y, Guo J, Chen H, Zhang R. Borneol increases blood-tumour barrier permeability by regulating the expression levels of tight junction-associated proteins. Pharm Biol. 2016;54(12):3009-3018.

73. Gonzalez-Mariscal L, Posadas Y, Miranda J, Uc PY, Ortega-Olvera JM, Hernandez S. Strategies that Target Tight Junctions for Enhanced Drug Delivery. Curr Pharm Des.

2016;22(35):5313-5346.

74. Shubbar MH, Penny JI. Therapeutic drugs modulate ATP-Binding cassette transporter-mediated transport of amyloid beta(1-42) in brain microvascular endothelial cells. Eur J Pharmacol. 2020; 874:173009.

75. Pan J, He R, Huo Q, Shi Y, Zhao L. Brain Microvascular Endothelial Cell Derived Exosomes Potently Ameliorate Cognitive Dysfunction by Enhancing the Clearance of Abeta Through Up-Regulation of P-gp in Mouse Model of AD. Neurochem Res. 2020.

76. Oikari LE, Pandit R, Stewart R, Cuni-Lopez C, Quek H, Sutharsan R, Rantanen LM, Oksanen M, Lehtonen S, de Boer CM, Polo JM, Gotz J, Koistinaho J, White AR. Altered Brain Endothelial Cell Phenotype from a Familial Alzheimer Mutation and Its Potential Implications for Amyloid Clearance and Drug Delivery. Stem Cell Reports. 2020;14(5):924-939.

77. Cheng Y, Haorah J. How does the brain remove its waste metabolites from within? Int J Physiol Pathophysiol Pharmacol. 2019;11(6):238-249.

78. Yang J, Zhang R, Shi C, Mao C, Yang Z, Suo Z, Torp R, Xu Y. AQP4 Association with Amyloid Deposition and Astrocyte Pathology in the Tg-ArcSwe Mouse Model of Alzheimer's Disease. J Alzheimers Dis. 2017;57(1):157-169.

79. Valenza M, Facchinetti R, Steardo L, Scuderi C. Altered Waste Disposal System in Aging and Alzheimer's Disease: Focus on Astrocytic Aquaporin-4. Front Pharmacol. 2019;10:1656.

80. Michinaga S, Koyama Y. Dual Roles of Astrocyte-Derived Factors in Regulation of Blood-Brain Barrier Function after Brain Damage. Int J Mol Sci. 2019;20(3).

81. Verkman AS, Smith AJ, Phuan PW, Tradtrantip L, Anderson MO. The aquaporin-4 water channel as a potential drug target in neurological disorders. Expert Opin Ther Targets. 2017;21(12):1161-1170.

82. Natale G, Limanaqi F, Busceti CL, Mastroiacovo F, Nicoletti F, Puglisi-Allegra S, Fornai F. Glymphatic System as a Gateway to Connect Neurodegeneration From Periphery to CNS. Front Neurosci. 2021;15:639140.

83. Zhang SL, Lahens NF, Yue Z, Arnold DM, Pakstis PP, Schwarz JE, Sehgal A. A circadian clock regulates efflux by the blood-brain barrier in mice and human cells. Nat Commun. 2021;12(1):617.

84. Mendelsohn AR, Larrick JW. Sleep facilitates clearance of metabolites from the brain: glymphatic function in aging and neurodegenerative diseases. Rejuvenation Res. 2013;16(6):518-523.

85. Dudvarski Stankovic N, Teodorczyk M, Ploen R, Zipp F, Schmidt MHH. Microglia-blood vessel interactions: a double-edged sword in brain pathologies. Acta Neuropathol. 2016;131(3):347-363.

86. Casano AM, Albert M, Peri F. Developmental Apoptosis Mediates Entry and Positioning of Microglia in the Zebrafish Brain. Cell Rep. 2016;16(4):897-906.

87. Ayata P, Badimon A, Strasburger HJ, Duff MK, Montgomery SE, Loh YE, Ebert A, Pimenova AA, Ramirez BR, Chan AT, Sullivan JM, Purushothaman I, Scarpa JR, Goate AM, Busslinger M, Shen L, Losic B, Schaefer A. Epigenetic regulation of brain region-specific microglia clearance activity. Nat Neurosci. 2018;21(8):1049-1060.

88. Daria A, Colombo A, Llovera G, Hampel H, Willem M, Liesz A, Haass C, Tahirovic S. Young microglia restore amyloid plaque clearance of aged microglia. EMBO J. 2017;36(5):583-603.

89. Loane DJ, Kumar A. Microglia in the TBI brain: The good, the bad, and the dysregulated. Exp Neurol. 2016;275 Pt 3:316-327.

90. Hammond TR, Robinton D, Stevens B. Microglia and the Brain: Complementary Partners in Development and Disease. Annu Rev Cell Dev Biol. 2018;34:523-544.

91. Hickman S, Izzy S, Sen P, Morsett L, El Khoury J. Microglia in neurodegeneration. Nat Neurosci. 2018;21(10):1359-1369.

92. Li Q, Barres BA. Microglia and macrophages in brain homeostasis and disease. Nat Rev Immunol. 2018;18(4):225-242.

93. Asai H, Ikezu S, Tsunoda S, Medalla M, Luebke J, Haydar T, Wolozin B, Butovsky O, Kugler S, Ikezu T. Depletion of microglia and inhibition of exosome synthesis halt tau propagation. Nat Neurosci. 2015;18(11):1584-1593.

94. Andreotti JP, Prazeres P, Magno LAV, Romano-Silva MA, Mintz A, Birbrair A. Neurogenesis in the postnatal cerebellum after injury. Int J Dev Neurosci. 2018;67:33-36.

95. Birbrair A, Sattiraju A, Zhu D, Zulato G, Batista I, Nguyen VT, Messi ML, Solingapuram Sai KK, Marini FC, Delbono O, Mintz A. Novel Peripherally Derived Neural-Like Stem Cells as Therapeutic Carriers for Treating Glioblastomas. Stem Cells Transl Med. 2017;6(2):471-481.

96. Santos GSP, Magno LAV, Romano-Silva MA, Mintz A, Birbrair A. Pericyte Plasticity in the Brain. Neurosci Bull. 2019;35(3):551-560.

97. Villasenor R, Kuennecke B, Ozmen L, Ammann M, Kugler C, Gruninger F, Loetscher H, Freskgard PO, Collin L. Region-specific permeability of the blood-brain barrier upon pericyte loss. J Cereb Blood Flow Metab. 2017;37(12):3683-3694.

98. Sweeney MD, Ayyadurai S, Zlokovic BV. Pericytes of the neurovascular unit: key functions and signaling pathways. Nat Neurosci. 2016;19(6):771-783.

99. Shackleton B, Ringland C, Abdullah L, Mullan M, Crawford F, Bachmeier C. Influence of Matrix Metallopeptidase 9 on Beta-Amyloid Elimination Across the Blood-Brain Barrier. Mol Neurobiol. 2019;56(12):8296-8305.

100.Zhang J, Li S, Li L, Li M, Guo C, Yao J, Mi S. Exosome and exosomal microRNA: trafficking, sorting, and function. Genomics Proteomics Bioinformatics. 2015;13(1):17-24.

101.Soria FN, Pampliega O, Bourdenx M, Meissner WG, Bezard E, Dehay B.

Exosomes, an Unmasked Culprit in Neurodegenerative Diseases. Front Neurosci. 2017;11:26.

102. Yang Y, Qin M, Bao P, Xu W, Xu J. Secretory carrier membrane protein 5 is an autophagy inhibitor that promotes the secretion of α-synuclein via exosome. PLoS One. 2017;12(7):e0180892.

103. Malm T, Loppi S, Kanninen KM. Exosomes in Alzheimer's disease. Neurochem Int. 2016;97:193-199.

104. Shi M, Sheng L, Stewart T, Zabetian CP, Zhang J. New windows into the brain: Central nervous system-derived extracellular vesicles in blood. Prog Neurobiol. 2019;175:96-106.

105. Ngolab J, Trinh I, Rockenstein E, Mante M, Florio J, Trejo M, Masliah D, Adame A, Masliah E, Rissman RA. Brain-derived exosomes from dementia with Lewy bodies propagate alpha-synuclein pathology. Acta Neuropathol Commun. 2017;5(1):46.

106. Saeedi S, Israel S, Nagy C, Turecki G. The emerging role of exosomes in mental disorders. Transl Psychiatry. 2019;9(1):122.

107. Nativio R, Lan Y, Donahue G, Sidoli S, Berson A, Srinivasan AR, Shcherbakova O, Amlie-Wolf A, Nie J, Cui X, He C, Wang LS, Garcia BA, Trojanowski JQ, Bonini NM, Berger SL. An integrated multi-omics approach identifies epigenetic alterations associated with Alzheimer's disease. Nat Genet. 2020;52(10):1024-1035.

108. Petermann-Rocha F, Gray SR, Pell JP, Celis-Morales C, Ho FK. Biomarkers Profile of People With Sarcopenia: A Cross-sectional Analysis From UK Biobank. J Am Med Dir Assoc. 2020;21(12):2017.e2011-2017.e2019.

109. Armando RG, Mengual Gómez DL, Gomez DE. New drugs are not enough-drug repositioning in oncology: An update. (1791-2423 (Electronic)).

DECLARATION: This chapter was authored by Jiachen Liu, Yunzhi Guo, Chengyue Zhang, Yang Zeng, Yongqi Luo and Gaiqing Wang published as "Clearance Systems in the Brain, From Structure to Function" in "Frontiers in Cellular Neuroscience",2022; 15:729706

Acknowledgments:

This work was supported by the grants from Region Program of Natural Science Foundation of China (**NO: 82160237**); Key Research and Development Program in Hainan Province (**NO: ZDYF2023SHFZ104**); General Program of Natural Science Foundation of Hainan Province (**NO: 822MS210**); Sanya Science and Technology Innovation Special Project (**NO: 2022KJCX24**) ; Natural Science Foundation of Sanya Central Hospital (**NO: SYZXYY202408**).

Publisher: Eliva Press Global Ltd

Email: info@elivapress.com

Eliva Press is an independent international publishing house established for the publication and dissemination of academic works all over the world. Company provides high quality and professional service for all of our authors.

Our Services:
Free of charge, open-minded, eco-friendly, innovational.

-Free standard publishing services (manuscript review, step-by-step book preparation, publication, distribution, and marketing).

-No financial risk. The author is not obliged to pay any hidden fees for publication.

-Editors. Dedicated editors will assist step by step through the projects.

-Money paid to the author for every book sold. Up to 50% royalties guaranteed.

-ISBN (International Standard Book Number). We assign a unique ISBN to every Eliva Press book.

-Digital archive storage. Books will be available online for a long time. We don't need to have a stock of our titles. No unsold copies. Eliva Press uses environment friendly print on demand technology that limits the needs of publishing business. We care about environment and share these principles with our customers.

-Cover design. Cover art is designed by a professional designer.

-Worldwide distribution. We continue expanding our distribution channels to make sure that all readers have access to our books.

-Marketing tools. We provide marketing tools such as banners, paid advertising, social media promotion and more.

www.elivapress.com

Printed in the USA
CPSIA information can be obtained
at www.ICGtesting.com
LVHW010523121024
793461LV00002B/3

9 789999 318327